Playing Sick

T0187690

Few life occurrences shaped individual and collective identities within Victorian-era society as critically as witnessing or suffering from illness. The prevalence of illness narratives within late nineteenth-century popular culture was made manifest on the period's British and American stages, where theatrical embodiments of illness were indisputable staples of actors' repertoires.

Playing Sick: Performances of Illness in the Age of Victorian Medicine reconstructs how actors embodied three of the era's most provocative illnesses: tuberculosis, drug addiction, and mental illness. In placing performances of illness within wider medicocultural contexts, Meredith Conti analyzes how such depictions confirmed or resisted salient constructions of diseases and the diseased. Conti's case studies, which range from Eleonora Duse's portrayal of the consumptive courtesan Marguerite Gautier to Henry Irving's performance of senile dementia in *King Lear*, help to illuminate the interdependence of medical science and theatre in constructing nineteenth-century illness narratives. Through reconstructing these performances, Conti isolates from the period's acting practices a lexicon of embodied illness: a flexible set of physical and vocal techniques that performers employed to theatricalize the sick body. In an age when medical science encouraged a gradual decentering of the patient from their own diagnosis and treatment, late nineteenth-century performances of illness symbolically restored the sick to positions of visibility and consequence.

Meredith Conti is Assistant Professor of Theatre at the University at Buffalo, SUNY, USA. A historian of nineteenth-century theatre and performance, Conti's work has appeared in the *Journal of American Drama and Theatre*, the *Journal of Dramatic Theory and Criticism*, *Studies of Musical Theatre*, and *Victorian Medicine and Popular Culture* (2015).

Routledge Advances in Theatre and Performance Studies

Performance and Phenomenology
Traditions and Transformations
Edited by Maaike Bleeker, Jon Foley Sherman, and Eirini Nedelkopoulou

Historical Affects and the Early Modern Theater
Edited by Ronda Arab, Michelle M. Dowd, and Adam Zucker

Food and Theatre on the World Stage
Edited by Dorothy Chansky and Ann Folino White

Global Insights on Theatre Censorship
Edited by Catherine O'Leary, Diego Santos Sánchez & Michael Thompson

Mainstream AIDS Theatre, the Media, and Gay Civil Rights
Making the Radical Palatable
Jacob Juntunen

Rewriting Narratives in Egyptian Theatre
Translation, Performance, Politics
Edited by Sirkku Aaltonen and Areeg Ibrahim

Theatre, Exhibition, and Curation
Displayed and Performed
Georgina Guy

Playing Sick
Performances of Illness in the Age of Victorian Medicine
Meredith Conti

Movements of Interweaving
Dance and Corporeality in Times of Travel and Migration
Gabriele Brandstetter, Gerko Egert and Holger Hartung

For more information about this series, please visit: https://www.routledge.com/Routledge-Advances-in-Theatre--Performance-Studies/book-series/RATPS

Playing Sick

Performances of Illness in the Age of Victorian Medicine

Meredith Conti

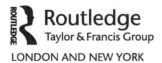
Routledge
Taylor & Francis Group

LONDON AND NEW YORK

First published 2019 by Routledge

2 Park Square, Milton Park, Abingdon, Oxon, OX14 4RN
605 Third Avenue, New York, NY 10017

Routledge is an imprint of the Taylor & Francis Group, an informa business

First issued in paperback 2020

British Library Cataloguing-in-Publication Data
A catalogue record for this book is available from the British
Library

Library of Congress Cataloging-in-Publication Data
A catalog record has been requested for this book

ISBN: 978-1-138-70311-7 (hbk)
ISBN: 978-0-367-73391-9 (pbk)

Typeset in Bembo
by Deanta Global Publishing Services, Chennai, India

For Milo and Vivian

Contents

Figures

Abbreviations

BRTC   Billy Rose Theatre Division Collections, New York Public Library for the Performing Arts at Lincoln Center

BL   British Library

HTC   Harvard Theatre Collection, Houghton Library, Harvard College Library

LOC   Library of Congress

V&A   Victoria and Albert Theatre and Performance Archives

Acknowledgments

When I first saw Alexandre Dumas fils's legendary creation Camille, she was projected onto the giant movie screen at Radio City Music Hall for the viewing pleasure of a red-headed orphan, a billionaire, his witty assistant, and a stray dog called Sandy. In the 1982 movie musical *Annie*, the characters watched as Greta Garbo's Camille, a courtesan stricken with pulmonary tuberculosis, died in the arms of the dashing Robert Taylor. Well, the adults watched; Annie had already fallen asleep, exhausted from all the Rockettes-fueled excitement. Like many young children of the 1980s, I became obsessed with Annie's tale of scrappy persistence and optimism. But Camille and her illness also left a lasting impression, and over the years she became part of a constellation of literary, artistic, and intellectual interests that gestured to my current role as a historian of nineteenth-century theatre and medicine. It seems only fitting that theatrical portrayals of Dumas's dying courtesan now occupy a prominent place in this book, a book that complicates dismissive readings of illness roles on the popular stage as merely sensationalistic by situating them within the era's medicocultural discourses.

Coincidentally, my mother's nickname for me as a young girl was "Camille." I was melodramatic from the womb.

This book has benefitted from the direct and indirect contributions of many remarkable people. *Playing Sick* began as a dissertation at the University of Pittsburgh, where a generous Andrew Mellon Pre-Doctoral Fellowship enabled me to conduct weeks of archival research at home and abroad. Bruce McConachie, Michael Chemers, Attilio "Buck" Favorini, and Kathleen George nudged me toward a sharper, meatier, and more articulate monograph without dictating the paths I took to get there. The project developed into its current incarnation in the summers between school years at James Madison University (JMU), where I held my first faculty appointment. Generosity of spirit, I came to discover, is native to the Shenandoah Valley, and the faculty, students, and staff of the School of Theatre and Dance initiated many thoughtful "check-ins" about the manuscript during my time there. A summer research grant from JMU's College of Visual and Performing Arts helped support the editing process, while the Center for Faculty Innovation's bi-yearly Scholarly Writers' Lockdowns offered precious days of writing time in quiet locations. During the final preparations of this manuscript, I joined the faculty at the University at Buffalo, SUNY (UB), a place of brave interdisciplinary collaborations and excellent institutional support for humanities scholars. I feel fortunate to call UB my new intellectual and creative home.

This book necessitated a number of research trips to libraries and archives in the United States and the UK. I say "necessitated," but that word misrepresents these excursions entirely; I delighted in my work and the outstanding archivists, librarians, and staff members that helped facilitate it. Edward Bishop introduced me to the Wellcome Library in London, perhaps the best repository for Victorian writings on medicine in the world. Kathryn Johnson, Elaine Pordes, and Tim Pye in the British Library's Rare Books and Manuscripts Reading Rooms provided skillful guidance, as did the librarians and the Commercial and Digital Development staff at the Victorian and Albert Museum's Theatre and Performance Archives, who continued to respond to my email inquiries with care and enthusiasm long after I had left the Blythe House. The hard-working research, circulation, and image reproduction staff at the Billy Rose Theatre Division (New York Public Library for the Performing Arts), the Harvard Theatre Collection (Houghton Library), the Folger Shakespeare Library, and the Library of Congress aided my stateside research and manuscript preparations. I am indebted to the Houghton Library's Mary Haegert, Susan Halpert, Emilie L. Hardman, Micah Hoggatt, and Dale Stinchcomb for their expert assistance through several stages of this project. At the Folger, LuEllen DeHaven and Abbie Weinberg joined gamely in my hunt for "THE Image" needed to complete this book's illustrations and celebrated with me when I found two additional images to include. Though archival research is often a solitary pursuit, regular interactions with genial and engaging librarians, administrators, custodians, security guards, and fellow researchers made it impossible to feel lonely.

Playing Sick matured (as do most book projects, I imagine) through a series of growth spurts, regressions, and plateaus. The penetrative insights of Aaron Tobiason helped this manuscript phase out of its awkward adolescence and into adulthood; for his editorial work and his collegiality (entirely established through electronic communications, no less) I am truly grateful. At Routledge, Ben Piggott, Kate Edwards, and Gabrielle Coakeley offered the kind of transparent and considerate publishing experience that academic scholars dream of having. My sincerest thank you to them and to the press's anonymous reviewers for their questions and encouragement. Several of the case studies contained herein were strengthened in conference working groups and panels, including those sponsored by the American Society for Theatre Research, the Mid-America Theatre Conference, the Literature and Pathology Conference (University of California, Davis), and the Northeast American Victorian Association. Portions of Part I's introduction were published within the article "'I am not suffering anymore': Tragic Potential in the Nineteenth-Century Consumptive Myth" in the *Journal of Dramatic Theory and Criticism* (fall 2009), and a modified version of Chapter 3 appears in *Victorian Medicine and*

Popular Culture, edited by Drs. Tabitha Sparks and Louise Penner (Routledge, 2015). *Playing Sick* received publication support from the American Society for Theatre Research's Brooks McNamara Publishing Subvention and the Julian Park Fund, College of Arts and Sciences, University at Buffalo.

My heartfelt appreciation goes to family members near and far, living and departed, who raised me to embrace rather than hide my love for nearly all things theatrical, historic, and macabre; in particular, thank you to Marian, Katherine, Michael, Rhian, and Peggy. Friends both inside and outside academia, many of whom are fierce, multi-hyphenate women of strength and grace, provided every type of support imaginable, from writing accountability to clarifying groupthinks. This book owes much to Ryan Conti, a human of warmth and patience who endured his share of inconveniences during its writing, and Milo and Vivian, who made sure I partook daily in restorative lightsaber battles, Lego builds, dance parties, and read-alouds.

Oscar Wilde once quipped that we like to rename our mistakes "experience." Though the temptation is great to Wilde-away my mistakes, I instead will apologize for any that you may find herein.

Introduction

The scene: A rooming-house at night. Clusters of sleeping lodgers overcrowd the room. Above the slumberous group hovers Typhus, whose work is interrupted by a disembodied voice:

> CHOLERA (*without*):
> Sister! Sister!
> TYPHUS:
>   I am here,
> Doing my work for to-morrow's bier.
> Nine and seven lie each in a row –
> Two are gone, and two will go.
>   CHOLERA (*enters*):
> Sister! Sister! you work too slow;
> For here, where the tide has left its slime
>   To mix with the filth of a hundred drains,
> And the hovels are rotting in damp and grime,
>   While the landlord is counting his daily gains,
>   And his slaves are groaning with chronic pains,
> You linger about, till famine and gin
> Must finish the work which you begin.
>   TYPHUS:
> Chide me not, Sister! My work is sure.
>   The days are many since last you came;
>   But you pass'd away, and your fearful name
> Was soon forgotten; but I endure.

The "sisters" then boast of dispatching unsuspecting humans by the scores; Typhus preys upon the poor, dirty, and undernourished, while Cholera claims to be an equal-opportunity assassin. But, Typhus avows, their carefree days are numbered: "The rich and the poor will both get wise; / And the Law will open its hoodwink'd eyes." Once that happens, "They will drain their streets, and build their schools, / And hunt us out." Cholera dismisses Typhus's fears, reminding her sister that "Twice warned, the fools / Still keep us here, and they still will keep" because "*Laissez-faire* still rules the land."[1] Entitled "Typhus and Cholera – An Eclogue," this allegorical *tête-à-tête* appeared in the September 24, 1853 issue of *The Times* of London, a year before the Broad Street cholera outbreak killed hundreds in the city's Soho district. Though *eclogue* is a short pastoral poem or dialogue, the conversation between these two epidemiological horrors is a scene fit for the Victorian playhouse. The author, identified only as "S. T.," provides the requisite stage directions; both diseases speak in rhyming couplets (a lyrical counterpoint to their grave exchange), and the piece concludes with a suitably dramatic moral: hesitation and negligence feed the plagues of humankind.

The Times was not alone in documenting, or dramatizing, the age's top health hazards. Indeed, in the Victorian news cycle three subjects were nothing short of omnipresent: politics, public health, and the theatre. The latter two claim the focus of this book. *Playing Sick: Performances of Illness in the Age of Victorian Medicine* reconstructs how actors embodied three of the era's most pervasive and provocative illnesses, placing them within the wider context of medicocultural discourses in order to highlight points of contact between medical science and the theatre. Illness has always been a collaborative, almost alchemical construct that blends biomedical, sociocultural, and individual theories and experiences, and actors' embodiments of illness participated in the forging of potent illness narratives in the nineteenth century. As Athena Vrettos offers in *Somatic Fictions: Imagining Illness in Victorian Culture*, "The ways in which [Victorians] talked about health and disease are not only issues of medical history, but also forms of cultural fiction making." In *Playing Sick*, I share Vrettos's focus on what she calls the "imaginative configurations through which Victorian culture understood illness."[2] Within a variety of cultural sites, nineteenth-century British and American citizens engaged in a perpetual dialogue about what it meant to be sick or healthy. Among the most trafficked of these sites was the theatre. Despite the abundance of related sources on illness and Victorian-era cultures emerging from the fields of literature, the history of medicine, and cultural studies, however, few full-length works of theatre scholarship examine how onstage representations of embodied sickness reinforced, subverted, or re-imagined salient constructions of illness, and none exclusively address the commercial stage, rife as it was with dynamic depictions of ill characters. *Playing Sick*'s three parts, each comprised of a pair of chapters, investigate performances of tuberculosis, drug addiction, and mental illness staged by mid- and late nineteenth-century actors in Britain and the United States.

An illness lived

Being sick, even very sick, can at times escape our notice. Infections eat away at healthy tissue, white blood cells attack cancerous cells, and we can go about our days, unsuspecting. Pain may be present, but invisible symptoms—fatigue, migraines, insomnia, or hallucinations—can also be managed or dismissed;

perhaps our bodies are talking, but we do not always listen. When the internal wars waged within an ill body become externalized, they demand to be reckoned with. Bruising, seizures, or sudden weight loss draw an illness out of the shadows; so too does the patient's voicing of suspicions—"something is wrong," or "I am not feeling like myself"—no matter how imprecisely or hesitantly uttered. Once the "something wrong" becomes labeled, the symptoms logged, cross-checked, and authenticated by a serious or life-threatening diagnosis, there is often no returning to a pre-illness state-of-being or knowing, even for those fully restored to health. Illness transforms.

And we rely on bodies to communicate this transformation, often to a fault. Bodies, we hope, will act as living topographical maps, magnifying and charting the microscopic battles playing out just beneath the surface. This is a prime reason why, even in the twenty-first century, we misinterpret or downplay illnesses that lack conspicuous markers ("but you don't *look* sick") and pathologize visually expressive non-illnesses, like pregnancy. Despite earnest efforts to engage in patient-centric diagnosis and treatment strategies, our dependence on the legibility of sick bodies and on empirically driven methods of evaluating human health can still result in detached, techno-centric healthcare, a system that treats human *bodies* but not always human *beings*. As we will discover, Victorian medical science approached healthcare in much the same way, albeit in a vastly different sociocultural moment. In many ways, *Playing Sick* is a book about bodies: healthy and ill, disguised and exposed, constrained and ungovernable. It is also a book about *perceiving* bodies during a period of hyper-vigilant anatomical monitoring, and not just via the formalized systems of institutionalized medicine. The majority of nineteenth-century medical disciplines worked within a "correlational" or "anatomo-clinical" model of disease, meaning that the external symptoms of illness were expressions of benign or malignant changes to the body's anatomical structures (tissues, organs, fibers, bones).[3] Western audiences developed over the course of the nineteenth century what Kirsten E. Shepherd-Barr calls the "diagnostic gaze," a new lens that recast theatrical spectators as amateur clinicians charged with discovering the causes of staged medical conditions.[4] The biocentric Victorian age distorted or dissolved some of the divisions separating the medical and theatrical domains, and this is particularly apparent in the ways Americans and Britons often perceived medical bodies as performative and performing bodies as medical.

Performances of illness operated at a nexus of artistic, scientific, and social modes of ideating and expressing "illness-as-lived," a helpful phrase from philosopher S. Kay Toombs that prioritizes the sentient experiencing of illness over its pathological definition.[5] Understanding this nexus is the overarching purpose of *Playing Sick*, which considers performances of illness staged between 1850 and 1899 for anglophone audiences in Britain and in the United States.[6] The number of diagnosable conditions from this period can easily overwhelm, but only a select few proved to be effective (and affective) dramatic devices on the late nineteenth-century stage. Three popular categories of staged illness— tuberculosis, drug addiction, and mental illness—transformed in response to and as part of three medical or scientific sea changes: the supplanting of the miasmatic theory of disease by germ theory; the medicalization of drug addiction; and the birth of modern psychology and psychoanalysis. The sexually transmitted disease syphilis will be addressed separately at the book's conclusion, both because it lacks a distinctly analogous shift in Victorian medical knowledge (its causative bacterium was not discovered until 1905) and because *fin-de-siècle* depictions of syphilis broke significantly from the precedents set by earlier illness roles. Each of the book's three parts analyzes landmark performances of illness in light of contemporaneous developments in medical and popular thought. My goals with this comparative approach are twofold. First, I seek to isolate from the period's acting practices a lexicon of embodied illness, which acquired meaning and force through rendering the sick body legible. Comprised of gestural and oral cues and using distinctive spatiotemporal signals, this lexicon was both durable and flexible, traversing geographic boundaries and those that defined theatrical genres. Through the externalizing of their characters' physical and emotional suffering, performers depicted illness as a consequential, life-altering experience, one that audiences could engage with both viscerally and empathetically. The efficacy of this imaginative transmission hinged not just upon the actors' choices, but their corporealities; critics often remarked upon the perceived fitness, maturity, and size of the actors' bodies as a way of validating or undermining their depictions. This emphasis on externalized suffering and "perform[ed] bodiliness," however, does not mean that such depictions lacked subtlety, ambiguity, or introspection.[7] Such a reading both devalues the body as a site of nuanced meaning(s) and assumes that an actor's commitment to physicalizing illness made psychological preparations for the role superfluous. Like Stanton B. Garner, Jr. and Katherine E. Kelly, I recognize the impact the natural sciences, germ theory, and the most crucial period of the medical field's professionalization had on the rapid expansion of theatrical realism and naturalism in the 1880s, but I also wish to highlight the incremental aesthetic shifts toward more unaffected performances of illness materializing throughout the latter half of the 1800s.[8] As we will see, many performers of illness roles blended romantic subjectivity with scientific objectivity, an approach that helped them convey both the mythic characteristics and medical realities of illness, though not with unqualified success. In this way, *Playing Sick* introduces fresh reference points from which to track developments in nineteenth-century acting methods.

Second, I aim to illuminate how commercial theatre helped generate influential constructions of diseases and the diseased. The case studies presented in *Playing Sick* exhibit unmistakable signs of responsiveness to shifts in medical knowledge and practice, both in their contributions to prevailing "imaginative configurations" of illness and in their explicit materiality. Actors including Ellen Terry, Richard Mansfield, and Clara Morris consulted physicians or studied the symptomatic behaviors of real sufferers. Arthur Conan Doyle, a medical man, wrote from a place of expertise about narcotics abuse when he brought Sherlock Holmes to life on the page and on the stage, and

Henry Irving deliberately trimmed *King Lear*'s script to frame and draw out Lear's madness. Critics enumerated the ways performed illnesses resembled those cataloged by medical science, and writings by physicians (like Dr. Cyrus Edson's 1983 editorial on performers' imprecise use of epileptic fits) betrayed the medical field's attentiveness to how actors played sick. Because of these examples and many others, I treat as axiomatic nineteenth-century medicine and theatre's mutual responsiveness.

Actors and audiences authenticated performances of illness not just through their embodied symptomatologies, but through the identity markers (both real and perceived) that gave them weight, shape, and context. Being ill in nineteenth-century society meant that you were a sick man or woman, and all that those distinctions implied. It meant that your nationality suggested to others whether you were especially vulnerable to illness and that your socioeconomic status determined if you were deserving of exhaustive therapeutic measures. Throughout *Playing Sick*, we will note prevalent associations of illness and ill persons to social identifiers: British and American critics associated Bernhardt's "Frenchness" obliquely with Marguerite's sensual, consumptive beauty in *La dame aux camélias*; censorious pundits of the era's mounting "drug problem" often stigmatized addicts as lower-class deviants, which Richard Mansfield reinforced in *Dr. Jekyll and Mr. Hyde* through Hyde's degeneracy; and binary constructs of the masculine and the feminine inspired a host of gendered archetypes of mental illness that then materialized in London's Lyceum Theatre.

Theatrical embodiments of illness in part redressed one of the detrimental outcomes of healthcare's systemic overhaul in the Victorian age: the rise of the paradoxically inconsequential patient. Over the course of the century, the institution of medicine ballooned in size and stature, bifurcated into specialties, improved its technological gadgetry, and swallowed up traditionally non-degreed professions (like gynecology's appropriation of midwifery). The expansion of physician authority and the public's increased faith in the findings of medical science encouraged a gradual decentering of the patient from her own diagnosis and treatment. Professional physicians of the positivist age sought to diagnose ailments by cataloguing and analyzing observable symptoms, preferably with the use of advanced technologies. The subjective illness testimonies of patients, then, served to authenticate clinical diagnoses rather than determine them, as they might have in earlier centuries. "[S]ymptoms became the means of determining the nature of the illness," note Claudine Herzlich and Janine Pierret. "The 'sick man' seemed to disappear from the medical cosmology as the clinical discourse began to take shape."[9] Many clinicians now assessed patients from a "professional" distance in order to disengage their sympathetic response to human suffering, and the common practices of quarantining and institutionalizing further reduced the visibility of the ill in society. The Victorian medical gaze often divested patients of subjecthood and dignity, and nowhere was this more evident than in the period's packed operating theatres, where performative surgeries showcased the skill, judgment, and poise of the surgeon-showman as the (usually) anesthetized and mute patient lay on a table or sat strapped to a chair, summarily draped or exposed as the procedure required. In short, the patient's unnatural dissociation from his or her own illness and its somatic expressivity was in fact a consequence of medicine's institutionalization.

I see nineteenth-century performances of illness as symbolically restorative in the sense of returning the (simulated) patient to a position of prominence and agency. Even on the commercial stage, where the primary objective was to entertain, performances of illness re-centralized and rendered visible, even consequential, the ill patient in ways unsurpassed by novelists, painters, and journalists. As a number of literature scholars concede, the lived experience of illness evades easy narrativization through language.[10] Likewise, the artist's brush could depict a single emblematic moment or mood within the illness-process, but the variable journey of an individual's experience of illness (over days, months, or years) challenges the medium of visual art. The difficulty of articulating experiential suffering with words or brushstrokes was partially ameliorated in theatrical enactments of illness. After all, theatre's very nature guarantees that when words or static images fail, bodies and voices fill the gaps of representation. Ephemeral and changeable, theatre resists essentializing the experience of illness by allowing multiple actors to embody and interpret illness roles in different spaces, times, and situations. This does not mean, however, that participating in theatrical reenactments of illness, as an actor or spectator, necessarily counteracts the disagreeable or traumatic repercussions of experiencing real illness. As Joseph Roach relates in *Cities of the Dead: Circum-Atlantic Performance*, most experiences of loss "through death or other forms of departure" instigate a form of surrogation by which "culture reproduces and re-creates itself." But attempts by "survivors" to fill the vacated spaces with "satisfactory alternates" rarely succeed, Roach explains, because "the fit cannot be exact."[11] If Roach's hypothesis is correct, imaginative configurations of illness were partly inspired by a collective need to locate suitable surrogates to fill the cavities forged by loss. Moreover, performances of illness need not be flattering portrayals to give prominence to the patient's experience. As played by Richard Mansfield, Dr. Jekyll's addiction was horrific, excessive, and ruinous, eliciting emotional and visceral responses from those who witnessed his undoing.

Playing Sick enters into a relatively new, yet rich, interdisciplinary field uniting theatre and medicine. The last twenty-five years of this scholarship have tended to focus on two periods of theatre-making. In the early modern period, Elizabethan and Jacobean stages registered a diverse collection of scientific approaches to treating illness, from humoral balancing to surgical procedures to homespun homeopathy, as well as a host of affiliated character types; this theatrical period remains the most studied by interdisciplinary historians.[12] The second centers on contemporary works that interface medicine, bioethics, personal illness narratives, and performance, inspired in large part by AIDS plays and pathographical pieces like Margaret Edson's 1995 play *Wit*.[13] *Performance Research*'s 2014 issue "On Medicine" and Alex Mermikides and

Gianna Bouchard's edited collection *Performance and the Medical Body* exemplify the field's growing attentiveness to medical performances operating outside of theatrical venues. The latter work brings together the scholarship of scientists, artists, and historians to interrogate within different sites and situations the "medical body," a form that is at once both an object (constrained and rendered passive by its clinical anatomization) and subject (active in its subjectivity, individuality, and heightened expressivity).[14]

Recent publication trends indicate that interest in nineteenth-century medicine and theatre is mounting. Leading the charge is Stanton B. Garner, Jr., who as the guest editor of a 2008 special issue of *Modern Drama* on medicine and theatre urged scholars to develop richer inquiries into such intersections within the last 125 years. Garner's own scholarship remains a model for those working in interdisciplinary arts research, and in the last decade an increasing body of scholarship (both published and presented) has critically advanced the conversation. Nevertheless, as with any burgeoning subject area, there is work to be done to redress omissions and diversify approaches. First, although scholars readily acknowledge the preeminence of the body in theatrical expressions of illness, many locate these bodies in the fixed texts of playwrights rather than in the phenomenological experience of performance. Together, these studies tend to represent the playwright as primary or sole generator of theatrical illness, an implication that obscures the complex collaborative processes at work in live performance, not to mention the ever-evolving relationship between playwright, performer, and spectator. In particular, scholars scrutinize the oeuvres of canonical giants like Ibsen, Strindberg, Zola, and Shaw through the lens of medical science, an invaluable method for interpreting early modernist playwriting that nevertheless sustains the dramatist-as-pathologist motif.[15] What I wish to call attention to is the gradual transfer of creative authority over the late nineteenth century, when realist and naturalist playwrights replaced actors as the chief engineers of onstage illness; I take up this topic in the book's conclusion. Second, if the naturalistic stage's association with medical science predominates in the extant literature, the proto-realist stage remains in relative shadow. The limited presence of nineteenth-century popular plays in studies of medicine and theatre implies (intentionally or not) that such works lacked the creative or intellectual responsiveness of the modern "legitimate" theatre and therefore have little to contribute to the meaningful topic of Illness in Theatre.

Scholars who do integrate studies of performance and late 1800s medicine tend to concentrate their research on theatrical expressions of mental illness. Of these, female portrayals of hysteria garner the most attention in influential works by Elin Diamond, Joanna Townsend, Elaine Aston, Anhki Mukherjee, and Kerry Powell, among others. Masculine performances of mental illness receive less consideration, though Jeffrey Richards and Michael Holroyd both describe actor Henry Irving's singular attraction to embodying mad characters, and Michael Schwartz includes performances of neurasthenia in his discussion of nervous conditions and the professional-managerial class. Benjamin Reiss, Kimberly Rhodes, Brant Wenegrat, Jonathan Marshall, and Rachel Fensham address the performativity of madness in non-theatrical sites, including nineteenth-century asylums.[16] Performances of contagion at times function as anecdotal support for critical deconstructions of nineteenth-century acting methods rather than being analyzed as influential expressions of illness, though Linda and Michael Hutcheon's *Opera: Desire, Disease, Death* profitably conceives of contagion, its corporeal markers, and its metaphors as central to operatic performances of disease. My work in Part I of *Playing Sick* is indebted to extent studies on the pathological and cultural constructs of tuberculosis in the nineteenth century, from Susan Sontag's seminal *Illness as Metaphor* to recent works by Clark Lawlor and Katherine Byrne, even as it proposes new approaches for analyzing consumption's performative impact.[17] To my knowledge, late nineteenth-century performances of drug addiction have not received any particular consideration, likely due to the infrequency of explicitly staged drug use in the period's plays; twentieth-century theatre offers far more instances. However, there have been several studies investigating nineteenth-century performances of alcohol addiction, including John W. Frick's *Theatre, Culture, and Temperance Reform in Nineteenth-Century America* and Amy E. Hughes's *Spectacles of Reform: Theater and Activism in Nineteenth-Century America*.[18] By prioritizing the performative and commercial over the textual and canonical, this book joins a growing collection of interdisciplinary histories centered on popular performance in the age of Victorian medicine.

Playing Sick diagnoses and analyzes embodied illness roles that operated both within and outside of the "science plays" genre so well catalogued by Shepherd-Barr.[19] Without physicians as central figures of the drama, plays like *The Lady of the Camelias*, *Sherlock Holmes*, and *The Bells* focused not on the interventions of institutionalized medicine or doctor-as-savior narratives, but on ill characters of consequence. In the case studies that follow, I hope to highlight the unique sociocultural work being done by actors performing illness in the latter half of the nineteenth century. In order to reconstruct these depictions, as well as identify the cultural currents by which they were transmitted to wider publics, this book incorporates theatre reviews, printed transcripts of scientific lectures, satirical cartoons, the memoirs of physicians and asylum superintendents, publicity stills of actors in illness roles, handwritten notes in prompt books, and other assorted materials. I acknowledge the challenges inherent in working with such disparate and tendentious artifacts; nevertheless, cultural fiction making happens in the interstices, and locating the charged, liminal spaces where constructs of illness form and re-form requires that comparable weight is given to cultural and medical theories, expressions, and commodities. I will use the term "medicocultural" throughout *Playing Sick*, first to persistently confront and dismantle the counterfactual binary of science and art, and second to emphasize that notions of illness are created by and through the continuous fusion of medical and cultural discourses.

The case studies employed in this book all took place in British and American theatres or both via transatlantic tours, though the actors were not always native performers. With the exception of Ibsen's *Ghosts*, I will only examine performances of illness in popular theatres (as opposed to the subscription houses that first produced the now canonical plays of Ibsen, Strindberg, Chekhov, and Zola). Shakespeare's prominent place in mainstream theatres' repertoires accounts for his inclusion in these analyses. When appropriate, I have endeavored to employ period-appropriate vocabulary to describe illnesses, medical procedures, anatomical structures, and other scientific phenomena. This adherence to the linguistic preferences of those living and writing in the nineteenth century at times occasions the citing of offensive terms. *Epileptic, paroxysmal, lame, paralyzed*: critics often used such words to describe a variety of performers' styles without a thought given to members of the disabled community. I do so now with caution and, I hope, economy. The phrase "Victorian medicine" appears throughout the book as shorthand for the scientific discoveries, institutional practices, specialties, and discourses that impacted the period's imaginative configurations of illness, including those on English-language popular stages. While "Victorian" implies (quite rightly) the centrality of British physicians, researchers, and establishments in the progression of late-century medical knowledge, I use "Victorian medicine" as a time-bound indicator of multinational trends in Western European and American medicine, whether they originated in Germany, France, the United Kingdom, or the United States. With an understanding of both its reductive connotations and its primacy in the nineteenth-century theatre, I have opted to call female performers "actresses" throughout.

Finally, I foreground the term "illness role" throughout this study to identify a distinctive subset of characters for which illness is an integral part, not as a means of displacing a character's other facets and functions. Dementia is a constitutive part of King Lear, of course, but his illness does not wholly eclipse his other qualities. Indeed, nineteenth-century actors reflected the complexities of "an illness lived" by integrating physical and psychological experiences of illness (pain, isolation, and despair, but also lightness, fellowship, and nostalgia) into characters that had pre-illness identities. Brant Wenegrat employs the term "illness role" differently in *Theater of Disorder*, using it to describe "a purposive behavior pattern consistent with a character in ill health" that patients assume, often with the assistance of their physicians, as a way of conceiving of, living with, or conveying their disorders to others.[20] Though *Playing Sick* locates illness roles on theatrical as opposed to metaphorical stages, I agree with Wenegrat's assertion that a medical diagnosis often brings with it behavioral expectations that reify, legitimate, and potentially stigmatize the patient's suffering. If suffering is useless in its passivity, as Emmanuel Levinas theorizes, submissive "in its hurt and its in-spite-of-consciousness," it is reasonable to speculate that a patient's performance of her illness role renders the suffering active and perhaps even productive.[21] In acknowledging the performative aspects of the illness-process I wish to avoid trivializing such experiences, and subscribe to the theory that the majority of the age's invalids were authentically ill and possessed no ulterior motives. And yet, illness is undeniably and fundamentally theatrical, related as it often was to identity transformations, interpersonal turmoil, questions of faith, and cycles of remission and relapse. The rapid institutionalization of the Victorian medical profession reduced patient agency to such a degree as to trigger a proliferation of compensatory expressions of illness across the visual, literary, and performing arts. Ultimately, stretching the illness-as-performance synthesis past its breaking point has the potential to oversimplify and distort what was a far more complex social condition.

An illness performed

In *Dance Pathologies: Performance, Poetics, Medicine*, a study on dance performances of feminine mental illness from *Giselle* to the ballets of *Bagatelles pour un massacre*, Felicia McCarren draws parallels between nineteenth-century medicine's "attempts to come to grips with how the body deploys 'idea' somatically" and dance's richly signifying visuality. The dancer's wordlessness, she argues, amplifies the moving body's power to speak, to create meaning through its "mute expressiveness."[22] While the theatre is rarely taciturn, McCarren's claim that performing bodies generated or revised cultural *ideas* of illness holds true for the nineteenth-century popular stage. Those who assumed the role of the consumptive Camille, for example, also devised and embodied a composition of tuberculosis itself. Using somatic, verbal, and spatiotemporal means, actors depicted the objectives—often irreconcilable, but at times compatible—of the illness and its human host, signaling to audiences the synchronous conflicts being waged on environmental, personal, and cellular levels.

Illness was but one in a repertoire of emotional and physical states-of-being performed by nineteenth-century actors. As such, illness roles must be considered in light of the methodologies, conditions, and expectations that governed acting. Bookended by the bold romanticism of the early nineteenth century and the meticulous naturalism of the *fin de siècle*, late 1800s theatre finds definition in its very lack of a singular dramaturgical or aesthetic hallmark. As with many periods, Victorian-era theatre was transitional and heterogeneous, with a wealth of genres and styles produced throughout Britain and the United States. English playhouses ran appealing but predictable repertoires consisting of melodramas, cup-and-saucer plays, light comedies and burlesques, Shakespearean revivals, and French translations, at times interspersed with musical interludes and *tableaux vivants*, depending upon the decade and venue. American theatres offered similar programs, adding plays by "native-born," non-indigenous playwrights into the rotation. The period's acting practices echoed the theatre's unique liminality, with a rich spectrum of acceptable methods in play at any given time. Some actors trained in eighteenth-century declamatory techniques, unable or unwilling to adapt to the changing tastes, became living totems to a bygone age. Others anticipated or heralded the naturalist turn. Still others embodied the period's transitional ethos by tempering the vivid emotionalism of the romantics with a more restrained psychological internality that eventually found its true expressive power at the century's end. Just as musicologist Carl Dahlhaus regards the compositions of Richard Wagner and his contemporaries as the "late flowering of romanticism in a positivist age," we can see in late nineteenth-century acting a paradoxical integrating of old and new, of the powerful but out-of-step romanticism mingling with more analytic approaches to character-building, inspired by the uncompromising positivism of industrialized modernity and the scientific age.[23] Historians cite the 1880s and 1890s as the formative decades of theatrical realism and naturalism because playwright-vanguards and advances in theatre technology transformed the situations, themes, language, *mise en scene*, and purposes of the Western stage, providing the superlative vehicles for naturalistic actors and necessitating the debut of the modern director. Nevertheless, this gradual shift began decades before, in stops and starts and within a number of cultural milieus, rather than materializing in a burst of creative innovation in Norway, France, or Russia. Premieres of social dramas and thesis plays in English-language theatres, not to mention the accelerated development of more realistic staging and acting techniques, signaled that the theatrical revolution brewing in continental Europe was also percolating at home.

The efforts of performers to externalize their ill characters' suffering reflect not just science's positivist priorities, but the entrenched practices of pre-realistic acting. As Joseph R. Roach and Gay Gibson Cima have detailed, performers of the eighteenth and nineteenth centuries physicalized the inner workings of the mind and spirit using a codified system of gestures, facial expressions, body positions, and blocking.[24] By doing so, they maintained the profoundly visual nature of the era's performing arts. In the early 1800s, actors learned this art of body mapping primarily through apprenticeship and personal study, though illustrated texts on the anatomy, functions, and appearances of human expression were published throughout the century, including works by nerve specialists, physiognomists, elocution experts, art historians, and famed naturalist Charles Darwin. Later in the century, new acting manuals established a "science of theatrical art," as did instructional courses in elocutionary and actor training schools, a burgeoning industry in the late 1800s.[25] The most well known of these systems was developed by François Delsarte, a French teacher of singing, acting, and aesthetics, who conducted painstaking investigations into the body's expressive anatomies and functions in an effort to observe and then teach the scientific principles of human behavior and expression. For Delsarte and his contemporaries, a person's spirit found articulation not in the words she speaks but in the way she physically moves through the world. "Gesture corresponds to the soul, to the heart; language to the life, to the thought, to the mind," wrote Delsarte in 1882. "The life and the mind being subordinate to the heart, to the soul, gesture is the chief organic agent."[26] Actors of the period calibrated the stage's gestural codes to suit a range of theatrical styles and characters, from the subdued bourgeoisie of cup-and-saucer dramas to the buffoonish sailors of Gilbert and Sullivan operettas.

Singing seamen notwithstanding, the pictorial nature of the period's theatre deemphasized, at least in part, the oratorical demands of acting. Still, performers regarded the breath and voice as one in an essential triumvirate of actor's tools, along with the body and the mind/spirit, to be formally trained or developed through performance. In a clear break from earlier declamatory or classical schools of acting, actors attempted to reproduce onstage the patterns and cadences of conversational speech, the better to articulate modern dramatic prose. Shakespeare's prominence in nineteenth-century repertoires necessitated at least a proficiency in delivering rhythmic verse; critics proved uncharitable to actors who struggled with meter (particularly those in England). The supple, well-modulated voice, natural in its lack of grandiloquence but elevated in its measured concessions to theatricality, became the preferred instrument for the nineteenth-century popular stage. For actors simulating illness, the voice and breath signaled a body or mind under duress. Coughs, stammers, sharp intakes of air, labored breathing, hysterical laughter: such vocalizations had the potential to reveal or punctuate the presence of illness. In some cases, an actor's own vocal shortcomings benefitted their illness roles. Henry Irving's stutter and idiosyncratic intonations, so often topics of ridicule in the popular press, helped manifest a mind traumatized by guilt, as in *The Bells'* Matthias, or a senile mind, as in King Lear.

Actors performing illness roles faced a task not dissimilar from their other parts: to convey the heightened stakes of the characters' suffering without compromising physical or mental control. Treatises on acting, including William Archer's *Masks or Faces? The Psychology of Acting*, an 1888 rejoinder to Denis Diderot's proclamations in *Paradoxe sur le comédien* (published in English in 1883), argued for a balance between emotions and technique. Both Roach and Lynn M. Voskuil offer nuanced histories of Diderot's impact on Victorian acting theories, but for our purposes a few points should be highlighted. Diderot's *Paradoxe* plots the mind and body on a shared continuum, which both breaks from the Cartesian mind–body duality and yet strangely reasserts the divisibility—or at least the potential remoteness—of the two in enacting theatrical roles. Diderot's actor exemplar engages in imaginative, impulsive discoveries in rehearsal and repeats until his actions and emotions become automatic, free of sensibility and deliberation. Onstage, the actor's mind is unemotional, open, and unencumbered, able to skillfully govern the performance without distraction.[27] Nineteenth-century theatre commentators, echoing Diderot, cautioned against an actor giving over to raw emotionalism without the taming influences of rehearsal, technical skill, rationality, and an awareness of the audience, but most disagreed with Diderot's assertion that empathetic sensibility and technical proficiency were mutually exclusive skill sets. Both Archer and English theorist and critic George Henry Lewes revised Diderot's formulation of the mind-body continuum into different articulations of what Archer calls dual or multiple "strata of consciousness," or more simply dual consciousness.[28] The notion of multiple selves operating concurrently in and through one body on different planes of consciousness would soon be taken up elsewhere, in the field of modern psychology. While the observations of Lewes and Archer remained primarily trained on English performers, Archer's *Masks and Faces* incorporated into his thesis American audiences and actors including Clara Morris, Charlotte Cushman, and Thomas A. Cooper.

Critics objecting to a performance of illness often registered their displeasure in terms of its failure to realistically represent a known medical condition and its impact on human experience. Illness roles, then, entered into and became central to a centuries-long dialogue, curated by theatre critics and theorists, about what constituted "real" onstage.[29] For some, "realistic" simply connoted a performance's *resemblance* to real life, not necessarily its rejection of theatrical artifice or sentimentality. Likewise, critics typically used the word "natural" to suggest one of following: the especial suitability of an actor to his part; the lack of discernable effort, strain, or grandiosity in an actor's choices; or the extent to which the audience seemed moved organically by an actor (rather than through the outmoded practice of making "points"). For Lewes, natural acting did not replicate real life, but refracted it using a filter:

> The supreme difficulty of an actor is to represent ideal character with such truthfulness that it shall affect us as real, not to drag down ideal character to the vulgar level. His art is one of representation, not of illusion. He has to use natural expressions, but he must sublimate them; the symbols must be such as we can sympathetically interpret, and for this purpose they must be the expressions of real human feeling; but just as the language is poetry, or choice prose, purified from the hesitancies, incoherences, and imperfections of careless daily speech, so must his utterance be measured, musical, incisive – his manner typical and pictorial.[30]

Lewes' understanding of truthfulness onstage, of acting "naturally," does not require duplicating the minute details of reality. Notes Voskuil, "Lewes here objects to a standard of verisimilitude that emphasizes the actual and the sensory at the expense of the imaginative."[31] An entirely artless performance, for Lewes and many in the theatregoing public, ceased to be art at all. The period's theatre reviews and acting treatises makes clear that the most esteemed performers avoided early-century "staginess" by employing the conventions of their craft (coded gestures, vocal techniques, stage movements, use of space, dramatic timing) not to demonstrate virtuosity and "emphasiz[e] the medium for its own sake," but to "materialize feeling."[32] Both Lewes and French actor Constant Coquelin took pains to differentiate between natural acting and the new fad of naturalism in articles published prior to the movement's arrival, with Coquelin declaring: "I am always on the side of nature, and against naturalism."[33] Naturalistic acting was, for those not persuaded by Zola's 1880 manifesto, the evocation of mundane, negligible, or base realities of human behavior in performance, or what Coquelin deemed "the exhibition of revolting hideousness, of pitiless and naked realities."[34] Though such colorful vitriol faded by the *fin de siècle* as aspects of naturalism infiltrated mainstream theatres, the potential of performances of illness to be deemed by audiences too graphic or indecorous extended into the twentieth century.

Archer's survey of acting obscures the differences in performance styles among British and American actors, though by the time of *Masks or Faces?*

publication, variances—both real and perceived—were less pronounced than earlier in the century. Edwin Forrest, the first influential American-born performer, initiated in the late 1820s a style of acting (referred to as the "heroic" or "American" school) that was robust, sonorous, fiery, and athletic. Though Forrest's acting was shaped in part by his admiration of English romantic actor Edmund Kean, the American school was the near antithesis of the classical English acting of the Kemble family or the dignified elegance of William Charles Macready. Forrest's largely working-class enthusiasts heralded their new stage icon as thrilling, unpretentious, and "American."[35] Prohibited by gender constraints from adopting the muscular athleticism of their countrymen, actresses of the antebellum American stage, including Cushman, Morris, and Matilda Heron, instead devised a style of performance typified by extreme emotionalism.[36] Even as British and American audiences celebrated the intelligence, diligence, and grace of mid-century tragedian Edwin Booth, the reputation of American actors as less polished and more demonstrative than their English competitors continued through the Victorian period. However, if American performers seemed more "undignified" in their expressivity than the English, they also appeared to nineteenth-century spectators and critics as more unfettered by custom and contrivances. Such impressions reaffirmed, for some Britons and Americans, fundamental disparities between the two body politics. "Our republic has been more than abundantly favored with material prosperity," declared American theatre critic William Winter in 1889, "yet it cannot be truthfully denied that as a people we are still deficient in gentleness and grace."[37] Historians have since located nineteenth-century American theatre in more nuanced territory, divorcing the vibrant, varied practices of American actors and audiences from outdated "second fiddle" narratives. Indeed, Amy Hughes's illumination of the "somatic spectacle[s]" in mid-century temperance melodramas aligns with the performances of illness I reconstruct here.[38]

Because performances of illness were composed using imbricated medical and theatrical influences, they invite us to reflect upon how the subsidiary discourses on disease and acting overlapped in the nineteenth century. What is remarkable is how analogous the period's narratives of illness and disease—recorded both in impersonal biomedical jargon and the private testimonials of the sick and dying—are to the period's performance theories and practices. Clearly, both challenged older notions of the human body as divisible into material and metaphysical parts, proposing instead a monistic human being whose mental states were fully embodied. This, coupled with medicine's faith in empirical research and the theatre's visual artistry, meant that "ideal" patients and actors provided clues to their internal states through external signs and signaling. Notions of internality and externality played out in other ways, too. In order to track disease pathologies, epidemiologists labored to identify where the seeds of illness were sown: in the internal makeup of the individual, an external or environmental factor, or a combination of both. In the case of tuberculosis, for example, science disproved the reputed internality of the disease with the discovery of the *tubercle bacillus*, a bacterium that invaded the body from the outside. The etiologies of tuberculosis, drug addiction, and mental illness transformed in the Victorian age, when external causes of disease—germs, addictive narcotics, traumatic events—gained widespread acceptance over internal factors like hereditary susceptibilities and moral defects. Meanwhile, nineteenth-century actors sought to balance, reconcile, and integrate internal impulses and external stimuli in performing their characters' emotions onstage, predicting the formal acting systems of Constantin Stanislavski, Michael Chekhov, and others. In this curious way, actors and epidemiologists both contemplated breaches of the body's barriers, though on vastly different scales and severities. Finally, those who endured illness and those who worked as theatre actors constituted two fringe groups operating on the peripheries of society. As such, patients and performers were described both in aggrandizing and demoralizing terms, scrutinized because of their spectacular bodies, mutable minds, and extended behavioral latitudes. The deliberate conflation of the female hysteric and late nineteenth-century actress, in particular, drew the hospital ward and theatrical stage together as analogous sites for the containment *and* exhibition of ungovernable women.

Part I of *Playing Sick* takes as its focus decades of consumptive suffering in the character of Marguerite Gautier/Camille, the consumptive courtesan of Alexandre Dumas fils's *La dame aux camélias*. During the play's tenure as a warhorse of the nineteenth-century stage, the discovery of a tiny but deadly microbe transformed tuberculosis from an inherited disease of extraordinary individuals to the contagious disease of the masses. This etiological shift, and the related supplanting of the miasmic theory of disease by germ theory, reframed Camille's illness and combatted, over time, the aestheticization of the "romantic" disease of consumption. The majority of nineteenth-century Camilles, I propose, complied with one of two dominant strains of performing consumption. Actresses who romanticized the courtesan's fatal affliction participated in the cultural prolongation of the "consumptive myth," or the fallacious belief that consumption was an inherited disease striking only the rich, beautiful, young, sensitive, or exceedingly talented. Another group of performers emphasized the graphic realities of tuberculosis as a contagious disease, thereby medicalizing her illness. Their explicit and uninhibited enactments of tubercular suffering loosened the consumptive myth's tight grasp on artistic representations of the disease. In Part I's second chapter, I turn to continental actresses Sarah Bernhardt and Eleonora Duse, whose corporealities, reputations, acting techniques, and foreignness served as compelling indexes of Marguerite's decadent lifestyle and terminal illness for anglophone critics and theatregoers.

Part II appraises early depictions of drug addiction in stage adaptations of *Dr. Jekyll and Mr. Hyde* and *Sherlock Holmes*, both of which coincided with institutionalized medicine's recoding of drug addiction as a disease. Richard Mansfield's fiendishly grotesque transformations in the double role of Jekyll/Hyde (1887) and William Gillette's embodiment of the cocaine-injecting Holmes (1899) presented *fin-de-siècle* audiences with three archetypal drug users: the reluctant victim, the criminalized fiend, and the controlled habitué. In *Sherlock Holmes*, Gillette's refined and intelligent detective self-administers hypodermic injections of cocaine, to the consternation of Dr. Watson and in full view of the audience, in order to stimulate his mental faculties. Holmes's drug use is socially acceptable, executed onstage by Gillette with control and panache, and the character's detecting skills are sharpened, not dulled, by the injections. In direct contrast to Gillette's performance, Mansfield's sensational rendition of substance abuse depended as much on his portrayal of two unsavory addicts as it did on his transformations from one to the other. Instead of liberating him from Victorian social mores, the vial of medicine Jekyll concocted to split his identity into halves robs him of joy, friendship, and agency. If Mansfield's Jekyll appeared as a remorseful, ensnared addict, his Mr. Hyde was an urban drug fiend, bestial and maniacal, even perhaps a personification of the drug itself.

From 1878 to 1899, actor-manager Henry Irving and his acting partner Ellen Terry performed a series of mental disorders ranging from masculine monomania (*The Bells*, 1871) to feminine hysteria (*Ravenswood*, 1890) for audiences at London's Lyceum Theatre, most to critical acclaim but some notably to public jeers. In Part III, I contend that the Lyceum's pictorial and physicalized method of enacting illness, widely celebrated at the beginning of Irving's management of the theatre, gradually lost favor as the birth of modern psychiatry and theatrical realism prompted more internalized, subtle approaches to acting. Moreover, both Terry and Irving's mad roles seemed to support medicocultural understandings of mental illness as essentially gendered. Madness became crucially feminized in the Victorian period, thereby normalizing women's experiences with mental illness and casting males with psychological conditions as effeminate, deviant, or broken. As these chapters make clear, critics and audiences viewed Terry's performances of feminine hysteria and madness in *Hamlet*, *Macbeth*, and *Ravenswood* as organic, alluring, and profoundly pathetic, whereas Irving's characters in *The Bells*, *Hamlet*, and *King Lear*, all of whom suffered from distinctive "mind disorders" or neuropathologies, were emasculated and denaturalized by their tragic mental states.

The brightest philosophical and critical minds of the last century have attempted to succinctly describe the transfiguring, holistic, enculturating experience of illness, of an illness *lived*: as pathology, as metaphor, as narrative, as phenomenological occurrence, as socio-ethical trauma, and countless other constructs. In its focus on an illness *performed*, the three parts of *Playing Sick* do not prioritize one particular theory of illness. Rather, I wish to highlight throughout how medical and theatrical conceptions of illness were endowed with similar anatomies in the late nineteenth century, a time of radical cross-disciplinary and cross-cultural transition. Both united the vestiges of romanticism (subjectivity, mythology, symbolism) with naturalism's core tenets (objectivity, reality, materialism). Both engaged in a profound and complicated discourse on what it meant to be a human under an embodied threat, as well as theorized on the external and internal causes of those threats. And yet, whereas the impact of the positivist revolution and the institutionalization of the medical profession reduced the authentic patient's agency and downplayed his illness narrative, actors recentralized simulated ill patients and rendered their voices, experiences, and materialities consequential. Through their expressive embodiments of suffering, theatre performers generated culturally salient constructions of illness and merit being counted among Keats, Baudelaire, Puccini, and Millais as cultural architects of nineteenth-century illness roles.

Notes

1 "Typhus and Cholera – An Eclogue," *The Times* (London), Sept. 24, 1853.
2 Athena Vrettos, *Somatic Fictions: Imagining Illness in Victorian Culture* (Stanford: Stanford University Press, 1995), 3.
3 Berrios and Freeman, "Dementia Before the Twentieth Century," in *Alzheimer and the Dementias*, ed. G. E. Berrios and H. L. Freeman (London: Royal Society of Medicine Services Ltd., 1991), 26.
4 Kirsten E. Shepherd-Barr, "The Diagnostic Gaze: Nineteenth-Century Contexts for Medicine and Performance," in *Performance and the Medical Body*, ed. Alex Mermikides and Gianna Bouchard (London: Bloomsbury Methuen, 2016), 37.
5 S. Kay Toombs, *The Meaning of Illness: A Phenomenological Account of the Different Perspectives of Physician and Patient* (Dordrecht, the Netherlands: Springer Netherlands, 1992), xvi.
6 Many nineteenth-century illness roles were performed well into the twentieth century, for example, William Gillette's Sherlock Holmes and several iterations of Camille/Marguerite Gautier.
7 Felicia McCarren, *Dance Pathologies: Performance, Poetics, Medicine* (Stanford: Stanford University Press, 1998), 15.
8 Stanton B. Garner, Jr., "Artaud, Germ Theory, and the Theatre of Contagion," *Theatre Journal* 58 (2006): 1–14; and Katherine E. Kelly, "Pandemic and Performance: Ibsen and the Outbreak of Modernism," *South Central Review* 25, no. 1 (Spring 2008): 12–35.
9 Claudine Herzlich and Janine Pierret, *Illness and Self in Society*, trans. Elborg Forster (Baltimore: Johns Hopkins University Press, 1987), 30. Recognizing that twentieth-century medical histories displaced the patient with near equivalency to nineteenth-century medical practice, Roy Porter's seminal 1985 essay "The Patient's View: Doing Medical History from Below" called on scholars to move beyond (and below) institution- and physician-centric medical histories and locate the voices, thoughts, and deeds of the patients. *Theory and Society* 14 (1985): 175–198.
10 See Vrettos, *Somatic Fictions*; Miriam Bailin, *The Sickroom in Victorian Fiction: The Art of Being Ill* (Cambridge: Cambridge University Press, 1994); and Jane Wood, *Passion and Pathology in Victorian Fiction* (Oxford: Oxford University Press, 2001).
11 Joseph Roach, *Cities of the Dead: Circum-Atlantic Performance* (New York: Columbia University Press, 1996), 2.
12 Stanton B. Garner, Jr. "Introduction: Is There a Doctor in the House? Medicine and the Making of Modern Drama," *Modern Drama* 55, no. 3 (Fall 2008): 311–328, 313.
13 Anne Hunsaker Hawkins uses *pathography* to describe "a form of autobiography or biography that describes personal experiences of illness, treatment, and sometimes death." *Reconstructing Illness: Studies in Pathography* (West Lafayette: Purdue University Press, 1993), 1.
14 Alex Mermikides and Gianna Bouchard, *Performance and the Medical Body*, eds. Alex Mermikides and Gianna Bouchard (London: Bloomsbury 2016), 12–13. Here Mermikides

and Bouchard are employing Jennifer Parker-Starbuck's notion of "medical body" from her 2014 book *Cyborg Theatre*. See also *Performance Research*'s robust issue "On Medicine" 9, no. 4 (2014) for scholarship on medicine and performance art.

15 Among these works are Shepherd-Barr, "The Diagnostic Gaze"; Katherine E. Kelly, "Pandemic and Performance"; Evert Sprinchorn, "Syphilis in Ibsen's *Ghosts*," *Ibsen Studies* (2004): 191–204; Amy Strahler Holzapfel, "Stringberg as Vivisector: Physiology, Pathology, and Anti-Mimesis in *The Father* and *Miss Julie*," *Modern Drama* 51, no. 3 (Fall 2008): 329–352; Stanton B. Garner, Jr., "Physiologies of the Modern: Zola, Experimental Medicine, and the Naturalist Stage," *Modern Drama* 43, no. 4 (Winter 2000): 529–542; and Charles A. Carpenter, "The Strategy and the Bacteriology: Scrutinizing the Microbe in Shaw's *Too True to Be Good*," *SHAW* 27 (2007): 135–155.

16 Elin Diamond, *Unmaking Mimesis: Essays on Feminism and Theater* (London: Routledge, 1997); Ankhi Mukherjee, *Aesthetic Hysteria: The Great Neurosis in Victorian Melodrama and Contemporary Fiction* (New York: Routledge, 2007); Joanna Townsend, "Elizabeth Robins: Hysteria, Politics, and Performance," in *Women, Theatre, and Performance: New Histories, New Historiographies*, ed. Maggie B. Gale and Viv Gardner (Manchester: Manchester University Press: 2000): 102–120; Elaine Aston, "'Studies in Hysteria': Actress and Courtesan, Sarah Bernhardt and Mrs. Patrick Campbell," in *The Cambridge Companion to the Actress*, ed. Maggie B. Gale and John Stokes (Cambridge: Cambridge University Press, 2007): 253–271; Kerry Powell, *Women and Victorian Theatre* (Cambridge: Cambridge University Press, 1997); Jeffrey Richards, *Sir Henry Irving: A Victorian Actor and His World* (London: Hambledon and London, 2005); Michael Holroyd, *A Strange Eventful History: The Dramatic Lives of Ellen Terry, Henry Irving, and Their Remarkable Families* (New York: Farrar, Straus and Giroux, 2009); Michael Schwartz, *Broadway and Corporate Capitalism: The Rise of the Professional-Managerial Class, 1900–1920* (New York: Palgrave Macmillan, 2009); Benjamin Reiss, *Theaters of Madness: Insane Asylums and Nineteenth-Century American Culture* (Chicago: University of Chicago Press, 2008); Kimberly Rhodes, *Ophelia and Victorian Visual Culture: Representing Body Politics in the Nineteenth Century* (Aldershot: Ashgate, 2008); Brant Wenegrat, *Theater of Disorder: Patients, Doctors, and the Construction of Illness* (Oxford: Oxford University Press, 2001); Jonathan Marshall, "Dynamic Medicine and Theatrical Form in the fin de siècle," *Modernism/Modernity* 15, no. 1 (January 2008): 131–153; and Rachel Fensham, "On Not Performing Madness," *Theatre Topics* 8, no. 2 (1998): 149–171.

17 Linda and Michael Hutcheon, *Opera: Disease, Desire, Death* (Lincoln: University of Nebraska Press, 1996); Susan Sontag, *Illness as Metaphor* (New York: Farrar, Straus and Giroux, 1977); Clark Lawlor, *Consumption and Literature: The Making of the Romantic Disease* (Basingstoke: Palgrave MacMillan, 2006); and Katherine Byrne, *Tuberculosis and the Victorian Literary Imagination* (Cambridge: Cambridge University Press, 2011).

18 John W. Frick, *Theatre, Culture, and Temperance Reform in Nineteenth-Century America* (Cambridge: Cambridge University Press, 2008); and Amy E. Hughes, *Spectacles of Reform: Theater and Activism in Nineteenth-Century America* (Ann Arbor: University of Michigan Press, 2012).

19 Kristen E. Shepherd-Barr, *Science on Stage: From Doctor Faustus to Copenhagen* (Princeton: Princeton University Press, 2006).

20 Wenegrat, *Theater of Disorder*, 4.

21 Emmanuel Levinas, "Useless Suffering," trans. Richard Cohen, in *Provocation of Levinas: Rethinking the Other*, ed. Robert Bernasconi and David Wood (London: Routledge, 1988): 156–167, 157.

22 McCarren, *Dance Pathologies*, 15 and 17.

23 Carl Dahlhaus, "Neo-Romanticism," *19th-Century Music* 3, no. 2 (1979): 97–105, 102.

24 See Joseph R. Roach, *The Player's Passion: Studies in the Science of Acting* (Newark: University of Delaware Press, 1985), 160–195; and Gay Gibson Cima, *Performing Women: Female Characters, Male Playwrights, and the Modern Stage* (Ithaca: Cornell University Press, 1996), 1–60.

25 Roach, *Player's Passion*, 165.

26 François Delsarte, *Delsarte System of Oratory*, 4th ed. (1882; reprinted New York: ESW, 1893), 465. Delsarte's Law of Correspondence, which explores the relationships of "tangible and intangible, outer and inner, movement and meaning," theorizes that a human's indivisible body houses cooperative "mental, emotional, and spiritual aspects of existence." Nancy Ruyter, *The Cultivation of Body and Mind in Nineteenth-Century American Delsartism* (Westport: Greenwood Press, 1999), 76. Such notions undergirded nineteenth-century acting techniques throughout Europe and North America, but beyond Delsarte's native France it was in the United States that his teachings took root, where former pupils Steele Mackaye and Genevieve Stebbins formed training schools founded on Delsartean theories and exercises after Delsarte's death in 1871.

27 Roach, *Player's Passion*, 152.

28 William Archer, *Masks or Faces? The Psychology of Acting*, in *The Paradox of Acting and Masks or Faces?*, intro. Lee Strasberg (New York: Hill and Wang, 1957), 184.

29 This conversation was spurred on in part by Charles Macklin and David Garrick, actors whose precise and individualized performances challenged the dominance of bombastic acting in the 1740s.

30 George Henry Lewes, *On Actors and the Art of Acting*, 2nd ed. (London: Smith, Elder and Co., 1875), 113.

31 Lynn M. Voskuil, *Acting Naturally: Victorian Theatricality and Authenticity* (Charlottesville: University of Virginia Press, 2004), 46.

32 Voskuil, *Acting Naturally*, 43.

33 Constant Coquelin, "Actors and Acting," in *Papers on Acting II: The Art of Acting, A Discussion by Constant Coquelin, Henry Irving, and Dion Boucicault* (New York: Columbia University Press, 1926), 36.

34 Coquelin, "Actors and Acting," 35. Naturalists in this sense were also called Zolaists in the 1870s and Ibsenites by the 1890s.

35 His critics countered that the actor's lack of refinement and control diminished his adaptability. The bloodshed of the Astor Place Riots in 1849 threw such debates into stark relief, as a presumed Forrest-Macready rivalry became the clarion call to working-class nativists to rail against the rise of an American pseudo-aristocracy and their British stage idols.

36 Morris was born in Canada, and Heron in Ireland.

37 William Winter, "The Actor," in *The Actor and Other Speeches, Chiefly on Theatrical Subjects and Occasions* (1891; reprint New York: Burt Franklin, 1970), 23.

38 Hughes, *Spectacles of Reform*, 10. See Rosemarie K. Bank, *Theatre Culture in America, 1825–1860* (Cambridge: Cambridge University Press, 1997); Richard Butsch, *The Making of American Audiences: From Stage to Television, 1750–1990* (Cambridge: Cambridge University Press, 2000); Bruce A. McConachie, *Melodramatic Formations: American Theatre and Society, 1820-1870* (Iowa City: University of Iowa Press, 1992); Tice Miller, *Entertaining the Nation: American Drama in the Eighteenth and Nineteenth Centuries* (Carbondale: Southern Illinois University Press, 2007); and Heather S. Nathans, *Slavery and Sentiment on the American Stage, 1787–1861: Lifting the Veil on Black* (Cambridge: Cambridge University Press, 2009).

Bibliography

Archer, William. *Masks or Faces?* In *The Paradox of Acting and Masks or Faces?*, 75–226. New York: Hill and Wang, 1957.

Aston, Elaine. "'Studies in Hysteria': Actress and Courtesan, Sarah Bernhardt and Mrs. Patrick Campbell." In *The Cambridge Companion to the Actress*. Edited by Maggie B. Gale and John Stokes, 253–271. Cambridge: Cambridge University Press, 2007.

Bailin, Miriam. *The Sickroom in Victorian Fiction: The Art of Being Ill*. Cambridge: Cambridge University Press, 1994.

Bank, Rosemary K. *Theatre Culture in America, 1825–1860.* Cambridge: Cambridge University Press, 1997.

Berrios, G. E. and H. L. Freeman. "Dementia Before the Twentieth Century." In *Alzheimer and the Dementias.* Edited by G. E. Berrios and H. L. Freeman, 9–27. London: Royal Society of Medicine Services Ltd., 1991.

Booth, Martin. *Opium: A History.* New York: St. Martin's Press, 1996.

Bouchard, Gianna and Martin O'Brien, eds. "Special Issue: On Medicine." *Performance Research* 19, no. 4 (2014).

Byrne, Katherine. *Tuberculosis and the Victorian Literary Imagination.* Cambridge: Cambridge University Press, 2011.

Carpenter, Charles A. "The Strategy and the Bacteriology: Scrutinizing the Microbe in Shaw's *Too True to Be Good.*" *SHAW* 27 (2007): 135–155.

Cima, Gay Gibson. *Performing Women: Female Characters, Male Playwrights, and the Modern Stage.* Ithaca: Cornell University Press, 1996.

Coquelin, Constant. "Acting and Acting." In *Papers on Acting II: The Art of Acting, A Discussion by Constant Coquelin, Henry Irving, and Dion Boucicault,* 5–42. New York: Columbia University Press, 1926.

Dahlhaus, Carol. "Neo-Romanticism." *19th-Century Music* 3, no. 2 (1979): 97–105.

Delsarte, François. *Delsarte System of Oratory,* 4th edition. New York: ESW, 1893.

Diamond, Elin. *Unmaking Mimesis: Essays on Feminism and Theater.* London: Routledge, 1997.

Fensham, Rachel. "On Not Performing Madness." *Theatre Topics* 8, no. 2 (1998): 149–171.

Frick, John. *Theatre, Culture, and Temperance Reform in Nineteenth-Century America.* Cambridge: Cambridge University Press, 2003.

Garner, Jr., Stanton B. "Artaud, Germ Theory, and the Theatre of Contagion." *Theatre Journal* 58, no. 1 (March 2006): 1–14.

Garner, Jr., Stanton B. "Introduction: Is There a Doctor in the House? Medicine and the Making of Modern Drama." *Modern Drama* 51, no. 3 (Fall 2008): 311–328.

Garner, Jr., Stanton B. "Physiologies of the Modern: Zola, Experimental Medicine, and the Naturalist Stage." *Modern Drama* 43, no. 4 (Winter 2000): 529–542.

Hawkins, Anne Hunsaker. *Reconstructing Illness: Studies in Pathography.* West Lafayette: Purdue University Press, 1993.

Herzlich, Claudine and Janine Pierret. *Illness and Self in Society.* Trans. Elborg Forster. Baltimore: Johns Hopkins University Press, 1987.

Holroyd, Michael. *A Strange Eventful History: The Dramatic Lives of Ellen Terry, Henry Irving, and Their Remarkable Families.* New York: Farrar, Straus and Giroux, 2009.

Holzapfel, Amy Strahler. "Strindberg as Vivisector: Physiology, Pathology, and Anti-Mimesis in *The Father* and *Miss Julie.* " *Modern Drama* 51, no. 3 (Fall 2008): 329–352.

Hughes, Amy E. *Spectacles of Reform: Theater and Activism in Nineteenth-Century America.* Ann Arbor: University of Michigan Press, 2012.

Hutcheon, Linda and Michael Hutcheon. *Opera: Desire, Disease, Death.* Lincoln: University of Nebraska Press, 1996.

Kelly, Katherine E. "Pandemic and Performance: Ibsen and the Outbreak of Modernism." *South Central Review* 25, no. 1 (Spring 2008): 12–35.

Lawlor, Clark. *Consumption and Literature: The Making of the Romantic Disease.* Basingstoke: Palgrave MacMillan, 2006.

Levinas, Emmanuel. "Useless Suffering." Trans. Richard Cohen. In *Provocation of Levinas: Rethinking the Other.* Edited by Robert Bernasconi and David Wood, 156–167. London: Routledge, 1988.

Lewes, George Henry. *On Actors and the Art of Acting*, 2nd edition. London: Smith, Elder and Co., 1875.

Marshall, Jonathan. "Dynamic Medicine and Theatrical Form in the fin de siècle." *Modernism/Modernity* 15, no. 1 (January 2008): 131–153.

Matos, Timothy Carlo. "Choleric Fictions: Epidemiology, Medical Authority, and *An Enemy of the People*." *Modern Drama* 51, no. 3 (Fall 2008): 353–368.

McArthur, Benjamin. *Actors and American Culture, 1880–1920.* Iowa City: University of Iowa Press, 2000.

McCarren, Felicia. *Dance Pathologies: Performance, Poetics, Medicine.* Stanford: Stanford University Press, 1998.

McConachie, Bruce A. *Melodramatic Formations: American Theatre and Society, 1820–1870.* Iowa City: University of Iowa Press, 1992.

Miller, Tice. *Entertaining the Nation: American Drama in the Eighteenth and Nineteenth Centuries.* Carbondale: Southern Illinois University Press, 2007.

Mukherjee, Ankhi. *Aesthetic Hysteria: The Great Neurosis in Victorian Melodrama and Contemporary Fiction.* New York: Routledge, 2007.

Nathans, Heather S. *Slavery and Sentiment on the American Stage, 1787–1861: Lifting the Veil on Black.* Cambridge: Cambridge University Press, 2009.

Porter, Roy. "The Patient's View: Doing Medical History from Below." *Theory and Society* 14 (1985): 175–198.

Powell, Kerry. *Women and Victorian Theatre.* Cambridge: Cambridge University Press, 1997.

Reiss, Benjamin. *Theaters of Madness: Insane Asylums and Nineteenth-Century American Culture.* Chicago: University of Chicago Press, 2008.

Richards, Jeffrey. *Sir Henry Irving: A Victorian Actor and His World.* London: Hambledon and London, 2005.

Roach, Joseph. *Cities of the Dead: Circum-Atlantic Performance.* New York: Columbia University Press, 1996.

Roach, Joseph. *The Player's Passion: Studies in the Science of Acting.* Newark: University of Delaware Press, 1985.

Ruyter, Nancy. *The Cultivation of Body and Mind in Nineteenth-Century American Delsartism.* Westport: Greenwood Press, 1999.

Schwartz, Michael. *Broadway and Corporate Capitalism: The Rise of the Professional-Managerial Class, 1900–1920.* New York: Palgrave Macmillan, 2009.

Shepherd-Barr, Kirsten E. "The Diagnostic Gaze: Nineteenth-Century Contexts for Medicine and Performance." In *Performance and the Medical Body.* Edited by Alex Mermikides and Gianna Bouchard, 37–50. London: Bloomsbury Methuen, 2016.

Shepherd-Barr, Kirsten E. *Science on Stage: From Doctor Faustus to Copenhagen.* Princeton: Princeton University Press, 2006.

Sontag, Susan. *Illness as Metaphor.* New York: Farrar, Straus and Giroux, 1977.

Sprinchorn, Evert. "Syphilis in Ibsen's *Ghosts*." *Ibsen Studies* 4, no. 2 (2004): 191–204.

Toombs, S. Kay. *The Meaning of Illness: A Phenomenological Account of the Different Perspectives of Physician and Patient.* Dordrecht, the Netherlands: Springer Netherlands, 1992.

Townsend, Joanna. "Elizabeth Robins: Hysteria, Politics and Performance." In *Women, Theatre, and Performance: New Histories, New Historiographies.* Edited by Maggie B. Gale and Viv Gardner, 102–120. Manchester: Manchester University Press, 2000.

Voskuil, Lynn M. *Acting Naturally: Victorian Theatricality and Authenticity.* Charlottesville: University of Virginia Press, 2004.

Vrettos, Athena. *Somatic Fictions: Imagining Illness in Victorian Culture.* Stanford: Stanford University Press, 1995.

Wenegrat, Brant. *Theater of Disorder: Patients, Doctors, and the Construction of Illness.* Oxford: Oxford University Press, 2001.

William Winter, "The Actor." In *The Actor and Other Speeches, Chiefly on Theatrical Subjects and Occasions*, 1–25. 1891. Reprinted. New York: Burt Franklin, 1970.

Wood, Jane. *Passion and Pathology in Victorian Fiction.* Oxford: Oxford University Press, 2001.

Part I
Performing consumption

1 Rosy cheeks and red handkerchiefs

Performing Camille's consumption before, during, and after the contagionist turn

On the evening of February 2, 1852, Madame Eugènie Doche returned from an early retirement to once again grace the French stage. According to theatre legend, the role that induced Doche to abandon her tranquil existence in England for Paris's Théâtre du Vaudeville was one that had been peremptorily rejected by no fewer than four leading French actresses, including the famed tragedienne Rachel. Alexandre Dumas fils' consumptive courtesan and "Lady of the Camellias," Marguerite Gautier, first appeared in the pages of *La dame aux camélias* (1848), a story of love, sacrifice, and redemption in decadent Paris. Dumas adapted his novel for the stage the following year, but repeated rejections by theatre managers to produce the work, along with casting difficulties and a censorship ban ordained by the Minister of the Interior, delayed the play's theatrical premiere for nearly three years. Finally, the renowned actor-manager Bouffé took up the play at the Vaudeville, despite his actors' protestations. When their lead actress refused to play Marguerite on moralistic grounds, Charles Fechter (who was to play Marguerite's lover Armand) sent the script to Doche.[1] Doche had been personally acquainted with Marie Duplessis, the young courtesan with whom Dumas had a two-year affair and whose glamorous lifestyle and premature death from tuberculosis inspired Marguerite's creation. She accepted the role.

Audience's flocked to the Vaudeville to see Doche's performance. She was, Grace Greenwood later declared in *The New York Times*, "by far the best representative of that anomalous, almost impossible, character," performing with "power and pathos" the role's defining illness, pulmonary tuberculosis. "She had no painful paroxysms of bronchitis, she swooned but once, and was temperate in her tears." Doche's much-admired restraint developed during rehearsals, which Dumas oversaw. When the actress punctuated Marguerite's speech with coughs like a chugging locomotive, Dumas warned her about being too "excessively pulmonic. 'I do so, Monsieur,' replied she, 'in order to die more rapidly.'"[2] Doche's tall body, porcelain skin, and graceful carriage, so similar to Duplessis' features, heightened her embodiment of the consumptive Marguerite. "I have heard persons," L.H. Hooper remarked, "who were present during her first representations of '*La Dame aux Camélias*,' expatiate on the effect produced in the last act by those white, slender, semi-transparent hands, and by the seeming fragility of the delicate frame, which every cough appeared to rack with painful violence."[3] Doche's Marguerite marked the birth of an enduring cultural icon and a moving portrait of terminal illness. Among those who witnessed Doche's performance were three artists who assured the character's perennial place in nineteenth-century repertoires: Guiseppe Verdi, who transformed Marguerite Gautier into Violetta Valéry in his opera *La traviata* (1853), and two actresses of relative obscurity, Jean M. Davenport and Matilda Heron, who became the earliest Camilles in the United States.

The theatrical sensation of *Camille* (as Marguerite Gautier's *La dame aux camélias* became titled) conquered the United States in the 1850s and Britain in the 1880s, the roughly thirty-year delay a result of the play's censorship by the Lord Chamberlain's office. The character's popularity eventually dipped in both countries during World War I, though the 1920s and 1930s saw successful revivals of the play headlined by Eva La Gallienne, Lillian Gish, and Tallulah Bankhead. *Camille*'s dwindling commercial appeal was partly the result of theatrical realism's rise; however, shifting artistic tastes were not the sole provocations of the play's decline. On the contrary, they worked in concert with landmark medical discoveries to redefine the pathology of the courtesan's tuberculosis and, ultimately, the role itself. In Part I's chapters, I will invest Camille's theatrical endurance with a deeper significance than that proposed in existing scholarship. The very fact that a number of *La dame aux camélias* adaptations survived tuberculosis's re-categorization as a contagious disease in 1882 attests to the play's warhorse status while also hinting at an underappreciated pliability. Far from simply satisfying the audience's appetite for melodramatic pathos, "woman-with-a-past" plot devices, and thwarted love affairs, Camille reigned as consumption's most famous victim, one whose tale made tragic sense of the disease's destabilizing senselessness.[4] Along with stage consumptives Little Eva (1852's *Uncle Tom's Cabin*) and Margaret Hartmann (1855's *Helping Hands*), Camille symbolically legitimated the illness-processes of tuberculosis's countless victims, albeit in ways that often sensationalized her medical condition. As David M. Morens writes in "At the Deathbed of Consumptive Art," because the era's scientists had yet to fully comprehend the etiological and epidemiological foundations of the disease, "it was left to the arts to make sense of misery and death in ways that turned otherwise senseless suffering into human dignity and hope, allowing consumption to reveal the innate worth even of prostitutes, the impoverished, and the socially outcast."[5] Despite her professional impropriety, Camille's delicate femininity in life and spiritual deliverance in death enabled her to operate as the sentimental surrogate for those whose lives were impacted either directly or obliquely by consumption. Though Camille's usefulness as a surrogate diminished with Robert Koch's discovery of tuberculosis's bacterial origins, she nevertheless sustained the more glorifying aspects of what Clark Lawlor calls the "consumptive myth" far into the twentieth century.[6] Like Terry Eagleton's conceptualization of the tragic art, which "shapes suffering into a significant pattern, containing it while rendering it agreeably intelligible," the consumptive myth—a performative construct that is both medical and extra-medical—deciphered, consolidated, and made meaningful the diverse experiences of those enduring the disease's bleakest realities.[7]

In what follows, I would like to consider the ways in which nineteenth-century embodiments of Camille engaged with contemporaneous medicocultural understandings of the disease that ends her life. I propose that two strains of performing Camille's illness thrived on the century's British and American stages. An older strain subsisted on Enlightenment and Romantic figurations of consumption as a gentle, dignified, beautiful, and ultimately purifying disease. A newer positivist-age strain disavowed tuberculosis's cultural aestheticization by foregrounding its physiological realities. Actresses in the former strain performatively reinforced the mythic representation of consumption imbedded within Dumas's script, while those who comprised the latter pushed against the text by presenting Camille as a flawed, earth-bound woman whose disease induces physical and psychical agony. These two strains were not apportioned neatly, as one might easily assume, on either side of Koch's 1882 discovery of the *Mycobacterium tuberculosis*. They existed concurrently and were often juxtaposed against one another, a fitting reflection of the discordance among specialists as to tuberculosis's etiology throughout the long nineteenth century. Claudine Herzlich and Janine Pierret best explain tuberculosis's conceptual duality:

> In the course of the nineteenth century, tuberculosis thus became bound up in two successive chains of signifiers: passion, the idleness and the luxury of the sanatorium, and a pleasure-filled life 'apart' on the one hand; the bacillus, the dank and airless slum, and exhaustion leading to an atrocious agony on the other. The disease therefore gave rise to a twofold discourse that both celebrated the consumptive and stigmatized the germ-carrier.[8]

It was within this dichotomous discourse that Camille operated as an icon of terminal illness on the nineteenth-century popular stage.

As Camille's depicters performatively engaged in tuberculosis's "twofold discourse," critics registered in rhetoric, tone, and aesthetic judgment consumption's etiological reclassification from inherited to contagious disease. In most cases, reviewers of mid-century Camilles preferred those who sanitized and sentimentalized her condition, while those writing at the *fin de siècle* honored more unadorned, realistic representations. The perceived "authenticity" of Camille's tubercular condition depended on not just the actress's onstage choices, but her physical resemblance to a late-stage consumptive. Performers not naturally endowed with the requisite waiflike figure or porcelain complexion often found themselves ridiculed by the era's predominantly male commentators, thereby linking each performer's efficacy as Camille to her own corporeality and perceived abstemiousness. The courtesan's provincial origins and affiliations with Paris's libertine *haut monde* also led *Camille*'s British and American critics to reference actresses' nationalities and personal lives as a way of legitimating their depictions.

After a primer on the disease's history and known pathology, this chapter details the signature components of the consumptive myth and its late-century foil, clinical tuberculosis, in order to identify the methods by which actresses romanticized or medicalized Camille's illness and contextualize critical responses to their performances. Chapter 3 investigates two landmark performances of the role by continental European actresses Sarah Bernhardt and Eleonora Duse, who performed *La dame aux camélias* in their native tongues for English-speaking audiences. Bernhardt's "Frenchness," fashioned not just by her nationality and francophone performances but through the mythic dimensions of her Parisian upbringing, authenticated her neo-romantic Marguerite for British and American critics. Italian-born Duse, whose naturalistic acting methods differed markedly from Bernhardt's, conveyed the gravity of Marguerite's illness without the graphic excess of other medicalizing performances. Together Bernhardt and Duse initiated new tactics for embodying Camille's tuberculosis, reviving *La dame aux camélias*'s tired reputation even as Koch's bacteriological findings began to dilute the disease's sentimental force.

The making of the consumptive myth

In pulmonary tuberculosis, rod-shaped *tubercle bacilli* enter the body through the inhalation or ingestion of microscopic air droplets expelled by an active tubercular.[9] Once inside the body they may lie dormant indefinitely, as is the case with the majority of those infected, or they may become activated, producing tiny white tubercles that deteriorate the delicate lung tissue. In prior centuries, physicians categorized tuberculosis by the rapidity of its progression; there were cases of swiftly advancing acute or "galloping" consumption, but typically it was a chronic illness with prolonged periods of health interrupted by critical relapses. No matter the pattern, tuberculosis can be fatal if left untreated, and is especially virulent in the immunosuppressed. The disease's early and mid-stage symptoms are not distinctly tubercular and could be mistaken for those of a common cold or stomach flu: modest weight loss, runny nose, pallor, persistent cough, and excessive sweating at night.[10] Indeed, the relative vagueness of these initial complaints ensured the neglect or misdiagnosis of many tuberculosis cases prior to the twentieth century. In the late stages of the disease, however, tuberculosis inscribes itself on the sufferer's body. The traits that comprised the tubercular appearance were crucial for nineteenth-century diagnosticians, as were the late-stage consumptive's wheezes, violent coughs, shortness of breath, joint pain, diarrhea, and expectoration of blood and lung matter. In his 1836 *Treatise on Consumption*, physician William Sweetser detailed the features of a terminal tubercular body: emaciation, a hollowed-out face, eyes shining from deep within their sockets, and thin, "retracted" lips:

> The chest in some instances—probably to adapt itself to the wasted state of the lungs,—becomes generally or partially contracted … the belly is

flattened and sunk … and all the comeliness, and pleasing symmetry of the human form are destroyed.[11]

It was the cadaverous appearance of late-stage tuberculars that furnished the disease with its most enduring monikers: "consumption," the "wasting disease," *phthisis* (Greek for "wasting"), and "the decline." Deaths from tuberculosis, usually due to respiratory failure, pulmonary hemorrhaging, or septic shock, were more often than not occasions of physical agony.[12] While tuberculosis was readily acknowledged to be endemic in Europe and North America, with one English physician boldly calculating in 1815 that one-fourth of the entire European population was consumptive, the disease resisted categorization as an infectious epidemic of the same ilk as cholera or smallpox.[13] Scientists and non-experts alike isolated tuberculosis from the inventory of stigmatizing illnesses by endorsing its mythic exclusivity, a centuries-old invention that ennobled consumptive victims and tranquilized their deaths.

Despite the nearly inextricable linkage between the consumptive myth and romanticism, crucial aspects of the myth significantly predate the nineteenth century. Two divergent but dialogic notions of consumption operated within the Renaissance; the first established the disease as a consequence of "love melancholy," and the second introduced the possibility of a mild consumptive deliverance to heaven for the innocent or religiously devout, echoing the established tradition of *ars moriendi*.[14] For Renaissance physicians, an imbalance of the humors precipitated consumption, and those with lymphatic temperaments were considered abnormally susceptible. This humoral conceit of consumption, too crude in its reliance on bodily fluids, surrendered during the Enlightenment to a more idealizing explanation, one that redefined the disease as a constitutional disorder targeting those of superior sensibility. This drastic revision hinged upon the period's paradigmatic fascinations with emotional delicacy (as a socially acceptable attribute of both men and women), aesthetic pulchritude, and the intricate workings of the brain and nervous system.[15] In addition to signaling a deep-rooted love melancholy, the languid sadness associated with consumptives could now also indicate a superfluity of refined sensibility, alleged to be an innate trait of well-bred families. Heredity, by extension, became a crucial component of the "consumptive diathesis," a constitutional trait or set of traits that predisposed individuals to developing the disease. The offspring of consumptive parents were thought to be phthisic from birth, whether or not they became ill. Conceived of as the inherited malady of the wealthy, the feminine, the youthful, and the melancholy, "tuberculosis was also a way of life full of luxury and leisure."[16] Nowhere was the link between consumption and indulgence stronger than in imperial Britain, where "consumption" referred both to an illness and a birthright of the blue bloods and bourgeoisie. Notes Susan Sontag, "TB is described in images that sum up the negative behavior of nineteenth-century *homo economicus*: consumption; wasting; squandering of vitality." Authenticating Sontag's assertion is a treatise by eighteenth-century physician Edward Barry that attributes

Great Britain's soaring rates of consumption, a "disease of indulgence," to the epicurean insatiability of Her higher-born subjects.[17] In this way, the deadly tuberculosis operated as an ambivalent endorsement of social progress and a flourishing Empire, even as it attacked the poor and malnourished in greater numbers than the wealthy.

European leisure classes soon fetishized the consumptive as a paragon of corporeal and sartorial beauty. The voluptuous female figure cherished for centuries as the model of physical perfection was starved in the late 1700s to replicate the consumptive female's wasting form: sunken chest, long willowy limbs and neck, and "winged" back (labeled thusly because of the severity with which the shoulder blades jutted out of an emaciated torso). For physician Benjamin Rush, women were more likely to develop consumption because of their "greater delicacy of constitution" and their unhealthy customs.[18] Women underwent relentless tight-lacing of corsets to achieve a diminutive waist, drank concoctions of lemon juice and vinegar to suppress hunger, replaced their heavy-fabric skirts with airy ensembles resembling the consumptive's bedroom shift, and cultivated public reputations as "bird-like" eaters.[19] The newly minted epitome of feminine beauty transformed life for fashion-forward women; not only was a near skeletal body the new mark of beauty and refinement, but feminine plumpness became equated with laziness and intellectual slowness. As Katherine Ott remarks, "The middle-class public thought robust health vulgar in a lady ... Albescence indicated not only a woman of leisure, unaccustomed to outdoor exertion, but also a delicate nature, coeval with death and ready to pass over at a sigh." Ironically, the extreme techniques employed to transform a healthy body into a consumptive-esque body likely fueled the tuberculosis epidemic. The popularity of "invalid-chic" continued unabated in the nineteenth century, when literary, theatrical, and visual depictions of consumptive-esque beauty proliferated, and "the image of pale, bed-ridden, wasting women and men quickened the pulse of Victorian[s]" on both sides of the Atlantic.[20]

By 1800, the consumptive myth was a sociocultural juggernaut, incorporating influences from the disease's newly formed affiliation with the Romantic Movement. The rechristening of consumption as the "romantic disease" sprung from two factors, one artistic and the other empirical. Consumption's "preference" for youthful victims of beauty and delicacy, as well as its unpredictable patterns of remission and relapse, rendered the disease a sublime, pathos-inducing device for inclusion in Romantic poetry, drama, literature, and art. Consumption inspired artistic meditations on premature death and dying, relinquished love, spiritual deliverance, subjectivity, and the sovereignty of nature, among other themes. Soon autumn supplanted spring as the preferred season for Romantic poets, the desiccated leaves and nipping frosts fitting metaphorical tributes to the wasting consumptive's final days.[21] The Romantics also commandeered the consumptive myth because of a stark reality: their brightest ambassadors were falling victim to the disease, including John Keats, Frédéric Chopin, Eugène Delacroix, Friedrich Schiller, and nearly the entire

Brontë family. Consumption was no longer just the romantic disease, but the disease *of* the Romantics. Because of their professional notoriety, passionate souls, and melancholic dispositions, Romantic artists became the iconic avatars of nineteenth-century consumption.

In order to reconcile the premature demises of the famed "wasting poets," many of whom hailed from the lower and middling classes, with the pre-existing aristocratic archetype of consumption, the myth expanded its class-bound definition of "superior." In the revised consumptive myth, a person endowed with exceptional intelligence, passion, or creativity was also suscep-tible to the disease, regardless of class. It was now possible, even probable, for a poet's mental overstimulation during an intense period of writing to arouse a dormant case of consumption.[22] Brilliance and creativity therefore came with costly price tags, and yet a diagnosis of consumption curiously legit-imated a scholar or artist's exertions, whether or not the fruits of their labors merited great acclamation. Similarly, in a conspicuous outgrowth of the dis-ease's Renaissance association with love melancholy, a passionate soul also left its owner vulnerable to developing consumption. The consumptive's fevers, sweating, and crimson cheeks, then, betrayed the presence of an ungovernable inner fire. Paradoxically, the overindulgence of these desires was thought to court consumption, but so too was the unnatural stifling of passion's incendiary impulses. "The romantic idea that the disease expresses the character is invari-ably extended to assert that the character causes the disease—because it has not expressed itself," argues Sontag. "Passion moves inward, striking and blighting the deepest cellular recesses."[23]

Perhaps the most staggering claim upheld by the consumptive myth was that its victims died painlessly. This premise, debunked by centuries of contrary reports, remained imperative to the disease's cultural efficacy throughout the nineteenth century. The perishing of consumption's "chosen" victims in phys-ical agony or psychological despair would diminish the disease's mythologizing exclusivity. Demoralizing deaths were expected of the nameless casualties of cholera, yellow fever, and other epidemic diseases, but not of those touched by the romantic disease. Though the pain-free death was an exclusive rite of pas-sage for consumptives, it was by no means an isolating ritual. "Everywhere and in all periods," write Herlich and Pierret, "it is the individual who is sick, but he is sick in the eyes of society, in relation to it, and in keeping with the modal-ities fixed by it."[24] Prior to the discovery of tuberculosis's communicability, the late-stage consumptive often spent his final days in a private sickroom sur-rounded by an intimate coterie of loved ones. Even the early seaside sanatoria constructed to accommodate wealthy consumptives forged their own inclusive communities of patients and personnel, a multilayered support system for the dying process. The reported ebb and flow of *spes phthisica*, a phenomenon that enjoyed widespread credibility in both the medical and cultural spheres, further corroborated claims that consumptives slipped gently into their eternal rest. Translated as "the hope of the consumptive," *spes phthisica* was a brief hallucinatory state in which consumptives underestimated the severity of their conditions and denied the nearness of death.[25] Under the spell of this "strange illusion," as Sweetser labeled it in his *Treatise*, "the sufferer is ofttimes cheerful, confident, buoyed up by a deceitful hope, when the disease has declared itself to all about him in language that cannot be misunderstood."[26] The *spes phthisica* then recedes, leaving behind startling mental clarity and a calm acceptance of their impending departure. As I have proposed elsewhere, *spes phthisica*'s pattern of ignorance to knowledge precisely replicates an Aristotelian recognition or *anagnorisis*; in this way the romantic myth of consumption permitted the consumptive's illness-process and eventual demise to be viewed within the context of tragedy.[27]

Consumption was, above all else, a disease of individuality, of exceptionalness, and (as no other epidemic diseases could reasonably claim) of transcendental purpose. The romantic myth's consumptives did not suffer through illness only to perish in anonymity, poverty, or disgrace; instead, even as the physical symptoms of tuberculosis threatened to restrict patients' self-sovereignty, the powerful cultural narrative validated their illness-processes and celebrated the very individualism that rendered them vulnerable to the disease. The disease also afforded consumptives a fair amount of behavioral latitude, as drastic mood swings were not only tolerated in tubercular patients, they were expected. This was especially true for women of the bourgeois classes, who were exempted from strictly proscribed codes of social conduct only during times of illness. Convinced of the restorative powers of fresh air therapy, physicians encouraged consumptives to relocate to healthier climes in the south of France or the Swiss Alps or, especially in the case of males, to take extended sea voyages. In these ways, mythic consumptives may have been robbed of physiological autonomy, but they were granted heightened agency.

Unmaking the consumptive myth

When physician and microbiologist Robert Koch announced to the Berlin Physiological Society on March 24, 1882 that he had discovered the pathogenic cause of tuberculosis, *Mycobacterium tuberculosis*, he delivered empirical proof of the disease's communicability.[28] Koch was not the first to argue that tuberculosis was contracted through person-to-person contact. Most notably, tuberculosis's known pathology had significantly expanded at the mid-century from Jean-Antoine Villemin's experiments with inoculating rabbits using tubercular tissue, demonstrating the disease's rightful place among society's most formidable threats. He published his findings in 1865's *Etudes sur la Tuberculosis*, but the medical community largely ignored Villemin's work until his results were corroborated by Koch's bacteriological evidence. Despite years of targeted speculation, both from experts and the wider public, the notion of non-contagious tuberculosis persevered tenaciously. Indeed, to the question "Is Consumption Contagious?" one 1889 treatise asserted that while many scientists had observed bacilli in the sputa of tuberculous patients, Koch's view that the bacilli caused tuberculosis was "not generally believed."[29]

If, as Nancy Tomes writes, "from 1865 to 1895 Western medicine underwent a virtual civil war over the truth of the germ theory," then tuberculosis can be regarded as the conflict's landmark battle.[30] In the largely positivist world of Victorian medicine, where ocular proof reigned as the most trusted method of determining truths, the "invisible enemies" that spread disease were immensely troubling entities. More palatable to Western scientists than germ theory was the miasmatic theory of disease, which proclaimed noxious air bearing particles of decomposed matter as the culprit for contagious diseases like cholera and plague. The miasmatic theory provided those concerned with contracting diseases with a behavioral directive: avoid noxious air to evade illness. The germ theorists, on the other hand, had no silver bullet to offer the anxious populace. Those hostile to the concept of microorganisms producing disease "were profoundly uncomfortable with the moral randomness they perceived in the germ theory," writes Tomes; "if contact with a microbe was the sole cause of disease, then living a virtuous, clean life did not necessarily protect one from its ravages."[31] Anti-contagionists were also wary of the germ theory's implicit undermining of the physician's craft and authority, as well as its discounting of social circumstances in the shaping of disease.[32] To combat these discomforts as well as stem the unhygienic practices that promoted the spread of microbes, germ theorists united with sanitation reformists. Though advancements in sanitation could not stop contagious disease epidemics, both groups argued, they could greatly lessen their impact. As the battle over germ theory's credibility waged on, the late-century experiments by Koch and French chemist Louis Pasteur identified species of microbes as etiologic agents for some of the most virulent diseases of the age, and between the late 1870s and the 1890s, bacterial sources were discovered for cholera, gonorrhea, anthrax, typhoid, scarlet fever, and, of course, tuberculosis. As Alcabes suggests of germ theory's eventual dominance, "The simplicity of the one-bug-causes-one-disease view was well suited to the mood of twentieth-century modernity."[33]

News that Koch, the newly ordained "hero of the empire," had identified tuberculosis's true pathology spread fairly quickly, as did the April 10 publication of his findings report, "The Etiology of Tuberculosis."[34] In less than a month, *The Times* of London and *The New York Times* announced Koch's landmark discovery to the English-speaking world. Though Koch's findings were not immediately or unanimously accepted, the microscopic *tubercle bacillus* contaminated nearly every component of the disease's mythic construction. The reclassification of tuberculosis as a contagious disease destroyed consumption's mythic, pathos-inducing exclusivity. The real bacterial tuberculosis was defined by its indiscriminate and indifferent nature, as the individualizing attributes of the uninfected populace were of little concern to the covetous bacilli. "No one asks 'Why me?' who gets cholera or typhus," remarks Sontag of contagion's arbitrary nature.[35] The stigma attached to such undesirable diseases now sullied tuberculosis's reputation, though the fact that tuberculosis activates in only a portion of those carrying the bacteria confirmed to some scientists the enduring validity of the consumptive diathesis.

"Tuberculosis picked out and killed a few Princes and it carried off more than one bejeweled, tender-hearted courtesan," concedes Thomas Dormandy, "but it slaughtered the poor by the million." With consumption's elitist predilections debunked, the new tuberculosis victim was "a creature of ignorance, poverty, and immorality, who seemed to deserve illness."[36] The disease's growing association with urban decay and insalubrious environs further tarnished its reputation, as did the body fluid now understood to most capably transmit tuberculosis from one human to another, sputum.[37] Instead of residing solely within the consumptive body (where the mythic disease was believed to be contained during its occupation, eventually expiring along with its host), the *tubercle bacilli* not only existed but thrived in outer environs, expertly breeching material and corporeal boundaries and waiting patiently in streets, in omnibuses, in carpets, and on skin and clothing for future victims (Figure 1.1). As the individuality and exclusivity of the consumptive victims

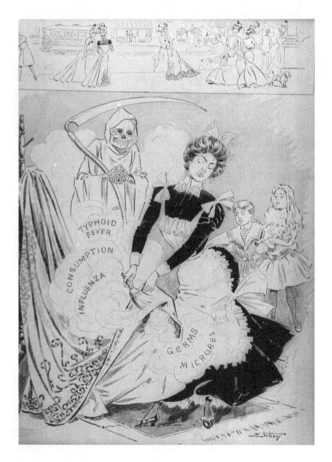

Figure 1.1 Communicable diseases spread by household and street dust. S. D. Erhardt. The National Library of Medicine.

waned, so to did the potential for a painless demise. Though antithetical reports of tubercular suffering had always been present, the gentle deaths "enjoyed" by consumption's romantic heroes were deemed now too extraordinary for contaminated millions.

Mythologized consumption was the disease of the individual. Clinical tuberculosis, however, was the disease of the anonymous masses. With the invention of streptomycin still sixty years away, isolation proved the most effective method of containing tubercular pathogens and their human hosts. In one of the most visible consequences of the consumptive myth's deterioration, impersonal contagious disease hospices replaced the private bedchamber and the wealthy seaside sanatoria as "proper" accommodations for tubercular patients, a cultural shift elegantly assessed in Eugene O'Neill's 1940 *Long Day's Journey Into Night*. If, as Pamela K. Gilbert claims, "the nineteenth century's twin terrors [were] the disintegration of the physical and social body," then quarantine, which lumped the infected together with no concern for economic or social disparities, was a decidedly mixed blessing. In a conspicuous sign that the scientific demythologizing of consumption had infiltrated the sociopolitical realm, *fin-de-siècle* France mandated a "declaration policy" that obligated doctors to register all tubercular cases with governmental authorities, a procedure that effectively "subordinated [individual rights] to the rights of others to be free from contagion."[38] The rise and fall of the nineteenth-century consumptive myth played out on American and British popular stages, both in dramaturgical changes to how tuberculosis operated as a plot device, a character trait, or a defining societal circumstance, and in performers' adjustments within consumptive roles like Camille.

Scripting consumption in Dumas's *La dame aux camélias*

"A Margaret Gauthier was as rare as a white blackbird," proclaimed American academic and writer Brander Matthews of Dumas's famed "Lady of the Camellias."[39] Central to Dumas's adapted play is Marguerite's transformation from a glamorous courtesan indifferent to love to a dying woman redeemed by self-sacrifice. When she falls for the respectable and naïve Armand Duval, Marguerite—who is already consumptive at the play's opening—abandons her life in wicked Paris for the provincial countryside, where the pair lives contentedly and in relative solitude. However, Armand's father soon arrives (unbeknownst to his son) to coerce Marguerite into ending the affair, fearful that Armand's relationship with a noted courtesan will forever tarnish the Duval name. A year after Marguerite's departure, she encounters a jilted and enraged Armand at a gambling party; her health declines rapidly following the altercation. The lovers are reunited on Marguerite's deathbed after Armand learns of his father's interference. She dies, absolved, in his arms. In Dumas's playscript and its subsequent English-language adaptations, Marguerite's eligibility for the ennobling disease of consumption is secured not by her occupation, but by her delicate beauty, passionate soul, and distinctive position as a sympathetic, somehow "moral" courtesan. Indeed, many of the period's dramatic critics took pains to distance the exceptional Marguerite from her indelicate sisters in sin, including one *Spirit of the Times* commentator who argued:

> There are, doubtless, in Paris, and even in the French portion of the city of New Orleans, numbers of females belonging to that type of woman intended to be represented by Dumas … [T]hey are women of education, great personal beauty, and possess extraordinary fascination of manners, and not unfrequently [*sic*] own every grace that adorn the female sex, except that priceless diadem, virtue.[40]

Marguerite's love for Armand further authenticates her as an idealized consumptive. As Théophile Gautier (who perhaps inspired Marguerite's surname) noted after witnessing *La dame aux camélias*'s 1852 premiere, both the courtesan's illness and passionate spirit—the latter stifled by Marguerite herself in order to avoid the occupational hazard of falling in love—are present but dormant in act one:

> [she] is not yet transformed by passion … But then as she begins to be troubled and then filled with real love, she becomes humble, shy, tender—and ill. She is consumed not only by love for Armand but also by the disease which consumes her body. And she knows it.[41]

Her suppression of these passions at the behest of Armand's father further aggravates the disease and ultimately leads to her death. However, Marguerite's consumptive vulnerability extends beyond her passionate soul. Though the stage adaptations make no mention of how Marguerite became consumptive, the novel implies that her illness was inherited from her dead mother. Additionally, the courtesan's lifestyle (leading to the conspicuous accumulation of material luxuries) is both a prime example of Sontag's "negative behavior of nineteenth-century *homo economicus*" and a character flaw with grave repercussions. As she succumbs to her disease Marguerite also sheds her earthly belongings until, in the play's final act, her austerely outfitted bedchamber matches her depleted corporeal form. Despite her impurity, Marguerite's status as the most beautiful, cultivated, and good-hearted *demimondaine* provides a place of superficial "good fortune" from which she tragically descends.

In Dumas's most overt acknowledgement of the consumptive myth, the transitory power of *spes phthisica* fuels the final act's climax. The scene opens on a feeble but lucid Marguerite, who appears to have made peace with her approaching death. Her demeanor shifts precipitously with the contrite Armand's arrival:

> Armand! I said this morning that only one thing could save me. I had given up hoping for it—and then you came. We must lose no time, beloved.

Life was slipping away from me, but you came and it stayed ... Nichette is to be married this morning, to Gustave. Let us go see her married ... Bring my outdoor things, Nanine, I want to go out.[42]

Marguerite's euphoria, however, is fleeting. After declaring to Armand "I want to live ... I must live," she grows introspective. "But if your coming has not saved me, nothing will, I have lived for love, now I am dying of it." Her remark is a simple *anagnorisis*, lacking sullenness or self-pity. Soon after, Marguerite dies.

Dumas's stage adaptation draws Camille's story even further into alignment with the consumptive myth through structural alterations and content changes. The novel's narrative jumps through time and utilizes a framing device, assaulting readers with a description of Marguerite's decomposing corpse, dug up from its grave at Armand's request, before flashing back to the spirited creature of his admiration. The play, however, follows a linear plot progression customary of the period's melodramas, eliminating the gravesite exhumation and the posthumous sale of Marguerite's belongings to pay off creditors. Dumas's script may require audiences to observe Marguerite's consumptive death just before the curtain falls, but it spares them the sobering sight of her disintegrating body, not to mention the cruelty with which her memory is dishonored in the novel. Even Marguerite's pain is sanitized and aestheticized for the stage; while Dumas's novel chronicles her consumptive decline and death over pages, with tortured cries, delirium, insomnia, fevers, and blood-spitting preceding the inevitable "last agony," the play's final scene features a tired but loquacious Marguerite giving the remainder of her money, along with sage bits of life advice, to her companions mere minutes before she dies.[43]

Playing the romantic disease

Because they largely avoided extensive stage directions and confessional monologues, Dumas and the many adapters of *La dame aux camélias* entrusted the task of rendering an affective portrait of illness to the play's lead performers, the majority of whom endorsed the consumptive myth. The romanticizing strain for performing Camille in the nineteenth century, built expressly upon the myth's central components, involved three key stanchions. First, actresses downplayed or purged Camille's more dissolute traits so as to purify her reputation and idealize her suffering. Theirs were Camilles of refined sensibility, virtue, and ethics, despite—and perhaps because of—the character's occupation as an elite sex worker. Second, the performers employed the fetishized optics of the consumptive appearance to entwine and consolidate Camille's beauty, declining health, and passionate spirit. Third, consumption's legendary gentleness was a linchpin of romanticizing performances of Camille. For actresses like Jean Davenport, Laura Keene, and Helena Modjeska, communicating the mildness of Camille's condition was an exercise in restraint. Graphic manifestations of tubercular suffering and death were antithetical to the consumptive myth, while sculptural poses, lyrical gestures, and the occasional fainting spell constituted the romanticized Camille's stage choreography, particularly in the play's earlier acts. Restraint was not, however, required to enact Camille's heightened sentimentality, nor the transcendental splendor of her *spes phthisica*. Such mythical endowments of consumption operated as performative tropes for many who played *Camille* in the nineteenth century.

Davenport, Keene, and Modjeska's efforts to bring *Camille* to anglophone audiences, of course, proceeded as part of separate career arcs. The first to perform *Camille* in the United States in 1853, Miss Jean M. Davenport (Lander) set the stage for decades of romanticizing portrayals of the courtesan. Born in England in 1829, Davenport was raised as a child performer. By 1849, the year she permanently relocated to the United States, Davenport had received glowing reviews in England, Germany, Holland, and the United States, and had studied music in Paris. From her informal but international training as a young actress, Davenport developed a highly refined acting style that was governed by what William Winter called a "thoroughness of impersonation, complete command of the essential implements of histrionic art, a fine intellect, a lovely feminine temperament ... and the controlling faculty of taste."[44] These characteristics were exhibited in abundance in Davenport's portrayals of Juliet, Cleopatra, Mary Stuart, and, of course, Camille. Laura Keene conducted a similar process of overzealous sanitization when she produced her own version of the play in 1856. Born in Westminster, England, as Mary Frances Moss, Keene took to the stage after the failure of her seven-year marriage to the Duke of Wellington's godson. As a novice to the profession, Keene learned the fundamentals of acting from the actress Emma Brougham and the famed Madame Vestris. One year after her British theatre debut, she moved to the United States and in 1853 became the country's first reputed actress-manager. As biographers have noted, Keene imbued roles with graceful femininity, intelligence, and personal charm, and Camille proved to be no exception.

The Kraków-born Modjeska's early life has been the subject of much speculation, as both her potential status as an illegitimate child of a Polish nobleman and her first marriage to her former (already married) guardian were later shrouded in secrecy by the actress and her managers. Modjeska performed in her native Poland for ten years, seven of which were spent as the lead actress at Warsaw's Imperial Theatre, before she and her second husband, Karol Bożenta Chłapowski, emigrated to California where they attempted to found a farming colony. The venture failed, however, and Modjeska returned to the stage, becoming one of the country's most acclaimed performers of classical roles. According to Benjamin McArthur, Modjeska's refined acting style corresponded most ably to the "classical school" of American performance, "characterized by a faultless declamatory delivery, controlled emotion, and a thoroughly dignified stage presence."[45] A cerebral actress rarely if ever given to shoddy or unstudied interpretations, Modjeska seemed to some evaluators a cold, calculated, and unemotional actress; others interpreted her efforts as dignified and realistic.

The conservative outcry against *La dame aux camélias*'s risqué themes expanded well beyond the borders Dumas's native France, most obviously in the Lord Chamberlain's decades-long censorship of the play in Britain. Because of this, artists who mounted productions of *Camille* in the United States and later in Britain purified the play's objectionable subject matter by deemphasizing Camille's profession and tempering the more distasteful aspects of tuberculosis. Davenport collaborated with writer John H. Wilkins to pen the first English-language adaptation of *La dame aux camélias* called *Camille, or, the Fate of a Coquette*, in 1853. As the title indicates, the play reduced Camille's moral misdeed from prostitution to flirtation, a revision that the *Spirit of the Times* claimed "does away with the objection raised against the French piece."[46] Keene, Davenport's fellow British expatriate, attempted to minimize public disapproval of *Camille* by reframing the play as an instructive nightmare from which Camille gratefully awakes in 1856's *Camille: a Moral of Life*. After first playing Camille in the United States in 1877, Modjeska debuted James Mortimer's *Heartsease* in 1880, the first adaptation of *La dame aux camélias* to circumvent British censorship. *Heartsease* implies that Constance (Mortimer's name for Marguerite/Camille) and Armand are engaged by the time they flee Paris for the French countryside. By diluting Camille's transgressions and highlighting her manifold virtues, English-language adaptations were among the most visible carriers of consumption's romantic mythology in the latter half of the nineteenth century. Framed by these myth-sustaining scripts, Davenport, Keene, and Modjeska reified in performance the conceits of romanticized consumption: an exceptional victim, whose worsening disease only enhances her beauty and allure, succumbs to a gentle, cathartic demise. Parsing out the methods by which these conceits were embodied helps us to trace the consumptive myth's performative contours.

An exceptional victim

Despite Camille's demotion from prostitution to coquetry in Davenport and Wilkins' *Camille, or the Fate of a Coquette*, the origin of her illness was little altered from Dumas's work: a constitutional susceptibility aggravated by a faulty behavioral choice—in the coquette's case, a full-tilt devotion to parties, flirting, and dancing. Only a handful of critics commented on *Camille*'s American debut, and those who did labeled Davenport and Wilkins's melodramatic adaptation as awkward and inferior to the French original. Given that Davenport expunged *Camille* of all sexual references, it is unsurprising that her embodiment gave little weight to Camille's amatory passions. "Mrs. Lander's purpose is always unmistakably pure and worthy," *The New York Tribune* affirmed of Davenport's approach. "If she fails at times to realize the fullest force of a passionate situation, it is apparently because of an excessive desire to guard herself against overstepping the perfect modesty of nature."[47] In vesting Camille with preternatural virtue, Davenport delighted some critics and vexed others. "Her rendering of the part," remarked George C. Odell generously, "was as chaste and elegant as such a performance could be," while *Appleton's Journal* pronounced her efforts "too stately, too cold, too much *au grand tragique*" for the diseased coquette.[48]

Like Davenport, Keene eliminated from Camille what she deemed to be unnecessary coarseness, vulgarity, and improper feelings and actions. But also like Davenport, Keene's elegant but inhibited Camille was left without the essential spark needed to ignite the quiescent disease: an impassioned spirit. Still, while the "it-was-all-a-dream" conceit may strike modern appraisers as somewhat absurd, *Camille: a Moral of Life* staged the consumptive's spiritual deliverance in death. In a supplemental scene, Camille (still dreaming) ascends to heaven to join her mother, presumably a tuberculosis victim herself. This apotheosis mirrors the final tableau of George L. Aiken's *Uncle Tom's Cabin* in which Little Eva appears in the clouds, clad in white and riding on the back of an ascending dove, to welcome Uncle Tom to heaven.[49] Keene's unambiguous allusion to *Uncle Tom's Cabin* linked her French Camille with America's most famous tubercular victim, Little Eva. In this way, Keene idealized Camille's suffering and rendered visible the familial origins of her tuberculosis, all the while satisfying the audience's appetite for spectacle and sentiment. That Camille awoke from this dream was likely a derivative of the eighteenth-century trend of rewriting tragic endings, and yet it also functioned as an optimistic converse of Dumas's original framing device. Whereas Dumas's novel bookended Marguerite's life with postmortem observations written by an unnamed narrator, Keene's play braced Camille's dream of death between restorative scenes of life.

"I can never understand why *Camille* is considered a bad play, when its moral is so pointed," Modjeska told the *Kansas City Journal* in 1884. "It is the terrible and sad lesson of a sinful woman purified by an honest love."[50] Eleven years prior to Modjeska's American debut in *Camille*, however, the actress refused to enact the role in the first Polish version of *La dame aux camélias* on moral grounds. The English-language adaptations Modjeska chose to produce in the United States and Britain, including the timid and wholesome *Heartsease*, downplayed the play's most objectionable themes. But it was her onstage efforts that prompted one critic to write: "it must be said that no actress has equally purified and ennobled the character of *Marguérite Gautier*, or as we call her, *Camille*."[51] Modjeska claimed in her autobiography to have returned to the role's original source, Marie Duplessis, for inspiration. Reading Arsène Houssaye's account of the famed courtesan as exceedingly cultured, refined, and delicate, Modjeska decided to "[follow] Houssaye's description" when creating her portrayal of Camille. "It pleased my imagination to present Camille as reserved, gentle, intense in her love, and most sensitive, – in one word, an exception to her kind," wrote the actress, echoing closely the tenets of the consumptive myth.[52] In an attempt to intervene in and perhaps remake the character's reputation, Modjeska resignified the role by positioning her Camille as a surrogate of the historical Duplessis and not Dumas's literary or theatrical creations. Favorable critical responses suggest Modjeska's romanticized Camille was among the most dignified and poetic to grace the popular stages in Britain and the United States. "There was no realism whatever," claimed the *Washington Post*: "It is, from beginning to end, a piece of pure ideality, imagination and poetic art worked by the most delicate and refined methods."[53] In Modjeska's conception, the wasting disease cleansed Camille of any lingering transgressive qualities, just as it revised Duplessis's significance within the archive of French romanticism. Boasting a performance style of studied elegance, balance, and attention to detail, Modjeska ennobled the famed tubercular without stripping her of all her spirited fervency.

The fetishized consumptive form

With its signature silhouette, color palette, and markings, the female consumptive form conveyed to those living in the 1800s the sufferer's fortune (privileged in class, intelligence, or character) and misfortune (afflicted with a chronic or terminal illness). In stage adaptations of *La dame aux camélias*, Camille's angelic beauty became an even more decisive indicator of the illness laying siege to her body, with actresses of all shapes and heights availing themselves of corsets, wigs, paints, powders, and ivory dressing gowns in order to replicate the late-stage consumptive's ethereal form and countenance. Davenport was only twenty-four years old when she first played Camille, a notable detail when considering that the character's most famous interpreters (Bernhardt, Duse, Morris) were all substantially older. Only one year older than Duplessis at the time of the courtesan's death, Davenport infused the role with a youthful innocence that older actresses could only attempt to replicate. An actress of medium height and build, with a round face, long nose, and wavy, chestnut brown hair, Davenport possessed few of the fabled physical traits so admired in Duplessis and in Madame Doche's Marguerite. However, unlike future reviews of *Camille*, in which the actresses' body measurements and complexions were stringently evaluated for their consumptive qualities, critics of Davenport's did not appraise her physical suitability to the role. It may be that Davenport's youthful appearance, rendered consumptive presumably by paints and corsetry, reduced the necessity for her to satisfy all of Camille's physical attributes.

Keene's appearance boasted "a graceful figure, features of classical outline, [and] bright sparkling eyes," according to *The New York Times*. William Winter's remark, that "in appearance she is almost seraphic," echoes the poetic descriptions of angelic beauty regularly applied to the period's consumptive sufferers.[54] Biographer John Creahan characterized Keene as "slight, graceful and willowy in her every movement, as if guided by the hand of the supernatural," suggesting that her body's sylphlike movements enabled the actress to more convincingly occupy the figure of a late-stage consumptive than Davenport. Indeed, the *Tribune*'s critic declared Keene's embodiment of Camille as expert as the role's originator, Eugènie Doche.[55] Like Keene, Modjeska possessed the thin figure suggestive of tubercular wasting and the delicate features and graceful comportment limned by the consumptive diathesis. "Her bodily presence is most attractive – the figure tall and graceful; the features mobile and expressive," attested *The Birmingham Daily Post*, while *Scribner's Monthly* pronounced her form as "spare, without being

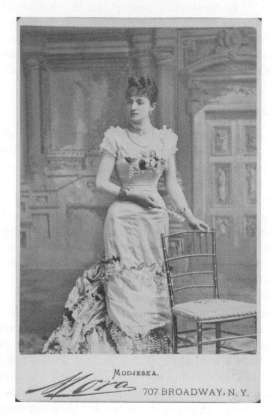

Figure 1.2 TCS 2 (Modjeska, Helena as Camille), Houghton Library, Harvard University.

thin; she is slender yet well knit, and endowed by nature with what painters call 'fine lengths,' that is to say, harmonious and noble proportions."[56]
Photographs of Modjeska's Camille/Constance evidence her fulfillment of
the consumptive's fetishized features: cinched waist, swan-like neck, porcelain skin, and deep-set eyes (Figure 1.2). For actresses and audiences, the
body was the chief signifier not only of the illness's presence, but of its
pathological progress. The consumptive myth transformed pain into beauty,
deterioration into glory.

Mythic mildness: Camille's decline and death

The romanticizing strain of performing Camille gave prominence to consumption's legendary gentleness. To exteriorize this paradoxical state of being
(of suffering sweetly, with purpose and largely without self-pity) actresses
devised an embodied lexicon of physical and vocal cues that drew upon the
nineteenth-century stage's pictorial aesthetics. Reviews, images, and memoirs

indicate that performers like Davenport, Keene, and Modjeska traversed the stage with graceful, arced crosses rather than cutting directly across the space, and moved in and out of sculptural poses fluidly. Audible symptoms of the disease, including shallow breathing, coughing, and a weakening capacity for speech, were subtly drawn. Camille, whose illness-process traces a bell pattern over the play's five acts (recovery from prior relapse, peak health, decline, and death), at times attempts to hide her symptoms from onlookers as part of a more comprehensive performance of untroubled conviviality. Occasional losses of balance, strength, or consciousness, however, splintered this façade and re-centered her illness. In such moments, actresses leaned on furniture or caregivers for support or melted onto chaise lounges, producing attractive, if not contrived, compositions of physiological weakening. Though act five's death scene could be played stoically (as was Keene's approach) or tearfully (as was Davenport's), a mild, cathartic passing was all but guaranteed for the era's sentimentalized Camilles.

Helena Modjeska proved the most virtuosic in upholding the consumptive myth's tenets as Camille lived with and succumbed to her disease. Hers was "the loveliest of Camilles" (*The New York Times*) in the 1870s and 1880s, a sympathetic and charming portrayal that was "finished and artistic to the highest degree" (*Aberdeen Weekly Journal*). Played in what the *Philadelphia Evening Bulletin* characterized "the quiet method [of acting] … which excludes all rant and tear, all high tones and all ferocious gesture," Modjeska's Camille appeared to critics on both sides of the Atlantic as sufficiently tasteful, if not a little too decorous for a queen of the *demi-monde*.[57] Honed through years of performing classical works in her native tongue and then in English, Modjeska' voice differentiated her cultured Camille from a sea of unexceptional portrayals. "She has a pure, sweet voice, full of agreeable modulations and bearing the faint flavor of a foreign accent which gives peculiar piquancy to her speech," declared the *Philadelphia Evening Bulletin*.[58] For a number of American and British critics, Modjeska's Polish accent (though it was not French) served as an adequate indicator of Camille's continental origins.[59] *The New York Times* commended Modjeska for avoiding the hectic vocalizations so prominent in Clara Morris's Camille: "the absence of agonizing paroxysms of coughing and choking and prolonged gasps for breath detracts not a whit from the merit of Mme. Modjeska's effort."

With the exception of act three, in which Modjeska—pushed to the edge of her emotional range—grew "angular and nervous" in her gestures in Camille's encounter with Monsieur Duval, the actress depicted Camille's suffering as delicate and poignant, never graphic.[60] Modjeska's contemporaries often played the first act of *Camille* for its contrasts: a lively and untroubled coquette charms visitors until her disease interjects itself by means of laborious breathing or a coughing fit. "Modjeska sounds a deeper note at once," the *Critic* advanced in 1882:

> As soon as she has touched the piano, her head falls with a sob. Her cough makes itself heard. Consumption is written on her face. Guests gather

round the table; broad jokes are bandied ... [but Camille] sits very pale and silent. Her mirth is evidently forced.[61]

Stifling (or *attempting* to stifle) her tubercular symptoms in mixed company, Modjeska's Camille prioritized the comfort of her friends over her own. In this way, her consumptive suffering was neither a manipulative theatrical 'reveal' nor a harrowing physical trauma. This shunning of tuberculosis's inconvenient or ugly realities continued through the drama, as Modjeska transitioned Camille from recovery to relapse to death.

Though she attested to spending many offstage hours mentally conceptualizing her roles, Modjeska's preparations for Camille did not include sickroom observations. "No, I do not walk the wards of hospitals to study death in its terrors," she once declared. "The plays were not written at a dying bedside."[62] Whether unaware of or resistant to embodying tuberculosis's effects on the terminal sufferer, Modjeska crafted a death scene that satisfied the consumption's mythic tenets while still providing plenty of audience-pleasing pathos. "In the final scene," described the *Birmingham Daily Post*, "where the poor girl lies dying, purified of the taint of her earlier life of vicious unreality ... cherishing the faith that [Armand] will yet come to her, the tender emotions were expressed with a nice sensibility and discrimination which belongs to the highest order of art."[63] Only a handful of critics interpreted Modjeska's death scene as medically accurate, with the *Aberdeen Weekly Journal* lauding (without evidentiary support) that "[T]he perception of the subtle symptoms of the dire disease which ends the heroine's life is astonishing even to doctors who have seen her."[64] The majority of critics, however, expressed relief that Modjeska's refined courtesan suffered and died in an elegant manner, with London's *Daily News* commending Madame Modjeska for avoiding "the customary painful minuteness" with which others enacted Camille's death.[65] Modjeska's tenure as the stage's most sympathetic Camille began in 1877 and extended through the 1880s, meaning that first, her Camille existed both before and after Koch's discovery of the *Mycobacterium tuberculosis*, and second, the performance matured as notions of realistic acting percolated, became systematized, and were put into increasing practice.

Perhaps the best evidence that Modjeska's embodiment perpetuated the consumptive myth is the intriguing shift in generic assumptions, about the play and its titular role, tendered by her British and American critics. As I have argued elsewhere, the centuries-long dominance of the consumptive myth in literature, the performing arts, and visual culture had much to do with its appropriation of the tragic genre's aggrandizing tenets.[66] The mythologized consumptive was conceived of as a tragic hero, both elevated and rendered vulnerable by one or more exceptional traits, fated to endure a fall that often precipitated an *anagnorisis*, or tragic recognition. Furthermore, the providential descent of the consumptive, like the tragic hero, was formulated to inspire fear and pity. "Camille, as Modjeska represents her," *The Critic* assured its readers, "is a figure of ancient tragedy rather than a mawkish creation of Dumas."[67]

Whether or not Modjeska intentionally guided *Camille* into the realm of tragedy, commentators acknowledged the presence of several of its markers in her performance. "Modjeska's Constance is no mere mercenary courtesan, but a loving, erring woman, whose *fall* apparently has resulted from the combined operation of strong impulses and weak guiding principles," volunteered the *Birmingham Daily Post*, "a creature, in fact, *more sinned against than sinning*, and to be *pitied* rather than condemned." This perceptual shift removed Modjeska's Camille from the melodramatic realm; instead, remarked George J. Jessop, "the imminence of fate in Modjeska's playing of the role … gave the play the power of the old Greek tragedies."[68]

Playing clinical tuberculosis

As Western medicine's contagionist turn transformed diseases like cholera, anthrax, and tuberculosis, *Camille*'s dominance on the popular stage continued, but not without skepticism or mockery. For decades the play's sentimentalized construction of Camille's disease largely paralleled prevailing medicocultural beliefs. Now *Camille* operated within, and persisted in spite of, a clear dissonance between the romantic myth of consumption and the clinical view of contagious tuberculosis. By 1886, one New York critic declared that audiences had finally "outgrown" the "morbid and unhealthy sentimentality" of plays like *La dame aux camélias*.[69] Changes to European and American theatre further antiquated *Camille*'s modes of character and plot development, and performers became more unwilling to romanticize the character's tubercular demise and death. "Audiences were beginning to demand realism as part of the act of perceiving in a theatre," writes Susan Bassnett, "hence the dying Marguerite Gautier came increasingly to be played as a consumptive, with the pale face and coughing of a sick woman rather than to be played as a tragic heroine *per se*."[70] Though this strain of performing Camille took hold in the 1880s and 1890s, its foundations can be found earlier in the century with the graphic consumptive performances of Matilda Heron and Clara Morris. For actresses like Heron, Morris, and Olga Nethersole, Camille's illness was far more than a mythic signifier of outer beauty and inner exceptionality. It was a physical and emotional crucible from which Camille never emerges.

Born in Ireland in 1830, Matilda Agnes Heron immigrated with her family to the United States in 1842. Soon after settling in Philadelphia, Heron's father died, leaving Matilda, her mother, and two sisters to seek an income from theatrical work while her brother Alexander entered the shipping business.[71] Reports differ as to whether the Herons were already a theatrical family or whether the sudden death of their patriarch pushed his female survivors to pursue stage careers, but it is clear she studied under the tutelage of English-born actor Peter Richlings. By 1854, Heron had completed engagements in many cities including New York, St. Louis, Pittsburgh, Sacramento, and San Francisco (where she performed opposite Edwin Booth). After seeing Doche's *La dame aux camélias* in Paris, the actress appeared in her own 1855

Camille adaptation, which she brought to New York's Wallack's Theater two years later. Heron's portrayal of the courtesan stunned audiences with its unprecedented naturalness and raw emotionalism, and the role became her most beloved and financially lucrative. Despite her early years of success as an actor and adapter of plays, Heron proved a poor money manager and died virtually penniless in 1872. Toronto-born Clara Morris's early life was a nomadic existence spent in the company of her single mother. The pair settled in Cleveland, where the untrained fifteen-year-old Morris debuted as a ballet girl at the city's Academy of Music. She was soon performing speaking roles as well as engaging in an affair with the company's married actor-manager. Morris moved with her mother to New York in 1870 to work at Augustin Daly's Fifth Avenue Theatre, where both actress and manager enjoyed immense success with sensational dramas like *Article 47* and *Madelein Morel*. Three years later while contracted at Albert Palmer's Union Square Theatre, Morris's notable turn in *Camille* gave especial prominence to the performer's maturing style as an emotional actress and a graphic interpreter of illness roles.[72] While at Palmer's, Morris began to suffer from protracted bouts of ill health and was prescribed morphine in 1876 for chronic pain, triggering a lifelong addiction to the drug. Though she did forge a profitable secondary career as a writer and lecturer, Morris's unquenchable morphine addiction, passé repertoire, and grueling schedule as a touring actress sabotaged her attempts to salvage her once-brilliant stage career.

Olga Nethersole was born in London's Kensington neighborhood to parents of Spanish and English heritage and received her education in England and Germany. The death of her father allegedly prompted Nethersole to pursue a stage career (although biographer Lavinia Hart conceded that sixteen-year-old Nethersole was also "badly stage struck"), and in 1887, she began her stage career in Brighton, followed in fifteen months by her London debut at the Adelphi.[73] Ambitious and intelligent, the actress received no formal training, but instead acquired the necessary skills of her craft while performing with provincial and urban troupes. Nethersole excelled at moments of dramatic intensity and could simulate a wide variety of emotions, but she was also an inconsistent artist, lacking the endurance and technical proficiencies required to perform complex or penetrative roles.[74] Though it became a valued part of her repertoire, Nethersole's Camille was not a career-defining role for the actress. Rather, it was one in a host of charismatic and sensational characters, including Floria Tosca, Carmen, Paula Tanqueray, and Sapho, for which Nethersole's abilities were particularly well suited. By the *fin de siècle* Nethersole's notoriety as a passionate and unfettered performer was secured by two daring theatrical exploits. First, she shocked audiences with an especially realistic kiss (known thereafter as the "Nethersole Kiss") in 1897's *Carmen*; then, three years later, her Sapho was carried upstairs by the play's male protagonist, prompting local authorities to close the production on the grounds of immorality. The matter was soon taken up in court, with Nethersole winning a favorable decision.

In order to demythologize tuberculosis, actresses like Heron, Morris, and Nethersole first resisted idealizing and elevating Camille to the status of tragic heroine. Their Camilles were earthbound creatures, flawed by carnal desires, fickle emotions, or unfinished manners. Within the framework of the consumptive myth, such indelicate Camilles were unsuitable. Within the framework of clinical tuberculosis, however, in which all strata of society were at risk for infection and in which the majority of tubercular patients were not of noble breeding or exceptional delicacy, such Camilles were quite appropriate. Second, performers manifested tuberculosis's symptomatology more gradually and consistently throughout the play's action, replicating tuberculosis's methodical process of destruction more accurately than their romanticizing peers. Labeled by critics as "hectic," "feverish," "sickly," and "morbid," the performances of Morris, Heron, and Nethersole strayed from custom by foregrounding Camille's tubercular suffering across the play's five acts. Third, actresses of the medicalizing group enacted tubercular deaths of disconcerting graphicness. Real deaths from tuberculosis only distantly resembled those tendered by the consumptive myth, with most terminal tuberculars experienced frightening moments of suffocation, extreme colic and joint pain, diarrhea, and feverish sweating before succumbing to a large hemorrhage or organ failure. Eschewing the fluttering gestures and beatific sighs of the romanticized Camille, actresses who medicalized Camille's illness categorically refused to enact painless, over-spiritualized deaths. Critical accounts suggest that Heron, Morris, and Nethersole presented similar versions of Camille's final moments. Though none of the three hastened around the stage with the speed and strength of the indefatigable Bernhardt, they all chose to keep Camille somewhat ambulatory. All selected moments for Camille to writhe in pain, cough, gasp, and struggle with speech, use Armand's body and furniture for physical support, and weakly collapse on the ground. Graphic, indelicate, and at times distressing to observers, such performances emphasized the pathological over the poetic, thereby disentangling Camille's disease from the consumptive myth.

An unexceptional tubercular

It is perhaps difficult to conceive of Camille as anything other than exceptional. Despite being a member of the Parisian *demi-monde*, she is ordained by Dumas as its unofficial queen; a professional courtesan who sells her body for security and material luxuries, Camille's fortitude, gracious heart, and premature death purify her. With the exception of Clara Morris's labored effort to present a virtuous, almost wholesome Camille, however, the women of the medicalizing group largely refused to idealize Camille as a mythic consumptive.[75] Instead, they presented her as a flesh-and-blood female, in equal possession of virtues and flaws, whose disease is neither tragic nor redemptive.

Heron portrayed Camille as an unassuming country lass whose provincial customs clashed with her occupation as a cosmopolitan plaything for the wealthy and desperate. Having partly sanitized her adaptation of Dumas's play for American audiences, Heron's acting in many ways pushed against her own script. As Barbara Wallace Grossman writes,

> The lusty physicality of [Heron's] performance made Camille seem common, even vulgar. According to the *New York Tribune*, she often walked brazenly with her hands on her hips and lifted the skirts of her ball gowns "as if she were entering a coach." One critic complained that she had turned Camille into an Irish washerwoman, while others objected to the coarseness of her interpretation.[76]

Those at *Flake's Bulletin* in Galvaston, Texas, found Heron's inelegant style too unmannerly for the legendary courtesan: "While admitting the wonderful art of Miss Heron's rendition, we objected to her roughness. Miss Heron seems not to know that Camille, though a woman, was always a lady by instinct and culture."[77] The newspaper's juxtaposition of the terms "lady" (noble, refined, and therefore exemplary) and "woman" (common, uncultivated, and therefore deficient) is particularly telling, for it highlights the metaphorical chasm that existed between the exceptional consumptive and the anonymous tubercular. As *Spirit of the Times*'s "Acorn" mused, "it is difficult to believe that a young man possessing the refinement that is supposed to belong to Armand, should be enamored of a woman displaying so many coarse, or at least, unfascinating [*sic*] traits of character."[78] Because of Heron's embodiment, lamented the *Philadelphia Inquirer*, "The world has been taught to regard 'La Dame aux Camelias' as a coarse unfortunate, who captivated the guilty creatures sitting at the play only by the force of her recklessness and her sufferings."[79] Heron's adaptation, the *United States Magazine* put bluntly, was a "catastrophe" fit for the hospital ward, not the stage.[80]

Of course, there were many who defended Heron's interpretation, including the actress herself. "'It is said that I expunged the most beautiful parts of Dumas' play, and introduced my own diseased fancies,'" Heron remarked:

> This is *not* so. After having witnessed in America different representations of the character[,] I went to Paris, where, for the first time I saw the true Camille, the reckless, erring, loving, hoping, sacrificing, despairing, repentant, *purified* woman. I saw the moral of the play in its *truth*—its terrible reality.[81]

Heron felt what American Camilles lacked was the role's "true" dimensionality and therefore played Camille as multifaceted and fallible. Perhaps Heron purposely coarsened Camille to conform to the populist ideologies of antebellum audiences, or perhaps a blunt, "anti-Victorian" Camille was the only one Heron's methods could devise.[82] Of Heron's lack of artifice, her advance man Fitz-James O'Brien wrote:

> She walked [into the apartment] easily, naturally, unwitting of any outside eyes. The petulant manner in which she took off her shawl, the

commonplace conversational tone in which she spoke to her servant, were revelations … Here was a daring reality.[83]

Adam Bandeau also vindicated Heron's vision of Camille in *The Vagabond*, arguing:

> She portrays a character exactly as it is, not without one touch of grace not its own, but with every touch of awkwardness belonging to it. She not only adds nothing, but subtracts nothing. She not only idealizes not, refines not, elevates not; she eliminates nothing of coarse or displeasing; she spares no harrowing thought, no disgusting minutiae; she is not only terrible in her lifelikeness, but at times offensive. And yet this very offensiveness adds to her thrall over you; you are held in spite of your dislike because of it.[84]

Accounts indicate that Heron periodically turned her back to the audience, an indecorous move on the 1850s stage that predicted the less ceremonious Camilles of Morris, Nethersole, and Eleonora Duse.

As was the case with her Sapho, Carmen, and Tosca, the Camille of Nethersole was guided by her excessive passions and thinly veiled carnality. "Nethersole," raved the obviously smitten Beaumont Fletcher, "is a ravishing bit of human loveliness, supple, voluptuous, opulent of physical graces; and these are sublimed with a melting tenderness and a vast hunger for a youthful trust to feed her own great love upon that is infinitely pathetic."[85] Nethersole's Camille—while characterized by a handful of reviewers as delicate and elegant—was nevertheless more unabashedly sensual than any of her counterparts. Indeed, some regarded her performance as unrefined and vulgar, with one critic complaining that "[her lovemaking] was too deliberate and overacted, thus leaving nothing to the imagination."[86] Furthermore, Nethersole compounded her Camille's flaws by depicting her as erratic, fickle, and at times even fatuous—qualities regarded by Victorians as being decidedly (and undesirably) female. In the estimation of *The Critic*'s reviewer in 1894, the actress's interpretation was "remarkable for the boldness and frankness of its opening scenes—although there never was an approach to vulgarity,—the passionate fervor of its love episodes[,] and the unaffected pathos of its suffering and despair." Nethersole's Camille, *The Critic* continued, underwent a significant conversion from "the imperious, impatient and reckless courtesan" of the earlier acts to the "simple, happy, trusting woman" of the third act, secure in her love of Armand but still resolutely sensual.[87] In this way, Nethersole distanced her Camille from the myth's more pristine, morally anchored consumptives as well as the new drama's controversial New Women: Nora Torvald, Hedda Gabler, and Paula Tanqueray.

Though Nethersole and her medicalizing peers resisted elevating Camille's reputation, the fetishized consumptive form remained a compulsory trait for those portraying tuberculosis onstage. Even after consumption's reclassification in 1882, there was no denying that the "wasting disease" often made walking skeletons of its human hosts, and theatregoers expected actresses to physically signify Camille's condition by whatever means were at their disposal. In 1898, one reviewer delighted in sending up British actress Margaret Fuller's less-than-wasting form:

> As you saw those powerful, muscular arms, you wondered how any tuberculous Marguerite Gunter [*sic*] could have owned them ... They showed you that Camille, in spite of her cough, was enjoying very good health – thanks for kind inquiries ... A healthier, buxomer, and more material Camille I have never seen. If she had cuddled poor Armand in those splendid bicycle arms of hers, you would have heard his bones creak.

Taking one last jab at Fuller's fullness, the critic quipped: "Here was a Camille that should have died from heart disease, or fatty degeneration, but never from consumption."[88] Fanny Davenport's shapely body also became the target of a number of editorial swipes, such as the *National Police Gazette*'s observation of her portrayals of Fedora and Camille: "Fanny is too decidedly Anglo-American in her physique and general style to do the skeleton drama of Bernhardt."[89] Newspapers soon circulated a derisive story (sometimes attributed to Davenport herself) that her Camille suffered from a fatal case of dropsy, not consumption. Only a few months before the actress's death from an enlarged heart in 1898, a Montana newspaper column entitled "All Actresses Dread Fat" blamed Davenport's poor health on the extreme weight loss regimen she initiated in the 1880s, presumably due to the rash of body-shaming *Camille* notices.[90] Clara Morris's progressive weight gain, too, disturbed the *St. Paul Daily News*'s critic, who remarked in 1890 that "something of the ridiculous creeps into being when we behold the dying Camille impersonated by a medium-sized woman who lingers near the 200-pound mark."[91]

Actresses in possession of consumptive-esque dimensions, however, at times fared little better in the presses. In appraising the Camille of Elizabeth Crocker Bowers, the *New York Herald* remarked, "she looked to the life a woman who was sacrificing her health to the excesses of a fast career, and it required no stretch of the imagination to believe her wasting away with consumption."[92] Such reviews, along with the brutal lampooning of Bernhardt's thinness by American cartoonists and commentators before her arrival in New York (addressed in the next chapter), demonstrate just how narrowly critics defined Camille's consumptive beauty. Late-century commentators, particularly those in the United States, entangled actresses' physical suitability for the role with culturally specific stereotypes of Western bodies. While Fanny Davenport's "too decidedly Anglo-American" body discredited her performance of tuberculosis, Bernhardt's slender figure became a signifier of her urbane, continental origins—and therefore her corporeal and geographical "nearness" to Marguerite—or of her Jewish heritage. Ultimately, the perceived "beauty" of the consumptive's wasting was a formidable cultural construct that failed to recede with the bacillus's discovery, even as *fin-de-siècle* clothing trends encouraged women to embrace a new silhouette, the hourglass.

Stages of suffering

In a post-Koch retrospective on the many renditions of Camille, the *Spirit of the Times* took comic aim at those that actresses who routinely downplayed Camille's tuberculosis until the play's final moments:

> [Some actresses] were uproarious bacchantes, rather than queens of the demi-monde, and bounced through the heart-breaking preliminaries of death with a jovial defiance that left upon our minds very serious doubts of their extinguishment in the last act, and despite all the illusion, we carried away a suspicion that the Dame aux Camelias, instead of lying white and weary in her last attire, was eating lamb chops and drinking warm stout in her dressing-room.[93]

In Dumas's script and its adaptations, Camille's illness is divulged within minutes of the opening curtain when her telltale cough pierces through the superficial chatter of her dinner guests. Later, the character swoons when dancing with Armand, and in act three, Camille admits to Monsieur Duval that she is not long for this world. For many actresses, these seemed to be the sole, playwright-authorized moments to demonstrate Camille's tubercular condition before act five's death scene, a formula that accomplished several things: it linked Camille's periods of good health with her love affair; it reinforced consumption's mythic gentleness; and it built dramatic tension through the erratic materialization and disappearance of symptoms. While it can be argued that Dumas's script intended to exploit the theatricality of "galloping" consumption's precipitous nature, such diagnoses were far outnumbered historically by cases of chronic consumption, in which the disease's symptoms progressively increased in intensity and duration.

Heron was the first to integrate tubercular symptoms throughout the course of *Camille*. Her sketch of the disease began subtly enough, as *Balou's Pictorial Drawing-Room Companion* reported: "Miss Heron had nothing to do at first but to enter superfinely [*sic*] and well dressed, cough and eat a lozenge."[94] Camille's cough, the most conspicuous feature of Heron's performed illness, worsened incrementally across the play's acts, signaling the acceleration of the disease and rendering the character's identity and illness indivisible from one another. "Matilda Heron limited her Camille to the courtezan [*sic*] and the consumptive," declared the *Philadelphia Inquirer*. Indeed, Heron's elaborate sufferings struck a number of critics as too morbid and pronounced. "If any body takes delight in tracing the cruel and insidious advances of a deadly and inexorable malady, they can do it in this play," *The Daily Ohio Statesman* quipped, "but who wants to go to see consumption?"[95] *The Vagabond*'s Badeau admitted to experiencing conflicted feelings as a witness to Heron's performance:

"The vulgarity of the earlier scenes in *Camille* is fearful in its faithfulness, but effective as well; the repulsiveness of the sick-bed is painfully real."[96] Badeau's perspective suggests why audiences flocked to Heron's *Camille*: her graphic composition of tuberculosis both thrilled and nauseated.

Following "the phthisicky example" set by Heron, Clara Morris based her embodiment of Camille's illness upon research and scientific observation.[97] As she later told Alan Dale, by consulting her own physician on tuberculosis's symptomatology,

> I learned … that there are two coughs peculiar to lingering consumption. One of them is a little hacking cough that interferes with the speech, and injures the throat; the other is a paroxysm brought on by extra exertion. I chose the paroxysm, and introduced it in the first scene, after I have been dancing.[98]

Morris's use of the term *lingering consumption* evinces her desire to enact the character's illness as progressive, nagging, and irreversible. To indicate the disease's constant presence in Camille's body, Morris also took to "gasping in 'little, pitiful spasms.'" Marveled *The Cleveland Leader* of Morris's unsparing work:

> "Acting?" It is not acting. When sinews are strung to their utmost with intensity of feeling; when the body writhes with anguish that is unmistakably real; when the hands spasmodically clutching at bosom and throat betray actual physical pain; when a genuine paroxysm of emotion shakes the whole frame like an aspen, delineation passes beyond the pale of acting and becomes – the acme of genius.[99]

Pathologized by critics as "convulsive," "painful," and "spasmodic," Morris's enactment of tubercular suffering surpassed even Heron's in its physical dynamism.[100]

Olga Nethersole also depicted the courtesan's health deteriorating slowly but painfully over the course of the play. For Beaumont Fletcher, who preferred Nethersole's Camille to all others:

> Bernhardt shows the ravages of the disease a little more pronouncedly [than Duse], but only Nethersole depicts the real tragedy of the dread torment wringing the fair young body inevitably to its grave. She does not overdo the pathological side of it, as does Miss Clara Morris, whose almost too convincing Camille has been dubbed "bronchial." Nethersole's innate refinement and artistic delicacy save her from that extreme, but by occasional writhen struggles with pain, and by her great pallor in the fourth act, and her tottering weakness in the last, she adds a terrible pathos to the double martyrdom of the girl upon the alter of her love and the rack of her disease.[101]

Like Morris, Nethersole studied the phthisic declines of real patients and achieved an impressive level of somatic and physiological detail, though her penchant for physical abandon was at times characterized by critics as messily chaotic or misguidedly self-indulgent. One Chicago reviewer noted that Nethersole's Camille was "nervous, restless, and in constant movement," and another chastised her for suffering too graphically.[102] Others regarded Nethersole's execution of Camille's suffering as mechanical and detached, a disparagement never directed at Morris.

Traumatic ends: Pathologizing the tubercular death

Actresses of the medicalizing strain of performing Camille took particular aim at the fabled gentleness of a consumptive death. No matter the adaptation, the phenomenon of *spes phthisica* always preceded Camille's death and her sickroom remained crowded with well-wishers (as opposed to the isolative TB hospital room); still, actresses had performative latitude in embodying the terminal effects of tuberculosis. Though both Heron and Nethersole composed death scenes of graphic detail that ranged around the whole bedchamber, Morris's represents a unique example of redoubled suffering, of actress and character simultaneously enduring pain and the responses such an exhibition elicits.

After witnessing Morris's Camille expire in her lover's arms, Sarah Bernhardt was reported to have said: "My God! this woman isn't acting; she is suffering."[103] Whether or not Bernhardt was praising or lampooning Morris's artistry is perhaps a moot point. What Bernhardt recognized in Morris's performance of illness was a body-and-soul commitment to enact Camille's tubercular demise. As with the courtesan's consumptive cough, Morris conferred with her physician in devising Camille's final moments, observing:

> Camille says at one time that all pain is gone. My doctor told me that this was on account of entire loss of the lungs. He cautioned me against saying much after that, and told me that the tubes of the throat could be used for a few words. I studied Camille in this manner.[104]

In addition to enacting the vocal incapacitation advised by her physician, Morris's movements indicated the presence of both localized joint pain and general physical enervation in Camille's body, with collapses and stumblings interrupting the actress's traverses across the bedroom. Sketches of Morris's last scene depict her "staggering" from couch to window and from window to vanity, "spasmodically clutching" nearby chairs for support. Staring into the mirror, her Camille discovers that tuberculosis has ravaged her beauty and she collapses onto the vanity, sobbing.[105] For most critics, Morris's performance teetered precariously on the line between admirable authenticity and harrowing nightmare. The *New York Daily Tribune* remarked that Morris's performance featured a wide array of "sick bed horrors and the physical accompaniments of death."[106] The *Spirit of the Times* concurred, stating that of "the most painful[ly] pulmonic" Camilles, Morris's rendition deserved top prize for explicitness: "There was a fascinating horror about the death of her Camille that drew us

back again and again to that sick chamber."[107] While a number of critics found
Morris's portrayal too clinical to be theatrically diverting, most conceded that
the dying consumptive's symptomology was, as a Boston reviewer remarked,
"wonderfully done,—horribly if you will"; in particular, Morris's vocal work
seemed painfully accurate: the "awful fallings away" of the voice weakened by
respiratory failure, a "hollow" and "spasmodic" cough, and the long pauses
between utterances.[108]

Though it is difficult to conceive of a performance that so brutally depicted
Camille's tubercular condition, Morris biographer Barbara Wallace Grossman
notes that only seven years after her *Camille* premiered, Morris out-suffered her
younger self. As the actress's own health precipitously declined and her morphine addiction escalated, she "took what the *Spirit of the Times* called 'the consumptive view of Camille,' emphasizing the character's illness and decline."[109]
Hers was now a performance of acute physical and emotional pain, perhaps
the only one the chronically afflicted actress could embody. At first, Morris's
ill health inspired sympathy among her theatregoing public. "People admired
her determination to perform whatever the physical cost and understood her
need to take 'restoratives' for sustenance," submits Grossman. "*The Spirit of the
Times* called her a 'remarkable little woman' for courageously completing the
engagement in spite of 'her wretched health," while the *Boston Daily Advertiser*
remarked that "any critic who had eyes and ears" could have gathered that the
actress was "wearily sick," but that Morris's talent in playing Camille easily
saved the evening's entertainment.[110] However, her drug addiction was made
very public in 1877 when a Chicago critic condemned the actress for taking
the stage while "saturated with morphia."[111] Even her admirers at *The Spirit of
the Times* stopped excusing her increasing deficiencies, writing "She has won
renown, the highest society is at her feet, why, therefore, should she drag
before us her shattered form, stricken by disease?" To such judgments Morris
responded via a letter to the *New York Sun*, in which she attempted to salvage
her feminine martyrdom as a suffering but dedicated artist: God has seen fit to
give me a brain as strong as my body is weak. It is true I have often acted when
wholly unfit for work, but even mine enemy will not accuse me of being actu-
ated by vanity.[112] Morris's declaration suggests it was not to her own pathologizing that she objected, but to the depletion of its romanticizing capacity.

Within a few short years, the reputed "Queen of Hearts" had become the
"Queen of Spasms," a moniker registering the shift in Morris's pathologizing process from humanizing to stigmatizing. Within this revised narrative,
Morris and her talent were trapped within a shattered body that rendered her
once electrifying performances disturbingly morbid. The actress's poor health,
which the public now speculated was at least partially self-inflicted, under-
scored all of her stage work. Instead of witnessing her legendary emotionalism,
audiences were recast as Morris's sickbed sentinels, intimately observing—for
a price—the actress's losing battle with her own pathological demons. Morris's
public debasement provides convincing support for what Kerry Powell has
labeled the "medicalizing" of Victorian actresses, a public process that framed

the woman of the theatre "in a rhetoric of pathology that both monitored and disarmed her subversive potential" while accommodating her broader behavioral latitude.[113]

The romanticizing and medicalizing strains of embodying Camille co-existed throughout the late nineteenth century. The former dominated in the earlier decades of English-language *Camille* productions and the latter grew more prominent in the years surrounding tuberculosis's medical reclassification and the rise of theatrical realism. I have employed the word "strain" to describe each of these major approaches to performing tuberculosis, first because of its microbiological implications and second because it suggests these categories were neither fixed nor binary. Rather, as part of *La dame aux camélias*'s stage evolution, the two strains expanded and contracted alongside shifting medical and theatrical trends. What often differentiated the mythologized and demythologized Camilles was not the absence or presence of tubercular symptoms; it was the degree to which actresses physicalized those symptoms. Performers almost always enacted Camille's consumptive cough, for example, but it was primarily those of the medicalizing strain that adopted a frequent, barking cough that doubled over the body, coupled with periodic wheezes and the use of blood-spattered handkerchiefs to signal the expectoration of lung matter. Critics, too, reflected in their appraisals and rhetoric the two strains of playing Camille, a pattern that would persist, though not without minor modifications, as two international stars reinvigorated the role and its medicocultural consequence in the century's final decades.

Notes

1 "The First Lady with the Camelias," *Theatre Magazine* 1 (Oct 1901): 14–16.
2 Grace Greenwood, "Five Camilles," *The New York Times*, Feb 21, 1875; and "Paris Letters," *Western Mail*, Feb 19, 1875.
3 L. H. Hooper, "The Adventures of a Drama," *Appletons' Journal*, Mar 22, 1873.
4 As a "fallen woman," Camille receives attention from Katie N. Johnson, *Sisters in Sin: Brothel Drama in America, 1900–1920* (Cambridge: Cambridge University Press, 2006); Nicholas John, ed., *Violetta and Her Sisters:* The Lady of the Camellias, *Responses to the Myth* (London: Faber and Faber, 1994); and Gwen Ursula Preston Jensen, "Matilda Heron and the Americanization of Camille" (PhD diss., University of Nebraska – Lincoln, 2003).
5 David M. Morens, "At the Deathbed of Consumptive Art," *Emerging Infectious Disease* 8, no. 11 (Nov 2011): 1353–1358.
6 Throughout these chapters I employ Clark Lawlor's terms "consumptive myth" and "romantic myth of consumption" from *Consumption and Literature: The Making of the Romantic Disease* (Basingstoke: Palgrave MacMillan, 2006).
7 Terry Eagleton, *Sweet Violence: The Ideal of the Tragic* (Malden: Blackwell Publishing, 2003), 169.
8 Claudine Herzlich and Janine Pierret, *Illness and Self in Society*, trans. Elborg Forster (Baltimore: Johns Hopkins University Press, 1987), 28.
9 F. B. Smith, *The Retreat of Tuberculosis, 1850–1950* (London: Croom Helm, 1988), 26–27. There is an extensive library of scholarship on tuberculosis. For scientific descriptions of tuberculosis as well as its cultural history in Western society (particularly Britain and the United States), see also David S. Barnes, *The Making of a Social Disease: Tuberculosis in*

Nineteenth-Century France (Berkeley: University of California Press, 1995); Barbara Bates, *Bargaining for Life: A Social History of Tuberculosis, 1876–1938* (Philadelphia: University of Philadelphia Press, 1992); Helen Bynum, *Spitting Blood: The History of Tuberculosis* (Oxford: Oxford University Press, 2012); Meredith Conti, "Tragic Potential in the Nineteenth-Century Consumptive Myth," *Journal of Dramatic Theory and Criticism* 24, no. 1 (Fall 2009): 59–82; Thomas M. Daniel, *Captain of Death: The Story of Tuberculosis* (Rochester: University of Rochester Press, 1997); Thomas Dormandy, *The White Death: A History of Tuberculosis* (New York: New York University Press, 2000); Georgina D. Feldberg, *Disease and Class: Tuberculosis and the Shaping of Modern North American Society* (New Brunswick: Rutgers University Press, 1995); R.Y. Keers, *Pulmonary Tuberculosis: A Journey Down the Centuries* (London: Baillière Tindall, 1978); Clark Lawlor and Akihito Suzuki, "The Disease of the Self: Representing Consumption, 1700–1830," *Bulletin of Historical Medicine* 74 (2000): 287–307; B. Meyer, "Till Death Do Us Part: The Consumptive Victorian Heroine in Popular Romantic Fiction," in *Journal of Popular Culture* 37, No. 2 (2003): 287–308; Katherine Ott, *Fevered Lives: Tuberculosis in American Culture Since 1870* (Cambridge: Harvard University Press, 1996); Barbara Gutmann Rosenkrantz, ed., *From Consumption to Tuberculosis: A Documentary History* (New York: Garland Publishing, Inc., 1994); Sheila M. Rothman, *Living in the Shadow of Death: Tuberculosis and the Social Experience of Illness in American History* (New York: BasicBooks, 1994); and Susan Sontag, *Illness as Metaphor* (New York: Farrar, Straus and Giroux, 1977).

10 Dormandy, *White Death*, 22.

11 William Sweetser, *Treatise on Consumption* (Boston: T.H. Carter, 1836), 72–73.

12 Lawlor, *Consumption and Literature*, 5. Tuberculosis deaths waned in the latter half of the nineteenth century before any effective treatments were introduced. A concrete explanation for this phenomenon has not been widely accepted, but improved nutrition, swifter diagnoses, and even "herd immunity" have all been cited by scientists as possible justifications.

13 Daniel, *Captain of Death*, 30.

14 Lawlor, *Consumption and Literature*, 36; For discussions of Renaissance views of consumption, see Lawlor, *Consumption and Literature*, 27–28; Barnes, *Making of a Social Disease*, 40; and Keers, *Pulmonary Tuberculosis*, 65.

15 Lawlor, *Consumption and Literature*, 44.

16 Herzlich and Pierret, *Illness and Self*, 24.

17 Sontag, *Illness as Metaphor*, 63 and 61.

18 Benjamin Rush, *The Family Physician, The Consumptives Guide to Health and Lady's Medical Companion*, ed. A.H. Flanders (Lowell: n.p., 1864), 64.

19 Dormany, *White Death*, 91.

20 Ott, *Fevered Lives*, 13.

21 Lawlor, *Consumption and Literature*, 2. See also Dormandy, *The White Death*, 85–100; and Hays, *Burdens of Disease*, 158.

22 Lawlor, *Consumption and Literature*, 116.

23 Sontag, *Illness as Metaphor*, 46.

24 Herzlich and Pierret, *Illness and Self in Society*, xi.

25 Meyer, "Till Death Do Us Part," 290.

26 Sweetser, *Treatise on Consumption*, 74.

27 Conti, "Tragic Potential," 71.

28 Daniel, *Captain of Death*, 80.

29 *Consumption: Cause and Nature by Rollin R. Gregg, M.D.; to which is added The Therapeutics of Tuberculous Affections by H. C. Allen, M.D.* (Ann Arbor, 1889), 183.

30 Nancy Tomes, *The Gospel of Germs: Men, Women, and the Microbe in American Life* (Cambridge, Harvard University Press, 1998), 28.

31 Ibid., 46.

32 Philip Alcabes, *Dread: How Fear and Fantasy Have Fueled Epidemics from the Black Death to Avian Flu* (New York: PublicAffairs, 2009), 96.

33 Ibid., 88.
34 Laura Otis, *Membranes: Metaphors of Invasion in Nineteenth-Century Literature, Science, and Politics* (Baltimore: Johns Hopkins University Press, 1999), 25.
35 Sontag, *Illness as Metaphor*, 38.
36 Dormandy, *The White Death*, 73; and Nan Marie McMurry, "'And I? I am in a Consumption:' The Tuberculosis Patient, 1780–1930" (PhD diss., Duke University, 1985), viii. Statistics revealed that the impoverished were contracting the disease at a rate of five times their wealthier counterparts.
37 Prohibition of spitting in public places was ordained in European and American cities for fear that "dry phthisical sputa sticking to the floor, clothing, etc., [which remains] virulent for a long time, if inhaled as dust into the lung" could cause tuberculosis. Hugo Engel, "The Etiology of Tuberculosis," *Philadelphia Medical Times* 12, no. 25 (Sept 9, 1882): 843–852.
38 Pamela K. Gilbert, *Disease, Desire, and the Body in Victorian Women's Popular Novels* (Cambridge: Cambridge University Press, 1997), 18; and Barnes, *Making of a Social Disease*, 104. Until streptomycin was approved for distribution in 1944, the treatment of tuberculosis patients remained relatively unchanged after the discovery of the tubercle bacillus.
39 J. Brander Matthews, *French Dramatists of the Nineteenth Century* (New York: Charles Scribner's Sons, 1881), 144.
40 Acorn, "Letter from 'Acorn'," *Spirit of the Times*, May 23, 1857.
41 Dormandy, *The White Death*, 70; and René Weis, *The Real Traviata: The Song of Marie Duplessis* (Oxford: Oxford University Press, 2015), 253.
42 Alexandre Dumas fils, *Camille (La dame aux camélias)*, trans. Edith Reynolds and Nigel Playfair, in *Camille and Other Plays*, ed. Stephen S. Stanton (New York: Hill and Wang, 1957), 105–164, 162.
43 Alexandre Dumas fils, *The Lady of the Camillias*, trans. and intro. by Edmund Gosse (New York: P.F. Collier and Son, 1902), 305–323. Bernadette C. Lintz sees the abundant references to fluids (tears, sputum, menstrual and expectorated blood, etc.) as essential tools in Dumas's depiction of "sexually transgressive women as diseased and contagious." "Concocting *La dame aux camélias*: Blood, Tears, and Other Fluids," *Nineteenth-Century French Studies* 33, no. 3&4 (2005): 287–307, 288.
44 William Winter, *The Wallet of Time; Containing Personal, Biographical, and Critical Reminiscence of the American Theatre*, vol. 1 (New York: Ayer Publishing, 1969), 232.
45 Benjamin McArthur, *Actors and American Culture, 1880–1920* (Iowa City: University of Iowa Press, 2000), 170.
46 Acorn, "Theatricals in Boston," *Spirit of the Times*, Oct 25, 1856.
47 *New York Tribune*, Feb 2, 1865.
48 George C. Odell, *Annals of the New York Stage*, vol. 6 (New York: Columbia University Press, 1931), 281; and Hooper, *Appletons' Journal*, March 22, 1873.
49 Bonnie Eckard, "Two Camilles, Matilda Heron and Clara Morris: Anti-Victorians on the Nineteenth-Century American Stage" in *Women's Contribution to Nineteenth-Century American Theatre*, eds. Miriam López Rodríguez and María Dolores Narbona Carrión (València: Universitat de València, 2011), 141–152, 144.
50 Bonnie Jean Eckard, "Camille in America" (PhD diss., University of Denver, 1982), 116.
51 Charles DeKay, "Modjeska," *Scribner's Monthly* 17 (Nov 1878–Jan 1879), 664.
52 Helena Modjeska, *Memories and Impressions of Helena Modjeska: An Autobiography* (New York: Macmillan, 1910), 356.
53 "Amusements," *Washington Post*, Jan 14, 1879.
54 *The New York Times*, June 20, 1886; and William Winter, *Vagrant Memories: Being Further Recollections of Other Times* (New York: George H. Doran Co., 1915), 46.
55 John Creahan, *The Life of Laura Keene* (Philadelphia: Ridgers Publishing, 1897), 99; and Vernanne Bryan, *Laura Keene: A British Actress on the American Stage, 1826–1873* (Jefferson, NC: McFarland, 1997), 65.

56   "Theatre Royal" *Birmingham Daily Post*, Oct 4, 1881; and "Modjeska," *Scribner's Monthly*, 664.
57   "Record of Amusements," *The New York Times*, Oct 1, 1878; "London Correspondence," *Aberdeen Weekly Journal*, May 3, 1880; and *Philadelphia Evening Bulletin*, Jan 29, 1878.
58   *Philadelphia Evening Bulletin*, Jan 29, 1878.
59   For critical responses to Modjeska's voice and accent, see "'Heartsease' at the Court," *The Examiner*, May 8, 1880; "Madame Modjeska at the Court Theatre," *Glasgow Herald*, Nov 24, 1881; "Theatre Royal: Madame Modjeska in 'Heartsease,'" *Birmingham Daily Post*, Oct 4, 1881; and "Yesterday's Theatricals," *Reynolds's Newspaper*, May 2, 1880.
60   "Record of Amusements," *The New York Times*, Oct 1, 1878.
61   "The Drama," *The Critic*, Dec 30, 1882.
62   Modjeska quoted in Eckard, "Camille in America," 107.
63   "Theatre Royal," *Birmingham Daily Post*, Oct 4, 1881.
64   "Our Ladies Column," *Aberdeen Weekly Journal*, June 7, 1880.
65   "The Theatres," *Daily News* (London), May 3, 1880.
66   Conti, "Tragic Potential."
67   "The Drama," *The Critic*, Dec 30, 1882.
68   "Theatre Royal," *Birmingham Daily Post*, April 14, 1885 (emphases mine) and Antoni Gronowiciz, *Modjeska: Her Life and Loves* (New York: Thomas Yoseloff, 1956), 162. Not everyone thought of Modjeska as a tragedian or Camille as a tragic figure. John Ranken Towse wrote in a short piece on the actress, declaring that "The woes of *Camille* never found a more graceful or more pathetic interpreter; but the awful imaginings of the despairing *Juliet* at the one supreme moment in the potion scene, demand powers of a different and higher order than any which she possesses." J. Ranken Towse, "Madame Modjeska," *Century Illustrated Magazine* 27, no. 1 (Nov 1883): 22–27.
69   "Amusements," *The New York Times*, Jan 5, 1886.
70   Susan Bassnett, "Eleonora Duse," in *Bernhardt, Terry, Duse: The Actress in Her Time* (Cambridge: Cambridge University Press, 1988), 138.
71   This summary of Heron's life was compiled using Bonnie Eckard, "Two Camilles," 147; and Jensen, "Matilda Heron and the Americanization of Camille."
72   The "emotional school of acting" in the nineteenth century implied both a talent for performing overly passionate or pathetic characters and a natural tendency toward such behaviors off the stage as well. I use the term only in the former meaning.
73   Lavinia Hart, "Olga Nethersole," *The Cosmopolitan: A Monthly Illustrated Magazine* 31, no. 1 (May 1901): 15.
74   "Olga Nethersole as Camille," *The Critic*, Nov 3, 1894.
75   In 1884, *The Cleveland Herald* stated the Morris did not attempt to hide any of Camille's "wicked and sinful" nature and presented the flawed character "as Dumas intended," but this interpretation seems at odds with other reviews that painted her Camille as sweet and virtuous (*Cleveland Herald*, April 17, 1884). It could be that Morris's performance of the role changed over time.
76   Barbara Wallace Grossman, *A Spectacle of Suffering: Clara Morris on the American Stage* (Carbondale: Southern Illinois University Press, 2009), 117.
77   "Amusements," *Flake's Bulletin*, Dec 7, 1867.
78   Acorn, "Letter from 'Acorn," *Spirit of the Times,* May 23, 1857.
79   "The Ex-Editor in New York," *Philadelphia Inquirer*, Dec. 1, 1895.
80   "Theatricals," *United States Magazine* 4, no. 5 (May 1857), 536.
81   "Matilda Heron's Opinion of Camille," *Daily Evening Bulletin* [San Francisco], May 28, 1857.
82   Eckard, "Two Camilles," 141.
83   Fitz-James O'Brien, *The Poems and Stories of Fitz-James O'Brien*, ed. William Winter (Boston: James R. Osgood and Co., 1881), 268.
84   Adam Badeau, *The Vagabond* (New York: Rudd and Carleton, 1859), 4.

85 Beaumont Fletcher, "Three Ladies of the Camellias," *Godey's Magazine*, May 1, 1896.
86 Eckard, "Camille in America," 153.
87 "Olga Nethersole as Camille," *The Critic*, Nov 3, 1894.
88 "Margaret Fuller is Quite Justified in Acting," unidentified newspaper clipping, March 23, 1898, Camille clippings file, HTC.
89 "Stage Whispers: The Prowling Robbers of the Square and Their Chosen," *National Police Gazette*, June 23, 1883.
90 "All Actresses Dread Fat," *The Anaconda Standard*, July 27, 1898.
91 "The Playhouse," *St. Paul Daily News*, Jan 28, 1890.
92 "The Stage," *New York Herald*, Oct 24, 1886.
93 "Causerie," *Spirit of the Times*, n.d., Camille clippings file, HTC.
94 "Miss Matilda Heron, The American Tragedienne, as 'Camille,'" *Balou's Pictorial Drawing-Room Companion*, April 4, 1857.
95 "The Ex-Editor in New York," *Philadelphia Inquirer*, Dec 1, 1895 and "Theater," *Daily Ohio Statesman*, Feb 26, 1858.
96 Badeau, *The Vagabond*, 4.
97 "Causerie," *Spirit of the Times*, n.d.
98 Alan Dale, *Familiar Chats with the Queens of the Stage* (New York: G.W. Dillingham, 1890), 365.
99 "Amusements: Academy of Music," *Cleveland Leader*, Dec 18, 1874.
100 Eckard, "Camille in America," 80 and 87.
101 Fletcher, "Three Ladies," 477.
102 Eckard, "Camille in America," 153–154.
103 "Amusements for the Week," *Tacoma Daily News*, Dec 27, 1890.
104 Dale, *Familiar Chats*, 365.
105 "A Bunch of Camellias," quoted in Eckard, "Camille in America," 80–81.
106 *New York Daily Tribune*, Nov 29, 1881.
107 "Causerie," *Spirit of the Times*, n.d.
108 "Music and the Drama," *Boston Daily Advertiser*, May 8, 1877.
109 Grossman, *Spectacle of Suffering*, 198.
110 Grossman, *Spectacle of Suffering*, 174; and "Music and the Drama," *Boston Daily Advertiser*, May 8, 1877.
111 "Clara Morris: Cupidity and Brutality—The Coming End," *New York Dramatic News*, Aug 25, 1877, quoted in Grossman, *Spectacle of Suffering*, 180.
112 *Spirit of the Times*, Sept 29, 1877; and "A Curious Letter from Clara Morris," *New York Sun*, n.d., quoted in Grossman, *Spectacle of Suffering*, 181 and 177.
113 Kerry Powell, *Women and Victorian Theatre* (Cambridge: Cambridge University Press, 1997), 38.

Bibliography

Alcabes, Philip. *Dread: How Fear and Fantasy Have Fueled Epidemics from the Black Death to Avian Flu*. New York: PublicAffairs, 2009.
Badeau, Adam. *The Vagabond*. New York: Rudd and Carleton, 1859.
Barnes, David S. *The Making of a Social Disease: Tuberculosis in Nineteenth-Century France*. Berkeley: University of California Press, 1995.
Bashford, Alison. "Foreign Bodies: Vaccination, Contagion, and Colonialism in the Nineteenth Century." In *Contagion: Historical and Cultural Studies*, edited by Alison Bashford and Claire Hooker, 39–60. London: Routledge, 2001.
Bassnett, Susan. "Eleonora Duse." In *Bernhardt, Terry, Duse: The Actress in Her Time*, edited by John Stokes, Michael R. Booth, and Susan Bassnett, 119–170. Cambridge: Cambridge University Press, 1988.

Bates, Barbara. *Bargaining for Life: A Social History of Tuberculosis, 1876–1938*. Philadelphia: University of Philadelphia Press, 1992.

Brown, Michael. "From Foetid Air to Filth: The Cultural Transformation of British Epidemiological Thought, ca. 1780–1848." *Bulletin of History of Medicine* 28, no. 3 (2008): 515–544.

Bryan, Vernanne. *Laura Keene: A British Actress on the American Stage, 1826–1873*. Jefferson: McFarland, 1997.

Bynum, Helen. *Spitting Blood: The History of Tuberculosis*. Oxford: Oxford University Press, 2012.

Conti, Meredith. "'I am not suffering anymore…': Tragic Potential in the Nineteenth-Century Consumptive Myth." *Journal of Dramatic Theory and Criticism* 24, no. 1 (Fall 2009): 59–82.

Creahan, John. *The Life of Laura Keene*. Philadelphia: Ridgers Publishing, 1897.

Dale, Alan. *Familiar Chats with the Queens of the Stage*. New York: G.W. Dillingham, 1890.

Daniel, Thomas M. *Captain of Death: The Story of Tuberculosis*. Rochester: University of Rochester Press, 1997.

De Kay, Charles. "Modjeska." *Scribner's Monthly* 17 (Nov 1878–Jan 1879): 665–671.

Dormandy, Thomas. *The White Death: A History of Tuberculosis*. New York: New York University Press, 2000.

Dumas fils, Alexandre. *Camille (La dame aux camélias)*. Trans. Edith Reynolds and Nigel Playfair. In *Camille and Other Plays*, edited by Stephen S. Stanton, 105–164. New York: Hill and Wang, 1957.

Dumas fils, Alexandre. *Camille. The Lady of the Camillias*. Translated by Edmund Gosse. New York: P.F. Collier and Son, 1902.

Eagleton, Terry. *Sweet Violence: The Ideal of the Tragic*. Malden: Blackwell Publishing, 2003.

Eckard, Bonnie Jean. "Camille in America." PhD dissertation. University of Denver, 1982.

Eckard, Bonnie Jean. "Two Camilles, Matilda Heron and Clara Morris: Anti-Victorians on the Nineteenth-Century American Stage." In *Women's Contribution to Nineteenth-Century American Theatre*, edited by Miriam López Rodríguez and María Dolores Narbona Carrión, 141–152. València: Universitat de València, 2011.

Engel, Hugo. "The Etiology of Tuberculosis." *Philadelphia Medical Times* 12, no. 25 (Sept 9, 1882): 843–852.

Feldberg, Georgina D. *Disease and Class: Tuberculosis and the Shaping of Modern North American Society*. New Brunswick: Rutgers University Press, 1995.

O'Brien, Fitz-James. *The Poems and Stories of Fitz-James O'Brien*. Edited by William Winter. Boston: James R. Osgood and Co., 1881.

Gilbert, Pamela K. *Disease, Desire, and the Body in Victorian Women's Popular Novels*. Cambridge: Cambridge University Press, 1997.

Gregg, Rollin R. *Consumption: Cause and Nature by Rollin R. Gregg, M.D.; to which is added The Therapeutics of Tuberculous Affections by H. C. Allen, M.D.* Ann Arbor, 1889.

Gronowicz, Antoni. *Modjeska: Her Life and Loves*. New York: Thomas Yoseloff, 1956.

Grossman, Barbara Wallace. *A Spectacle of Suffering: Clara Morris on the American Stage*. Carbondale: Southern Illinois University Press, 2009.

Herzlich, Claudine and Janine Pierret. *Illness and Self in Society*. Trans. Elborg Forster. Baltimore: Johns Hopkins University Press, 1987.

Jensen, Gwen Ursula Preston. "Matilda Heron and the Americanization of Camille." PhD dissertation. University of Nebraska–Lincoln, 2003.

John, Nicholas, ed. *Violetta and Her Sisters: The Lady of the Camellias, Responses to the Myth*. London: Faber and Faber, 1994.

Johnson, Katie N. *Sisters in Sin: Brothel Drama in America, 1900–1920.* Cambridge: Cambridge University Press, 2006.

Keers, R.Y. *Pulmonary Tuberculosis: A Journey Down the Centuries.* London: Baillière Tindall, 1978.

Lawlor, Clark. *Consumption and Literature: The Making of the Romantic Disease.* Basingstoke: Palgrave MacMillan, 2006.

Lawlor, Clark and Akihito Suzuki. "The Disease of the Self: Representing Consumption, 1700–1830." *Bulletin of Historical Medicine,* 74 (2000): 287–307.

Lintz, Bernadette C. "Concocting *La Dame aux camélias*: Blood, Tears, and Other Fluids." *Nineteenth-Century French Studies* 33, nos. 3-4 (2005): 287–307.

Matthews, J. Brander. *French Dramatists of the Nineteenth Century.* New York: Charles Scribner's Sons, 1881.

McArthur, Benjamin. *Actors and American Culture, 1880–1920.* Iowa City: University of Iowa Press, 2000.

McMurry, Nan Marie. "'And I? I am in a Consumption:' The Tuberculosis Patient, 1780–1930." PhD dissertation. Duke University, 1985.

Meyer, B. "Till Death Do Us Part: The Consumptive Victorian Heroine in Popular Romantic Fiction." *The Journal of Popular Culture* 37, no. 2 (2003): 287–308.

Modjeska, Helena. *Memories and Impressions of Helena Modjeska: An Autobiography.* New York: Macmillan, 1910.

Morens, David M. "At the Deathbed of Consumptive Art." *Emerging Infectious Disease* 8, no. 11 (Nov 2011): 1353–1358.

Odell, George C. *Annals of the New York Stage.* Vol. 6. New York: Columbia University Press, 1931.

Otis, Laura. *Membranes: Metaphors of Invasion in Nineteenth-Century Literature, Science, and Politics.* Baltimore: Johns Hopkins University Press, 1999.

Ott, Katherine. *Fevered Lives: Tuberculosis in American Culture Since 1870.* Cambridge: Harvard University Press, 1996.

Powell, Kerry. *Women and Victorian Theatre.* Cambridge: Cambridge University Press, 1997.

Rosenkrantz, Barbara Gutmann, ed. *From Consumption to Tuberculosis: A Documentary History.* New York: Garland Publishing, Inc., 1994.

Rothman, Sheila M. *Living in the Shadow of Death: Tuberculosis and the Social Experience of Illness in American History.* New York: BasicBooks, 1994.

Rush, Benjamin. *The Family Physician, The Consumptives Guide to Health and Lady's Medical Companion.* Edited by A. H. Flanders. Lowell: Flanders, 1864: n.p.

Smith, F. B. *The Retreat of Tuberculosis, 1850–1950.* London: Croom Helm, 1988.

Sontag, Susan. *Illness as Metaphor.* New York: Farrar, Straus and Giroux, 1977.

Sweetser, William. *Treatise on Consumption.* Boston: T.H. Carter, 1836.

Tomes, Nancy. "Epidemic Entertainments: Disease and Popular Culture in Early-Twentieth-Century America." *American Literary History* 14, no. 4 (2002): 625–652.

Tomes, Nancy. *The Gospel of Germs: Men, Women, and the Microbe in American Life.* Cambridge: Harvard University Press, 1998.

Towse, J. Ranken. "Madame Modjeska." *Century Illustrated Magazine* 27, no. 1 (Nov 1883): 22–27.

Wald, Priscilla. *Contagious: Cultures, Carriers, and the Outbreak Narrative.* Durham: Duke University Press, 2008.

Weinstein, Arnold. "Afterword: Infection as Metaphor." *Literature and Medicine: Contagion and Infection* 2, no. 1 (Spring 2003): 102–115.

Weis, René. *The Real Traviata: The Song of Marie Duplessis*. Oxford: Oxford University Press, 2015.

Winter, William. *Vagrant Memories: Being Further Recollections of Other Times*. New York: George H. Doran Co., 1915.

Winter, William. *The Wallet of Time, Containing Personal, Biographical, and Critical Reminiscence of the American Theatre*. Vol. 1. New York: Ayer Publishing, 1969.

2 Foreign invasions

The transatlantic consumptives of Sarah Bernhardt and Eleonora Duse

By the 1880s, a seemingly endless wave of Camilles had inundated American theatres for nearly thirty years. British spectators, however, had yet to bear witness to the courtesan's tale of redemptive suffering until *Heartsease*, James Mortimer's translation of *La dame aux camélias*, was approved for its English premiere in 1880. This imbalance of exposure, as well as the distinctive cultural sensibilities at play in both countries, impacted how British and American audiences received new Camilles in the nineteenth century's final decades. Moreover, as we discovered in Chapter 1, twinned paradigm shifts recalibrated approaches to (and critical evaluations of) Camille's onstage decline and death: the contagionist turn in medical science and the realist turn in European and American theatre. This tangle of theatrical and extra-theatrical frameworks intervened in conspicuous ways in the transatlantic Marguerite Gautiers of performers Sarah Bernhardt and Eleonora Duse.

While Bernhardt in many ways perfected the romanticized approach to Marguerite Gautier, her death scene ventured into more macabre territory than Jean Davenport, Helena Modjeska, and their peers. The naturalistic Duse took a different tack with Marguerite, challenging the aestheticization of tuberculosis and drawing the courtesan's physiological sufferings inward instead of pictorializing them, an interpretation befitting what some have labeled nineteenth-century medicine's "Bacteriological Revolution."[1] This comparative approach also throws into relief the gradual changes to English-language *Camille* criticism as the century came to a close. As a general rule, commentators of the 1880s and 1890s attended to Camille's illness more assiduously than mid-century writers. Whereas earlier reviews of *Camille* prioritized the play's redemptive love story in assessing an actress's skill in the role, later notices dedicated considerable time to analyzing her persuasiveness as a terminally ill woman, often fortifying their claims with modern scientific explanations or personal anecdotes of witnessing a loved one's tubercular decline. Furthermore, press coverage—and in particular that of publications from the United States—intermingled materialistic, moralistic, and nationalistic critiques of the actresses themselves with those aimed at Dumas's courtesan. Because Bernhardt and Duse only played *La dame aux camélias* in their native tongues, anglophone audiences read Marguerite's illness primarily through the actresses' bodies and vocalities.[2] Bernhardt and Duse's physical forms, foreignness, personal lives, and perceived health, therefore, became integral factors in appraising and authenticating their performances of tuberculosis. At a time when physicians, social reformers, and politicians labored to publicly divest tuberculosis of its pernicious sentimentality, Bernhardt and Duse remolded the role's contours to fit their artistic principles, methodologies, and own insights into Marguerite's disease.

The sublime and the grotesque in Bernhardt's neo-romantic Camille

> There have been Camilles material to the last endurable degree of realism, laden with the pungent odors of dissolute joy, not redeemed by love, but seeming to drag to the depths of sin the love that hovered over them like a benediction. The character has, on the other hand, been poetized, made beautiful, and given an aspect not its own, a condition more harmful than the sensual; but it remained for Bernhardt to give it that spiritual ideality which proclaims the ascendance of soul despite the influence of physical environments.
>
> *The Daily Inter Ocean*, April 28, 1887[3]

For many who witnessed it, Sarah Bernhardt's Marguerite Gautier was a theatrical revelation. Fusing the aesthetic principles of early nineteenth-century romanticism and *fin-de-siècle* symbolism together with the classical French school of drama and the pantomimic excess of the Boulevard theatres, Bernhardt succeeded where other Camille actresses had failed: she created a "soiled dove" that was simultaneously impassioned and pure. Not only did the role occupy an esteemed position in Bernhardt's repertoire for over four decades, hers became the definitive interpretation against which all other Camilles were judged. Generations of theatre scholars have sought to historically deconstruct Bernhardt's performance in the hopes of ascertaining just how it captivated thousands of playgoers and inspired critics to label it "the finest piece of acting of our time" or, on rarer occasions, "an apotheosis ... of bawdry."[4] However, because Bernhardt's Marguerite (like many other acting efforts contained in this book) is not often recognized as a performance of illness, many scholars fail to sufficiently dissect Bernhardt's method of staging consumption or acknowledge its centrality to her success in the role. Bernhardt's embodiment of Marguerite did not fully adhere to the aesthetic prescriptions implicated within the romanticized consumptive myth *or* its late nineteeth-century rival, the medicalized, epidemiologic view of tuberculosis. Instead, Bernhardt's neo-romantic depiction of Marguerite's consumption bore subtle markings of clinical tuberculosis's escalating influence, particularly in her elaborate death scene. As is suggested by the *Daily Inter Ocean*'s remarks above, the actress eschewed both the explicitly graphic and cloyingly beatific approaches to Marguerite and her illness, and in their place presented a character whose oppressive earthly confines could not inhibit her spiritual transcendence.

The actress's nearly forty-five-year tenure as Marguerite, beginning in 1880, was the longest in the stage character's history, with decades of critical reviews charting changes to Bernhardt's perceived health, appearance, stamina, and commitment to the role. Even as *fin-de-siècle* critics declared *La dame* an artifact of a bygone era, in 1896 Bernhardt launched a revamped production in 1840s dress (the time period of Dumas's novel) with favorable results. As her acting methods matured, Bernhardt shunned the stark French naturalism of the Théâtre Libre but warmed to symbolist modes of performance; as such, she was poetic and modern, the superlative combination for playing the pathos and pathology of the role.[5] These methodological and aesthetic juxtapositions, I contend, enabled Bernhardt to articulate tuberculosis's mythic and clinical dimensions. As Gerda Taranow offers in her study of Bernhardt, Dumas's courtesan exemplifies Victor Hugo's romantic formation of the sublime and the grotesque, or human nature's commingling of the dark and the light, the ugly and the beautiful.[6] Taranow situates Marguerite within a larger discussion of the actress's *premier courtisane roles*, a useful strategy that nevertheless underappreciates Bernhardt's performance of tuberculosis was in itself a conspicuous expression of Hugo's Sublime/Grotesque dyad. As such, the longevity of Bernhardt's neo-romantic portrait of love, loss, and rebirth can be explained, at least in part, by its performative bridging of the disease's mythological past and its clinical present.

To understand the discordant judgments of Bernhardt's work in general and in *La dame aux camélias* in particular, it is helpful to characterize how British and American audiences regarded France's provocative theatrical export. Even before she set sail for England and the United States, Bernhardt was the subject of much speculation and ridicule in the countries' presses. Though England was not without its fervent Bernhardt detractors, her 1879 season at London's Gaiety Theatre with the Comédie-Française cemented her reputation as a stage star of supreme magnetism, intelligence, and emotional depth; "her genius is beyond dispute," declared the *London Illustrated News* in an otherwise measured evaluation of three Comédie-Française actresses performing at the Gaiety.[7] Indeed, Bernhardt was treated as a celebrity nonpareil by elite Victorians: Oscar Wilde honored her disembarkation at Folkstone by laying a trail of lilies before her, Britain's aristocratic and moneyed families commanded private recitals, and her paintings and sculptures were given a public exhibition in Piccadilly. Her subsequent American tour in 1880 and 1881, however, inspired inconsonant media reports from the adulatory to the damnatory. In her meticulous study of Bernhardt's first tour of the United States, Patricia Marks attributes many of the disparities in critical responses, ticket sales, and Bernhardt's social calendar to the regional, religious, economic, and size differences in her host cities. Whereas Boston audiences met Bernhardt's arrival with a puritan reserve that eased over time, French-settled St. Louis proved a profitable and welcoming host; small-town critics in the South and Midwest often adopted a "cheeky, provincial tone" to report on Bernhardt's foreign repertoire and social customs, a tactic Marks describes as "a type of reverse snobbery that tries to deflate elitism by democratizing it."[8] While Bernhardt's entrepreneurship prevented her easy commodification by business associates and audiences, her ambitions also left her vulnerable to character attacks—misogynistic and anti-Semitic critiques disguised by only the thinnest of veils. Nevertheless, Bernhardt's 51-city tour was largely triumphant, and eight subsequent visits to the United States secured Bernhardt's standing as one of the American stage's most popular and celebrated guests.

Bernhardt's idiosyncratic public persona (much of which was self-generated via media interviews, publicity photos, and folkloric memoirs) was a fusion of facts, inferences, exaggerations, and lies. Some in the United States and England, however, employed Bernhardt's sensationalized past as a way of authenticating her interpretation of Marguerite. As the illegitimate daughter of a Dutch-Jewish courtesan and a sexually liberated woman with a history of love affairs, Parisian-born Bernhardt could, critics implied, empathize closely with Marguerite; similarly, English-language press coverage on Bernhardt suggested that her lack of Victorian propriety, while distasteful on principle, released the actress from the inhibitions regulating others of her sex, as did her decadent Frenchness. "Her private life has certainly not been an exaltation of womanhood; it rather has been a degradation of the holiest sentiments and most sacred ideals of domestic and social virtue," noted one reviewer, "but it has been a frank, undisguised life, speaking its own warning to society and holding aloof from imposture."[9] Bernhardt molded each of her characters to accommodate her own personality, a common practice for nineteenth-century actors that drew contradictory responses in the 1880s and 1890s. "She does not enter into the leading character," George Bernard Shaw once wrote scornfully of the actress; "she substitutes herself for it." *The Times*'s J. Comyns Carr defended Bernhardt's individualized methods more generously, remarking that "it is the richness of that personality vibrating in response to every deeper experience that gives its final stamp to the creation."[10] Indeed, for one New York reviewer, Bernhardt's Marguerite captivated precisely because the actress never vanished into the role: "The pleasure which we get from seeing [Bernhardt] as Marguerite Gautier is doubled by that other pleasure, never completely out of our minds, that she is also Sarah Bernhardt."[11] Whether Bernhardt was particularly suited to the role of Marguerite by virtue of her strange and sordid past or whether the actress's own magnetic personality overwhelmed the character is a matter of opinion. As two mythic entities, Bernhardt and Marguerite were intertwined to such a degree that in 1890 the *New Haven Evening Register* expressed outrage that the actress planned to embody the Virgin Mary in a French passion play:

> *Camille* as the Virgin Mary! The woman who has never, up to within a few weeks, appeared in a play to which mothers could take their children, depicting the mother of the Christ ... We hope that for once Paris will frown upon this adventurous *Camille*. Art has its limits.[12]

In many ways, Bernhardt's performance of consumption began decades prior to playing Marguerite. The young Sarah was convinced she would perish of the romantic disease, and as an adult, Bernhardt closely observed tuberculosis's symptomatology as she cared for her sister Régine, who succumbed to the disease at age 21. Arthur Gold and Robert Fizdale note that that in her (often fantastical) autobiography *My Double Life*, "Bernhardt speaks of herself as a consumptive who spat blood, fainted frequently, and suffered agonizing bouts of exhaustion." After a particularly severe bout of coughing blood in 1870, Bernhardt's physician directed her to "take the cure" at the mountainous spa town of Eaux-Bonnes, near Bordeaux.[13] In a March 1873 letter to lover Jean Mounet-Sully, Bernhardt conveyed herself in a manner strikingly like her most famous character:

> My beloved Jean: I collapsed at the rehearsal, overcome by fits of cough-ing and spitting blood, and had to be carried to my carriage by Messrs Petter and Feuillet. I am in bed. I beg you my adored one, come to see me. It would give me so much pleasure ... Please forgive me for all the trouble I've caused you ... You must overlook a great deal.[14]

A true testimony to her espousal of the consumptive myth, Bernhardt conceived of her own tubercular-esque sufferings as confirmation of her creative genius, tireless dedication to her craft, and passionate soul. In the end, Bernhardt's adolescent premonition that she would contract tuberculosis had some merit, though not how she imagined. In 1915, doctors amputated Bernhardt's right leg, which had been causing her extreme pain since she injured it jumping from a parapet in Victorien Sardou's *La Tosca* years prior. The pathologist's examination of her leg revealed "Carious bone, fresh necrosis, numerous areas of caseation: tuberculosis of the joint, amputation fully justified."[15] The rest of Bernhardt's body, however, showed no signs of the disease.

Labeled "statuesque" and "majestic" by admirers, Bernhardt's body was tall and thin, endowments that signaled Marguerite's phthisical condition in per-formance. Her slenderness, which by late 1800s standards bordered on emacia-tion, inspired a wealth of visual and literary travesties depicting the actress as amusingly or repulsively thin. "Sarah Bernhardt successfully appeared last night in a new part at the Théâtre Français," one *Puck* humorist teased in 1880, the same year Bernhardt premiered her portrayal of Marguerite. "It was as the broom-stick of one of the witches in *Macbeth*. She is physically admirably fit-ted for the role."[16] Some American cartoons moved beyond satire to depict Bernhardt as abhorrently skeletal, observes Marks, disfiguring her "so that she is no longer an icon of fertility and regeneration, but rather an icon of death" and insinuating that "what lies beneath the charm and costumes ... [is] only thinness, or nothingness"[17] (Figure 2.1).

As Bernhardt aged her frame became considerably less willowy, a transforma-tion that several critics implied reduced her consumptive appearance and appeal. "[S]he has begun to lose her abnormal thinness and with it some of that won-derful *chatterie* which was her characteristic," lamented *The Times*, while *The Era* announced of Bernhardt's 1892 Marguerite that "the ethereal figure of twenty years ago has expanded."[18] In addition to the younger Bernhardt's reed-like

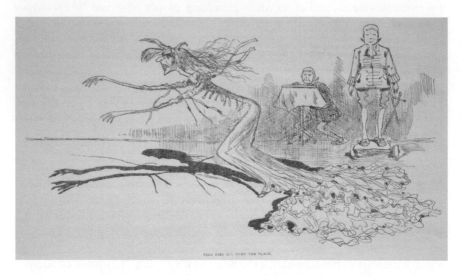

Figure 2.1 "Sarah dies all over the place." *Chic* November 17, 1880. Library of Congress.

figure, the actress's face boasted a pleasing blend of romantic features often asso-ciated with consumption: rosebud mouth, wide-set, shining, and feline-like eyes, a long nose framed by pronounced cheekbones, and pale skin, which she enhanced with white powder. Bernhardt was also widely rumored to paint on the telltale hectic flush of the consumptive. "Those charming roseate effects which French painters produce by giving flesh the pretty color of strawberries and cream ... are cunningly reproduced by Madame Bernhardt," wrote Shaw in his withering critique of the actress.[19] A head of abundant, frizzy, red-blonde hair framed Bernhardt's face; she typically pinned up her unruly mane or, if portray-ing distraught or morally dissolute characters, permitted it to spill down her back. In her memoirs, Ellen Terry described Bernhardt in fittingly consumptive terms:

> as transparent as an azalea, only more so; like a cloud, only not so thick. Smoke from a burning paper describes her more nearly! She was hollow-eyed, thin, almost consumptive-looking. Her body was not the prison of her soul, but its shadow.[20]

Bernhardt's costumes further augmented Marguerite's physical decline: extrav-agant corseted gowns in the play's early acts gave way to the fifth act's diapha-nous bedroom sheath in virginal white. That Bernhardt's body, by itself and as a proxy for Marguerite's tubercular form, provoked such antithetical responses (was it exquisite or monstrous?) appears at first glance a curious matter. And yet, if conceived of as an embodied articulation of tuberculosis's problematic aestheticization at the dawning of the bacteriological age, Bernhardt's con-tested appearance strengthens the linkage of her *La dame aux camélias* to Hugo's notion of the sublime and the grotesque.

Anglophone audiences also looked to Bernhardt's body, and to the full vision of her embodiment, to "translate" what the courtesan's foreign tongue left enigmatic or incomprehensible. Edmund Rostand once christened Bernhardt "the princess of stage movement" and "queen of postures," titles that, for most of *La dame*'s critics, Bernhardt's embodiment of Marguerite capably upheld. A master technician who once lectured in Delsartean fashion that "gesture should always precede speech," and who often blocked intricate choreography into her dialogue during rehearsals, Bernhardt was regarded by a minority of critics as an insincere manipulator of audience emotions.[21] In her recent analysis of Bernhardt's affective provocations of nineteenth-century audiences, Sharon Marcus offers the term "exteriority effects" (a refashioning of literature scholar Felicity Nussbaum's "interiority effects") to describe Bernhardt's methods of externalizing her characters' thoughts and emotions. For Marcus, Bernhardt's prominent exteriority effects included "mobility" (near-constant body movements and perambulations), "framing" (the focused isolation of a single moving body part), "tempo control" (deliberate vacillations in speed, both in speech and movement), and "hyperextension" (as in Bernhardt's use of her spine's suppleness to replicate the period's coveted "S" curve) (Figure 2.2).[22] Bernhardt's somatic expressivity electrified audiences, even as it was suspected by critics to be the work of a diligent craftswoman. "She was trained to be a conscious artist," offers Robert Horville. "And the critics insist[ed] with enthusiasm on the control which accompanied [Bernhardt's] passionate outbursts."[23] Particularly effective were

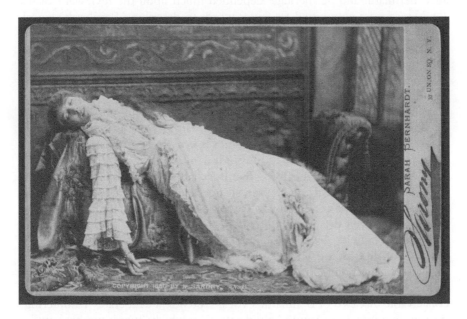

Figure 2.2 TCS 2 Bernhardt, Sarah as Marguerite Gautier in 'La dame aux camélias', Houghton Library, Harvard University.

the actress's undulating arm gestures, which Taranow describes as originating not in the elbows but the shoulders, and her habit of turning her back on the audience (a defiant act for someone trained in French classicism). In contrasting Marguerite's spindly, brittle body and hollowed visage with curved stage crosses and dramatic, fluid gestures that bordered on extravagant, Bernhardt achieved what Cornelia Otis Skinner termed "an exquisite frailty."[24] As Bernhardt's choreography often united feminine elegance with animalistic sensuality, a striking number of critics described Bernhardt's onstage actions and gestures as cat-like. "We wonder not at her fondness for feline parts," remarked *The Bristol Mercury and Daily Post*, "for there is something feline in the grace and character of her movements." An anonymous American critic proclaimed: "Elephantine power she has not, but she has the terrible force of the tigress as well as the insinuating grace of that royal mistress of the jungle."[25] While some reviews chastised Bernhardt for her almost incessant movement as Marguerite, accounts of her acting suggest she was equally compelling in rare moments of stillness. According to Bernhardt admirer Théodore de Banville, "she is so well-equipped to give expression to poetry that, even when she is immobile and silent, one feels that her movement, like her voice, obeys a lyrical rhythm."[26] As John Stokes writes, Bernhardt's *La dame* was "the most phantasmal display of her physical presence," a haunting but lyrical somatic spectacle.[27]

Bernhardt's francophone performance lent her Parisian courtesan especial validity for British and American audiences. Whether this honored or disparaged Bernhardt and her heritage depended much upon the reviewer's biases. *La dame*'s critics committed far fewer words to describing Bernhardt's vocality than they did her physicality, but early voice recordings and reports of her elocutionary techniques are abundant. Her celebrated voice was classically trained at the Conservatoire and later matured during her tenure at the Comédie-Française. Called the *la voix d'or*, or "the golden voice," by Victor Hugo, Bernhardt's instrument was expressive and versatile. In comparing the Camilles of Nethersole, Duse, and Bernhardt, critic Beaumont Fletcher gives his best vocal reviews to Dame Sarah: "Bernhardt's voice is unsurpassed anywhere. Though she chants with it, it never grows elocutional or unnatural. And though it is like a strain of music, like music it has fearful guttural dissonances for its anger."[28] It is likely that Bernhardt's voice utilized two systems of declamation taught at the Conservatoire: *chant*, a rhythmic style highlighting the musicality of verse through variations of pitch and rhythm, and *vérité*, which emphasized the text's content over its lyricism. By her own account, Bernhardt's individualized technique "intensif[ied] the sonorous music of verse, the melody of the word, as well as the music and melody of thought," an integrative approach appropriate to Dumas's poetic Marguerite, whose façade in the early acts is one of insouciance, charm, and mellifluous banter.[29] It is conceivable that two of Bernhardt's vocal crutches, a deliberate "hammering" staccato (her *voix de rage*) and a "rapid patter" in which "words tumbled out" at a breathtaking pace, were enlisted in acts three and four, as passions, conflicts, and illness threaten to mar Marguerite's carefully constructed artifice.[30] Even Bernhardt's most apparent vocal defect, a nasal thinness that at times failed to sustain the thunderous fury of roles like her acclaimed Phédre, was uniquely suited to depict Marguerite's pulmonary and muscular decline. Bernhardt simulated the late-stage consumptive's hoarse cough, and yet there is no indication that Bernhardt's vocal work became inordinately hectic. As was the case with Modjeska's crisp, sweet, and carefully modulated vocality, Bernhardt's golden voice disassociated her sublime Marguerite from the unrefined Camilles of actresses less proficient in the art of elocution.

In a playful mock circular advertising "The Great French Dier," the satirical magazine *Puck* enumerated six Bernhardtian deaths that the actress could produce "on the Shortest Notice": The Adrienne, The Frou-Frou, The Camille ("a die of paroxysmally emotional character … highly recommended for matinée wear"), The Donna Sol, The Phedre ("a die of classic and severe shade"), and The Sphinx ("a crawly, sensational die" with "foamy variations").[31] Humorous it may be, but "The Great French Dier" in fact affirms that Bernhardt's onstage deaths were neither generically drawn nor indistinguishable from one another, though she was later accused by a French critic of recycling some of her *La dame* choreography for her *Fédora* death scene.[32] As Marguerite, Bernhardt called on her pantomimic strengths—and presumably her lifelong preoccupation with the romantic disease—to choreograph a tubercular death that was both tender and distressing. Whereas Keene, Davenport, and Modjeska resolutely upheld the mythologized view of consumptive deaths as lachrymose but peaceful departures from the material world, Bernhardt's heroine experienced a less quixotic demise.

The final scene opened, as it always does, on Marguerite's sickroom. Bernhardt's Marguerite lay motionless in bed, hair loosened from its pins, cheeks flushed with fever, lips rosy. With her first line, "Nanine, donne-moi a boire, veux-tu?" ("Nanine, give me a drink, will you?"), moaned softly and without fully opening her eyes, Bernhardt spelled Marguerite's decline in health since her public shaming at the hands of Armand in act four. "All through this last act," observed *The Era*, "Madame Bernhardt suggests in some wonderful way – entirely without either 'realism' or unreality – the nearness of death. You feel, as in Maeterlink's *L'Intruse*, that the strange visitor is at the door." Following Armand's return, the phenomenon of *spes phthisica* propelled Bernhardt's Marguerite from her bed and into a state of hyperactivity, during which she commanded Nanine to ready her for an outing. As with most depictions of *spes phthisica*, Marguerite's vitality evaporated and she regained her reasoning, growing quiet, contemplative, and finally euphoric. *The Era* characterized it as "a *euthanasia*, a swansong, a perfect end … She lifts her arms, her face is upturned, she stands reaching upwards to heaven, she is transfigured, quite a divine light of love illuminates her, her beautiful eyes, her smile."[33] With her *anagnorisis* complete, Bernhardt's Marguerite was ready to die.

The silence that accompanied Bernhardt's intricately choreographed death deepened the audience's reliance on the language of her body; no coughs or gasps punctuated the hushed proceedings. This pantomime, however, was not a solitary venture, as Bernhardt's dying sequence required the intimate physical contact of Marguerite and Armand's bodies. Biographer May Agate's description of the scene details the actors' weight-sharing and partner work, as well as Bernhardt's arm movements:

> For a period, she always stood up just before the final collapse which occurred in Armand's arms, on an embrace. She had her right arm (the downstage one) round his neck, and in her hand she held a handkerchief – death as indicated by her hand opening and quivering convulsively – the handkerchief fluttering to the ground. The arm then slipped of its own weight from Armand's neck, first slowly along his shoulder, then dropped suddenly over the edge to her side – and you knew she was gone. Armand, feeling her grow heavy and inert in his arms, moved away to peer into her face, keeping tight hold of her other hand, this jerked her backward, and the next moment she fell to the floor, where she lay still.[34]

For much of this final sequence Bernhardt's face was pressed to her fellow actor's chest. Because of this, her arm's reflexive tremors and slow descent (courtesy of Bernhardt's "framing" and "tempo control" exteriority effects) became the principal signifiers of the body's internal failures, while the courtesan's waving and releasing of the handkerchief—not bloodstained, but pure white—marked her surrender to the disease. Taranow's description of the scene, based upon theatregoers' recollections as well as the 1912 silent film of *La dame*, elaborates on Bernhardt's final fall to the floor, a semicircular pivot and collapse that Armand (Lou Tellegen in the film) broke by catching her and placing her on the ground.[35] With her rotation, Bernhardt's back turned toward the audience, compelling audiences to read Marguerite's death not solely in her face, but in her body's performed release of muscular tension. As Bernhardt continued to play Marguerite in the 1890s, she lengthened the time between the lovers' initial embrace and her collapse to the floor so that the pantomimed death occupied more time in her *La dame* than in other actresses' adaptations. Dumas's text easily accommodated her preference.

If accounts of Bernhardt's *La dame* are to be believed, the actress engaged every limb, muscle, and sinew to convey the breakdown of Marguerite's material body. Her death scene rarely struck critics as inordinately graphic or crude, and some named hers the most realistic of the period's ailing Camilles. With actresses like Clara Morris startling audiences with (reputedly) spontaneous expressions of Camille's suffering, critics engaged in a Diderotian debate as to whether Bernhardt's death scene emanated from the heart or the intellect. Whereas the *New Orleans Picayune* pronounced it "as near to real death as one can approach in health and live," the *Pall Mall Gazette* conceded in a largely favorable 1881 review that "One or two of the effects on which, quite needlessly, the actress insists smack of artifice, and may possibly be decried as tricks," citing Bernhardt's habit of leaning against Armand long after Marguerite's organs failed, falling only when "that support is withdrawn." Fourteen years later, *Bristol Mercury and Daily Post* contrarily claimed:

> Of course, Marguerite was made up for the final scene, but no stage trick could contrive the transfiguration of her face, which recovered all its old beauty in the joy of Armand's return, and then had the gaunt pallor, the cavernous eyes of a dying woman. She was, of course, so real because she loses herself in the part, and unless we are greatly mistaken she was more than once like our own Ellen Terry wiping away real tears caused by the sorrow she was expressing.[36]

For her part, Agate authenticated Bernhardt's work by way of an anecdote: her old family physician endorsed the death scene as medically accurate. After noting in post-Koch alarm that visitors of Marguerite's bedchamber encountered a host of dangerous bacteria ("Everything she touches is infected"), the doctor attested that Bernhardt's final collapse, which took about thirty seconds, accounted for the failure of the spinal cord to support the body's weight after the heart stopped beating.[37] Dr. L. L. Seaman, physician-in-chief of New York's Charity Hospital, judged Bernhardt's death differently, stating in 1883 that Bernhardt had "seven ways of dying, and all of them were totally unlike anything he had ever seen" in his medical career.[38] Whether or not Bernhardt's death was a 'realistic' reconstruction of a tubercular demise, her embodiment of Marguerite inextricably linked the sublime and the grotesque, yoking the failure of the consumptive's corporeal body to the transcendental deliverance of her soul in ways unmatched by other performers.

The myth unmasked: Eleonora Duse's naturalistic Marguerite

> We are sorry for the man who saw sixty-four Camilles. After the first four or five times the play, excellent creation that it is, becomes a bit gloomy. Tuberculosis is not pleasant, no matter how charming the victim. But if he did really see sixty-four Camilles we believe he miss the best one if he did not see Mme. Duse.
>
> *Life*, March 5, 1896[39]

Italian actress Eleonora Giulia Amalia Duse began acting at the tender age of four when she joined her family's acting troupe.[40] As an adolescent traveling player, Duse "guarded jealously the secret of her youth" and assembled a surprisingly mature and diverse repertoire of roles; at age fourteen she played Shakespeare's Juliet in Verona's open-air theatre. Word of Duse's theatrical triumphs in Naples, Florence, and Venice spread through the continent, and soon she was playing engagements in major cities across Europe. Following an 1885 tour in South America, Duse founded her own theatre company, and in 1893 she appeared for the first time in the United States and England. By this time Duse's armory of roles (Marguerite Gautier, Fedora, Frou-Frou, Magda) bore a striking resemblance to that of Bernhardt. The dissimilarities in their acting methods, however, were pronounced and well-documented. If Bernhardt excelled in exteriorizing her characters' heightened passions, Duse was lauded for her naturalism, responsiveness, and quiet emotion. As Hugo Whittmann declared of Duse in 1923, the year before her death, "everything about her was genuine, truly conceived and truly represented in spirit and in action ... She exhibited not a breath of affectation."[41] Cynics, however, viewed the actress's perceived lack of artifice to be an equally synthetic presentation of theatrics to those of her more demonstrative peers. For fellow actor and Duse biographer Eva le Gallienne, Duse was neither artless nor formulaic: her seemingly spontaneous actions and ability to speak lines as if her character had never uttered them before were "part of a highly disciplined concept of the role and of the play, executed with such truth and such superlative skill that it seldom varied from one performance to the next."[42] Duse appeared in the United States in 1893, 1896, 1903, and 1923 to 1924 and in London in 1893, 1905 to 1906, and 1923, with *La dame aux camélias* (listed at times as *La Signora delle Camelie* or *Camille*) opening or anchoring many of her nineteenth-century engagements. Duse's later years were marked by critical successes in "New Woman" dramas by Henrik Ibsen, Arthur Wing Pinero, and Maurice Maeterlinck, exhaustive international touring, mentoring of younger artists, and persistent health problems. The actress succumbed at age sixty-five to pneumonia while on tour in Pittsburgh. Several biographers have named tuberculosis, her mother's cause of death, as the source of Duse's lifelong pulmonary complaints, though this remains conjecture.[43]

A reluctant public figure, Duse largely avoided interacting with journalists and well-heeled admirers unless she felt it furthered one of two projects: to elevate the status of Italian theatre or to enhance her reputation as an audacious pioneer of naturalism. Her observers, however, contrived alternative narratives, consolidating Duse's poor health and her predilection for overwork into a modernist portrait of New Womanhood, not unlike those she composed onstage. "Duse has created her own style," noted fellow Italian actress Adelaide Ristori, "through which she effectively becomes the woman of modern times, with all her complaints of hysteria, anaemia and nerve trouble and with all the consequences of those complaints; she is, in short, the fin de siècle woman." Ristori counted Dumas's mid-century Marguerite Gautier as part of Duse's collection of "abnormal" women, "with all their weaknesses, quirks, unevenness, all their outbursts and languor," along with Pinero's Aubrey Tanqueray and Sudermann's Magda, which both premiered in 1893.[44] In Duse's hands, Ristori's inventory implies, Marguerite could not help but be a modern creature.

Duse's Marguerite was a true departure from all previous incarnations—an "absolutely new 'Camille'" alleged *The Washington Post*—and perhaps the only portrayal that can be labeled "realistic" in a Stanislavskian sense.[45] In Duse's hands, Marguerite spoke, moved, suffered, and died with a quotidian naturalness that defied artistic precedents and de-fetishized the female consumptive's body. "Mme Duse does not try from any point of view to make Camille extraordinary," wrote *The North American*'s George Rogers, who like many other late-century critics signaled that Duse uncoupled Marguerite's tuberculosis from her extra-occupational virtues and legendary beauty.[46] Despite reports of a nervous excitability that infused Duse's death scene, critics applauded the actress's "subtle finesse" in the role. "To audiences accustomed to seeing actresses roll on the floor in violent hysteria and weep great tears," wrote the *New Haven Register*, "Duse's rendition might have seemed tame." The actress "rarely raised her voice above an ordinary conversational tone, and never resorted to the frenzied gestures or motions which most actresses find requisite to the expression of grief or anger," announced New York weekly *The Critic*.[47] Duse's Marguerite was not the frivolous, glittering treasure of the *demi-monde*, but a guarded woman of wit and reason, aware of (and perhaps resigned to) her deteriorating health. Even as Armand's love renewed Marguerite's spirit, it was with a world-weary hesitancy that Duse's heroine pursued the romance. In her 1893 assessment of "Signora Duse" as Marguerite, *The Critic* contributor Mary Cadwalader Jones contended:

> To put it roughly, the part of the Dame aux Camelias is usually played as though Marguerite were either a young person of refinement whose lines have fallen in unfortunate places, or else a courtesan who has somehow managed, until she meets Armand, to escape a great passion. Signora Duse brings her before us as a girl of the people who has drifted into or chosen an easier life than that to which she was born, and who accepts its drawbacks without question until she feels that she is loved for herself alone.[48]

Like Matilda Heron, Olga Nethersole, and others of the medicalizing strain, Duse divested Marguerite and her disease of their mythic exceptionalness, but not through graphic displays of physical and emotional suffering. Rather, her unidealized portrait of Marguerite refrained from aestheticizing the disease, an approach befitting of tuberculosis's new etiology as an indiscriminate bacteriological illness.

Duse once likened theatricality to a "poisoned coat" that immobilizes and pollutes the theatre.[49] As part of her crusade against artifice, she eschewed many of the nineteenth-century actress's customary adornments: wigs, heavy stage makeup, extravagant costumes, and—perhaps most revolutionarily—corsets. Such contrivances, she felt, hobbled the actress's ability to communicate intimately and truthfully to audiences while endowing with inordinate value her hyper-constructed appearance. In her 1896 study of the art of "La Duse," Laura Marholm Handsson reported:

> Just as Duse never acted anything but what was in her own soul, she never attempted any disguise of her body. Her own face was the only mask she wore when I saw her act ... No jewel glittered against her sallow skin, and she wore no ornament on her dress; there was something pathetic in the unconcealed thinness of her neck and throat.[50]

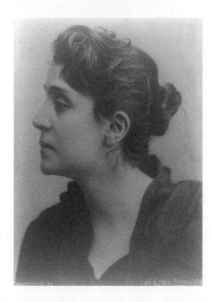

Figure 2.3 Eleonora Duse, 1893. Copyright by Carl and Theo Rosenfeld. Library of Congress.

The actress's rejection of the tight-lacing corset—itself a means for replicating the consumptive's wasting torso—coincided with the dress reformers' campaign against the garment for its negative health impacts (including a probable link to tuberculosis's precipitous rise in Europe and the United States). That Duse embodied without a corset the theatre's most famous consumptive, a courtesan whose job security depended upon her sexual attractiveness, perhaps points not just to her artistic asceticism, but her own chronic respiratory troubles. Duse's abundant chestnut-colored hair, deep-set eyes, and slim frame (that Ristori speculated was *fausse maigre*) sufficed to indicate Marguerite's condition (Figure 2.3).

Though it was rumored she "powdered up" to accentuate her paleness, Duse performed nearly her whole repertoire sans external ornamentation, including *La dame*. Duse's own unadorned body and face, then, lacked the disease's angelic markers: the pink cheeks, rosebud lips, and dewy complexion. Of Duse's singular approach, a number of critics expressed astonishment and gratitude. "She seems to have no powder or paint on her face," remarked the *New York World*. "Its colors, the flush of excitement or the gray pallor of suffering, seem to be the colors of life."[51] Justin Huntly McCarthy of *Gentleman's Magazine* concurred, noting:

> Her pale, powerful face, that disdains the traditional adornment of the stage, its crimsons and whites and blacks, is so endowed with expression that by it alone, were she silent and motionless, she could, we may well believe, convey all the purposes of the drama which for the time she seems to live.[52]

Not all were stirred by a plain-faced Marguerite, however, which some critics took variously as a sign of Duse's eccentricity, her egotism, her indifference to the realities of Marguerite's profession (for what French courtesan would be caught without her paints?), and her ignorance to the discernable effects of tuberculosis. George Barlow of London's *Contemporary Review* reproached Duse for "so despis[ing] the art of make-up that she comes to the [death] scene with her face presenting precisely the same as it did during the previous four acts of the drama."[53] We can only speculate on how conscious Duse was of subverting the fetishized optics of tuberculosis with her more unvarnished portrait of Marguerite's illness. For Helen Sheehy, Duse's refusal to wear makeup, wigs, and restrictive undergarments served a larger purpose:

> [She] stood metaphorically naked in front of her audiences. At the same time Freud was developing his theories of the unconscious, and Ibsen was exploring the unconscious in his plays, Duse was giving flesh to those ideas onstage. The era's harsh new electrical lighting illuminated every nuance of her acting, which was startling, disturbing, new – artistic and erotic.

George Bernard Shaw, who penned an extensive comparison of Bernhardt (who he disparages with characteristic zeal) and Duse (who he lionizes), encouraged theatregoers to count Duse's wrinkles using their opera glasses, as "they are the credentials of her humanity; and she knows better than to obliterate that significant handwriting beneath a layer of peach-bloom from the chemist's." By understanding and internalizing her characters' lived experiences, Shaw intimated, the "ambidextrous and supple" Duse could appear different in every role.[54]

Duse's somatic and performative techniques further distorted the notion that consumptive sufferers were endowed with a feminized, spiritual grace. Supplanting the meandering crosses, fleeting sculptural poses, and delicate, fluttering gestures of the romanticized Camilles were the secular, unorthodox movements of Duse's Marguerite. With no corset to constrict her mobility, the actress "could 'curl up like a cat' on the sofa, or stretch full length with her arms over her head, even cross her legs like a man."[55] Of whether stillness or restlessness was Duse's most forceful spatiotemporal mode reviewers disagreed, and her voice, untrained and natural in tenor and volume, drew neither great acclaim not condemnation, though anglophone critics regularly satirized her Italian. In a striking departure from tradition, Duse changed Marguerite's chaste kiss of her lover's brow at the end of act three to a kiss on his mouth. Believing it the last time she will see Armand, Marguerite "wants to leave all her love on his lips," wrote Duse biographer Arthur Symons, an approach to the scene that resisted veiling the couple's sexual relationship with a quasi-maternal brow kiss.[56] Duse's critics, most of them writing after tuberculosis's reclassification as a contagious disease, seemed to overlook the health implications of such a kiss.

In 1893's "Disease and Death on the Stage," published in the *North American Review*, New York City's health commissioner Dr. Cyrus Edson disparaged actors who "have failed to learn what are the physical symptoms, the movements of the body or parts of it, that invariably follow certain causes of death." Among the most egregious offenders, Edson stated, are the actresses who embody Camille:

> Camille is supposed to die of consumption and the death comes from hemorrhage of the lungs. Now, in point of fact, the action of the body following hemorrhage of the lungs has nothing dramatic about it. If the blood vessel which breaks is very large there may be a semi-convulsion resulting from shock. Otherwise, the death comes from loss of blood that pours from the mouth or from strangulation; that is, the lungs fill with blood, so that the sufferer cannot breathe. But such a death as this would not satisfy the demands of the stage, or what are believed by many persons to be those demands, and we therefore see Camille in strong convulsions. It is the old story of the galloping horse once more.

Because few actors study the physiological manifestations of fatal illnesses, assumed Edson, they relied upon violent symptoms of epilepsy to signify death in its many forms. "But exactly why the symptoms of epilepsy should have become the conventional symptoms of heart disease, of consumption, of poisoning, of death by violence – in short, of every death on the stage – I do not quite understand."[57] That the provocative modifiers "spasmodic," "convulsive," and "paroxysmal" appeared with some regularity in *Camille* reviews corroborates the physician's claims.

"Has Dr. Edson seen … Duse in this rôle?" asked *The Critic* in its response to the article. "[She] dies so quietly that the audience would not know that she was dead if they did not see the curtain slowly descending on this impressive scene."[58] Likely due both to the timing of her British and American engagements (less than ten years after Koch's discovery) and Duse's modern acting, medical and non-medical commentators regularly appraised the accuracy of her Marguerite's consumptive decline and death. On this point, reviewers' opinions were split, and not along British and American lines. Duse was either the most authentic stage consumptive to grace the nineteenth-century stage, or the least. Those without medical degrees often cited intimate knowledge of consumptive deaths to validate their assessments of Duse, such as American actress Maude Harrison's claim that "[Duse] has met that death somewhere in her life! for I saw a dear one die of consumption once, and the going away was much as Duse portrays it in Camille's death."[59] George Barlow similarly contextualized what he deemed to be Duse's inappropriate perambulations in the play's final scene:

> Those who have had the misfortune to witness deaths from consumption will realise the utter impossibility of nearly every action and movement of Signora Duse during the last act of 'Camille.' … It has evidently never crossed her mind that consumption means a slow, or rapid, wasting away of the organism, and that in the last stages of this terrible illness the prominent

symptom of the patient is excessive, extraordinary weakness, including, of course, complete incapacity for any prolonged muscular effort.[60]

Among Duse's most controversial choices was her refusal to simulate the consumptive cough. *The Washington Post* applauded it, as well as Duse's avoidance of other graphic symptoms of tubercular decline, for "she struck the happy medium between extreme staginess and realism."[61] Beaumont Fletcher, however, pilloried Duse for what he regarded as her highly deficient performance of Marguerite's disease. Bristling at the Italian actress's "ridiculous appearance of entire good health" throughout the play, particularly her exclusion of the tubercular cough, Fletcher implied that Duse's rendition failed to reflect the audience's evolving understanding of tuberculosis's realities.[62]

A wider survey of critical responses to Duse's Marguerite, however, implies that the actress was by no means neglecting the character's illness. Rather, her Marguerite's "appearance of entire good health" was just that: an appearance, devised and performed for the benefit of the courtesan's many devotees. Fletcher's own description of the play's party scene confirms such a claim:

> In the first act in the episode, where [Marguerite] is overcome with faintness during the dance, Duse indeed pauses before she begins to dance, falls back into Armand's arms, is led straight to the divan, buries her head in it for a moment, then rises with the cold grimness of an elderly woman.[63]

Duse's portrayal drew tremendous power from her Marguerite's deliberate suppression of tubercular suffering across the five acts. When examined in this light, Duse's death scene, though certainly subtler than Morris's or even Heron's, cannot be categorized as a romanticized portrait of consumption. Rather than telegraphing Marguerite's advanced condition through an elaborate somatic spectacle, Duse depicted a woman straining to conceal her pain: fingers repeatedly touching the hair at the nape of her neck, she perambulated the sickroom as if afraid to stop moving. Marguerite's final moments, then, were those of bittersweet release, in which the character permitted herself to drop her façade of resiliency and acknowledge the disease's dominance within her body. Even the critical Fletcher concedes:

> at the very moment of death Duse's art eclipses the others. She is huddled limply in Armand's arms and keeps repeating his name more and more feebly until her voice dies quite away. But her hands still caress his hair weakly, with deathless love; then they pause, quiver in one last struggle with fate, and slip slowly away. Suddenly her arms drop into outstretched rigidity, her head rolls forward, and she is dead.[64]

While the *New Haven Register* argued that "Duse has divorced the famous death scene from all that horrible realism which has made it a picture of terror to sensitive natures," Duse's naturalistic performance in fact offered an alternate realism, one that was just as combative against the fallacies of the consumptive myth as other more graphic portrayals.[65]

Camille and the death of consumptive sentiment

Of the many public and private battlegrounds on which Bernhardt and Duse waged their presumed rivalry, *La dame aux camélias* was perhaps the most conspicuous. Despite Duse's disaffection for the script, both she and Bernhardt deemed the role too important to their repertoires to jettison, with Bernhardt habitually reviving the play when ticket sales flagged. Just as the consumptive myth and clinical tuberculosis were foils, so too were the Marguerites of Bernhardt and Duse. Incarnating Victor Hugo's sublime and grotesque manifesto, Bernhardt's neo-romantic approach to Marguerite profited from the actress's conscious aestheticization of the disease, while Duse's naturalistic performance, defiant in its originality and its refusal to reproduce consumption's mythic features, de-fetishized the character's tubercular condition. Both Marguerites suffered, but the placement and purpose of their sufferings differed. Externalized by Bernhardt's body, Marguerite's consumptive pain and mental anguish radiated outward, generating a composition of somatic excess that was sculptural, lyrical, and provocative. Duse's Marguerite, in contrast, purposively suppressed her illness's symptoms until her dying body could no longer contain them. By shifting the locus of the character's suffering into the hidden recesses of the body and mind, Duse's performance was no less consumptive than Bernhardt's. Rather, the actress challenged paradigmatic models of tubercular suffering and the iconic beauty of the wasting female form, vestiges of the romantic myth of consumption. The internality of Marguerite's subtly expressed illness, then, signaled not just Duse's naturalistic methods; it mirrored the imperceptibility of tuberculosis's true etiological agent, the contagious *Mycobacterium tuberculosis*. In their transatlantic stagings of *La dame*, the actresses' bodies, nationalities, and personal histories exerted appreciable force on the character's illness narrative, authenticating their portrayals for audiences and critics accustomed to decades of Anglicized and Americanized Camilles.

In an 1886 essay in *The Nineteenth Century*, Nestor Tirard remarked that Victorian scientific developments were robbing illnesses of their poetic sentimentalism:

> Every disease when first discovered has its picturesque aspect, but the progress of science gradually robs it of this, and destroys its artistic value ... We all know too much about them; they are deprived all romance ... [This] is true of consumption; once a favourite, it is now being neglected. The glittering eye, the hectic flush, the uncertainty of its lingering course, have been depicted again and again; but ... all the symptoms are so well known at present that the subject is painful, if not actually of no value.[66]

Tirand's point is both accurate and misleading. Tuberculosis remained a compelling feature in early twentieth-century English-language plays by Eugene

O'Neill, Sean O'Casey, and George Bernard Shaw, whose *The Doctor's Dilemma* (1906) derides the overblown theatrics of the previous century's stage consumptive, and *Camille* revivals continued into the 1930s.[67]

Still, the disease had lost much of its romantic poignancy and dramatic treatments of the disease dwindled in number, perhaps a fitting denouement for a disease that had less impact on the population with each passing year. Twentieth-century playwrights typically depicted tuberculosis as an indiscriminate threat to all social classes; stage tuberculars were still *individuals*, but they were not granted *individuality* through their suffering. In 1908, a *New York Times* column commended the Museum of Natural History's tuberculosis exhibit for providing visitors with "a complete object lesson" in the grave realities of the disease and methods of prevention and cure. With public dialogues about tuberculosis now safely housed in a building of science and not a theatre, the writer celebrated the death of tuberculosis's sentimental leverage:

> It is well that the influence of the poets and the pseudo-poets should no longer lend a false glamour and charm to a disease so horrible. The people now have the means of knowing all about consumption, how to prevent it, how it may be cured. And they know that it possesses no sort of poetical charm.[68]

Perhaps because of their generous stores of "poetical charm," consumptive heroines (Camille queen among them) proved resilient in the face of scientific obsolescence. Indeed, artists have adapted Camille's iconic tale of love, illness, and spiritual deliverance to new genres, mediums, and spaces, from Tennessee Williams' allegorical *Camino Real* (1953) and Charles Ludlam and the Ridiculous Theatre Company's subversive *Camille: A Travesty on La dame aux camélias* (1973), to 1963's *Marguerite and Armand*, a narrative ballet choreographed for Rudolf Nureyev and Margot Fonteyn, and numerous film and television productions both faithful (1936's *Camille* starring Greta Garbo) and refashioned (2001's *Moulin Rouge!*). These transposed Camilles, however, perform different dramaturgical and cultural work than their predecessors on the nineteenth-century popular stage. As low tuberculosis-incidence countries, present-day Britain and the United States no longer play host to epidemic levels of tuberculosis cases; because of this, Camille's suffering as a white female consumptive of relative privilege, once so culturally salient and correlative to nineteenth-century medical discourses, now fails to retain its sense of urgency. Honored and parodied in equal measure, Camille endures not as a performative surrogate for the terminally ill but as a symbol of idealized womanhood, beautiful in its many contradictions.

Notes

1 Medical historian Michael Worboys recently challenged the notion of a British Bacteriological Revolution, citing the gradual and uneven shifts in medical knowledge and procedures as proof that the 1880s were part of a larger biomedical movement. "Was There a Bacteriological Revolution in Late Nineteenth-Century Medicine?" *Studies in History and Philosophy of Biological and Biomedical Sciences* 38, no. 1 (Mar 2007): 20–42.

2   English-language librettos were often provided for spectators, though Americans who had seen countless *Camille* adaptations likely followed the action without using them.

3   "Amusements," *Daily Inter Ocean,* Apr 28, 1887.

4   P.C., "The Theatre," *Speaker,* July 6, 1901; and *The Times,* Jan 14, 1888, quoted in Patricia Marks, *Sarah Bernhardt's First American Theatrical Tour, 1880–1881* (Jefferson: McFarland, 2003), 99.

5   John Stokes, "Sarah Bernhardt," in *Bernhardt, Terry, Duse: The Actress in Her Time* (Cambridge: Cambridge University Press, 1988), 15.

6   Gerda Taranow, *Sarah Bernhardt: The Art Within the Legend* (Princeton: Princeton University Press, 1972), 195.

7   "Three of the Principal Actresses of the Comedie Francaise," *Illustrated London News,* June 7, 1879.

8   Marks, *Sarah Bernhardt's First American Tour,* 143 and 144.

9   Unidentified newspaper clipping, Camille Clippings File, HTC. Additionally, her notorious habit (whether authentic or feigned) of sleeping in a coffin in order to better understand her tragic roles as well as her own mortality boosted Bernhardt's macabre public persona, recommending her as the paramount interpreter of the terminally ill Marguerite.

10 Quoted in William Weaver, *Duse: A Biography* (Orlando: Harcourt Brace, 1984), 128; and J. Comyns Carr, "Mme. Sarah Bernhardt: A Personal Impression," *The Times* (London) Oct 11, 1913.

11 "A Vivisection of Sarah Bernhardt's Art," *Current Literature* 53, no. 4 (Oct 1912).

12 "Camille as the Virgin Mary," *New Haven Register,* Feb 19, 1890.

13 Arthur Gold and Robert Fizdale, *The Divine Sarah: A Life of Sarah Bernhardt* (New York: Knopf, 1991), 120; and Ruth Brandon, *Being Divine: A Biography of Sarah Bernhardt* (London: Secker and Warburg, 1991), 133.

14 Letter from Sarah Bernhardt to Jean Mounet-Sully, quoted in Gold and Fizdale, *Divine Sarah,* 106.

15 Caroline De Costa and Francesca Miller, "Sarah Bernhardt's Missing Leg," *Lancet,* July 25, 2009.

16 Robert Horville, "The Stage Techniques of Sarah Bernhardt," in *Sarah Bernhardt and the Theatre of Her Time,* trans. and ed. Eric Salmon (Westport: Greenwood Press, 1984), 45 and 46; and "Bogus!!!," *Puck,* Dec 1, 1880.

17 Marks, *Sarah Bernhardt's First American Theatrical Tour,* 29.

18 "Madame Sarah Bernhardt at Her Majesty's," *The Times* (London), April 30, 1886; and "La Dame Aux Camelias," *The Era,* June 25, 1892. Even an anonymous American critic remarked "Mme. Bernhardt has grown stouter; or it would be better to say, perhaps, is not quite so slender as she was." "Bernhardt in Camille," unidentified newspaper clipping, Camille clippings file, HTC.

19 George Bernard Shaw, "Duse and Bernhardt," *Saturday Review* (June 15, 1895), reprinted in *The Collected Works of Bernard Shaw,* v. 13 (New York: 1931), 158.

20 Ellen Terry, *Ellen Terry's Memoirs* (New York: G.P. Putnam's Sons, 1932), 168.

21 Rostand and Bernhardt quoted in Horville, "Stage Techniques," 47 and 51.

22 Sharon Marcus, "Sarah Bernhardt's Exteriority Effects," *Modern Drama* 60, no. 3 (Fall 2017): 296–321, 302 and 305.

23 Horville, "Stage Techniques," 43.

24 Taranow, *Sarah Bernhardt,* 123; and Cornelia Otis Skinner, *Madame Sarah* (Houghton Mifflin, 1967): 166.

25 "Prince's Theatre: Mme. Sarah Bernhardt," *The Bristol Mercury and Daily Post,* June 27, 1895, and unidentified newspaper clipping. Such characterizations of Bernhardt echoed George Henry Lewes's description of the famed French actress Rachel as a "panther."

26 Quoted in Horville, "Stage Techniques," 45.

27 Stokes, "Sarah Bernhardt," in *Bernhardt, Terry, Duse,* 53.

28 Beaumont Fletcher, "Three Ladies of the Camellias," *Godey's Magazine*, May 1, 1896.
29 Bernhardt, *V'Art du théâtre* (Paris, 1923), 125, trans. Taranow in *Sarah Bernhardt*, 6.
30 Bonnie Jean Eckard, "Camille in America," (PhD diss., University of Denver, 1982), 139–140.
31 "The Great French Dier," *Puck*, Dec 1, 1880.
32 Taranow, *Sarah Bernhardt*, 93.
33 "La Dame Aux Camelias," *The Era*, June 25, 1892.
34 "La Dame Aux Camelias," *The Era*, June 25, 1892; and May Agate, *Madame Sarah* (New York: Benjamin Blom, 1969), 131.
35 Taranow, *Sarah Bernhardt*, 95.
36 *New Orleans Picayune*, u.d.; "Reappearance of Mddle. Sarah Bernhardt," *Pall Mall Gazette*, June 13, 1881; and *Bristol Mercury and Daily Post*, June 27, 1895.
37 Agate, *Madame Sarah*, 131.
38 "Way People Die," *The Times* (Owosso, Mich.), Aug 10, 1883.
39 "Amusements," *Daily Inter Ocean*, April 28, 1887; and Metcalfe, *Life*, March 5, 1896.
40 This summary of Duse's life and career was compiled using: Helen Sheehy, *Eleonora Duse: A Biography* (New York: Knopf, 2003); Weaver, *Duse: A Biography*; J. Ranken Towse, "Eleonora Duse," *Century Illustrated Magazine* 49, no. 1 (Nov 1895), 130; Jeanne Bourdeux, *Eleonora Duse: The Story of Her Life* (Whitefish: Kessinger, 2005); Georg Brandes, "Eleonora Duse," *The Living Age*, Oct 15, 1926; and Eva le Gallienne, *The Mystic in the Theatre: Eleonora Duse* (Carbondale: Southern Illinois University Press, 1973).
41 Hugo Whittman, "Eleanora Duse," *Living Age*, Nov 24, 1923.
42 Le Gallienne, *Mystic in the Theatre*, 21.
43 Sheehy and Le Gallienne both state that Duse's mother Angelica died of tuberculosis in 1875. Descriptions of Duse's final moments of life, taken from companion Désirée von Wertheimstein's account, seem to authenticate the medical phenomenon of *spes phthisica*, with a reinvigorated Duse insisting "We must move! We must leave! Do something! Do something!" before dying ten minutes later. Weaver, *Duse: A Biography*, 361; and Sheehy, *Eleonora Duse*, 321–322.
44 Adelaide Ristori, quoted in Bassnett, "Eleonora Duse," in *Bernhardt, Terry, Duse*, 137.
45 "The Italian Camille: Duse Depicts the Marguerite Gautier of Dumas," *The Washington Post*, Feb 18, 1896.
46 George Rogers, "An Italian Camille," *The North American* (Philadelphia), March 15, 1893.
47 Franklin Fyles, "Theatrical News in Gotham," *The Washington Post*, April 24, 1904; "Duse in a New Camille," *New Haven Register*, April 21, 1896; and "The Drama," *The Critic*, Feb 29, 1896.
48 Mary Cadwalader Jones, "Signora Duse," *The Critic*, Feb 4, 1893.
49 Duse quoted in Stark Young, "Sense About Duse," *Theatre Arts Monthly* 23, no. 4 (1939), 279–282.
50 Laura Marholm Handsson, "Eleonora Duse: The Italian Actress and Her Art," *Current Literature* 19, no. 4 (Apr 1896), 287.
51 "The Return of Eleonora Duse," *New York World*, July 27, 1896.
52 Justin Huntly McCarthy, "Pages on Plays," *Gentlemen's Magazine* (July 1893).
53 George Barlow, "French Plays and English Audiences," *The Contemporary Review* 64 (July 1, 1893): 171–181, 178–179.
54 Sheehy, *Eleonora Duse*, 116; and George Bernhard Shaw, quoted in Weaver, *Duse: A Biography*, 128. Duse's legendary rejection of stage makeup is called into question by reports of theatre personnel seeing her applying powder with an expert hand. However, it is clear that she avoided heavily painting her face with rouge and eye makeup.
55 Sheehy, *Eleonora Duse*, 110.
56 Arthur Symons, *Eleonora Duse* (New York: Benjamin Blom, 1969), 65.
57 Cyrus Edson, "Disease and Death on the Stage," *North American Review* (Aug 1893), 160.
58 "The Stage Idea of Disease and Death," *The Critic*, Aug 12, 1893, 107.

59   "Duse, Teacher," *Boston Daily Advertiser*, March 24, 1896.
60   Barlow, "French Plays and English Audiences," 178–179.
61   "The Italian Camille," *The Washington Post*, Feb 18, 1896, 3.
62   Fletcher, "Three Ladies," 484.
63   Ibid.
64   Ibid., 486.
65   "Duse in a New Camille," *New Haven Register*, April 21, 1896, 3.
66   Nestor Tirard, "Disease in Fiction," *The Nineteenth Century* 20, no. 116 (October 1888): 579–591, 578.
67   See George Bernard Shaw's *The Doctor's Dilemma* (1906), Sean O'Casey's *The Plough and the Stars* (1926), and O'Neill's *The Web* (1913), *The Straw* (1919), and *Long Day's Journey into Night* (1940). Giacomo Puccini's 1896 *La bohème* joined *La traviata* and 1881's *Les contes d'Hoffman* as operas featuring heroines presumed to be dying of tuberculosis.
68   "Tuberculosis and Sentiment," *New York Times*, Dec 15, 1908.

Bibliography

Agate, May. *Madame Sarah*. New York: Benjamin Blom, 1969.

Barlow, George. "French Plays and English Audiences." *The Contemporary Review* 64 (July 1, 1893): 171–181.

Bassnett, Susan. "Eleonora Duse." In *Bernhardt, Terry, and Duse: The Actress in Her Time*, edited by John Stokes, Michael R. Booth, and Susan Bassnett, 119–170. Cambridge: Cambridge University Press, 1988.

Bourdeux, Jeanne. *Eleonora Duse: The Story of Her Life*. Whitefish: Kessinger, 2005.

Brandon, Ruth. *Being Divine: A Biography of Sarah Bernhardt*. London: Secker and Warburg, 1991.

Eckard, Bonnie Jean. "Camille in America." PhD dissertation. University of Denver, 1982.

Edson, Cyrus. "Disease and Death on the Stage." *North American Review* 157 (Aug 1893): 160–169.

Gold, Arthur and Robert Fizdale, *The Divine Sarah: A Life of Sarah Bernhardt*. New York: Knopf, 1991.

Handsson, Laura Marholm. "Eleonora Duse: The Italian Actress and Her Art." *Current Literature* 19, no. 4 (Apr 1896): 287.

Horville, Robert. "The Stage Techniques of Sarah Bernhardt." In *Sarah Bernhardt and the Theatre of Her Time*, trans. and edited by Eric Salmon, 35–67. Westport: Greenwood Press, 1984.

Le Gallienne, Eva. *The Mystic in the Theatre: Eleonora Duse*. Carbondale: Southern Illinois University Press, 1973.

Marcus, Sharon. "Sarah Bernhardt's Exteriority Effects." *Modern Drama* 60, no. 3 (Fall 2017): 296–321.

Marks, Patricia. *Sarah Bernhardt's First American Theatrical Tour, 1880–1881*. Jefferson: McFarland, 2003.

Shaw, George Bernard. "Duse and Bernhardt." *Saturday Review* (June 15, 1895). Reprinted in *The Collected Works of Bernard Shaw*, v. 13. New York: W. H. Wise, 1931.

Sheehy, Helen. *Eleonora Duse: A Biography*. New York: Knopf, 2003.

Skinner, Cornelia Otis. *Madame Sarah*. Boston: Houghton Mifflin, 1967.

Stokes, John. "Sarah Bernhardt." In *Bernhardt, Terry, Duse: The Actress in Her Time*, edited by John Stokes, Michael R. Booth, and Susan Bassnett, 13–64. Cambridge: Cambridge University Press, 1988.

Stokes, John, Michael R. Booth, and Susan Bassnett. *Bernhardt, Terry, Duse: The Actress in Her Time*. Cambridge: Cambridge University Press, 1988.

Symons, Arthur. *Eleonora Duse*. New York: Benjamin Blom, 1969.

Taranow, Gerda. *Sarah Bernhardt: The Art Within the Legend*. Princeton: Princeton University Press, 1972.

Terry, Ellen. *Ellen Terry's Memoirs*. New York: G.P. Putnam's Sons, 1932.

Tirard, Nestor. "Disease in Fiction." *The Nineteenth Century* 20, no. 116 (October 1888): 579–91.

Weaver, William. *Duse: A Biography*. Orlando: Harcourt Brace, 1984.

Worboys, Michael. "Was There a Bacteriological Revolution in Late Nineteenth-Century Medicine?" *Studies in History and Philosophy of Biological and Biomedical Sciences* 38, no. 1 (March 2007): 20–42.

Young, Stark. "Sense About Duse." *Theatre Arts Monthly* 23, no. 4 (1939): 279–288.

Part II
Performing drug addiction

3 Early dramaturgies of drug addiction in stage adaptations of *Dr. Jekyll and Mr. Hyde* and *Sherlock Holmes*

As the nineteenth century drew to a close, the roster of human health threats expanded to include the very substances physicians relied upon to alleviate suffering: pharmaceutical drugs. A number of scientists reported observing withdrawal symptoms and intensifying tolerances among opium users as early as the 1700s, but the budding concept of drug addiction—a formal attempt to define and treat what had variously been labeled "inebriety," "habituation," and "dependency"—rapidly matured at the *fin de siècle*. Readily available at the corner chemist's (and sometimes without a prescription, depending on the apothecary's scruples), drugs like morphine, chloral hydrate, and cocaine dosed sections of the populace, including an unprecedented number of pleasure-seeking habitués. The invention of the hypodermic needle in 1853 by Alexander Wood of Scotland and Charles-Gabriel Pravaz of France transformed the way drugs were dispensed, and the widespread sale of hypodermic kits in the 1870s and 1880s made self-administering injections easy and, particularly for middle and upper-class women, fashionable. Institutional medicine's grasp on drug use grew tenuous at best, but in the 1880s, physicians established the disease model of addiction, which asserted that a drug enslaved its consumer by altering the body's physiology or biochemistry. In relabeling habitual drug consumption a diagnosable illness, the medical establishment rendered itself indispensable in the diagnosing and treating of addiction. The founding of the *Journal of Inebriety* in the United States in 1876 and the *British Journal of Addiction* in 1884 affirm the Victorian-era medicalization of compulsive drug use, as well as the persistent etiological and etymological slipperiness of drug concepts, categories, and terminologies.[1] By 1910 the disease model of addiction, founded primarily on the work of German physicians, had "fully matured" in Britain and the United States, and soon demand mounted for legislation that would regulate the manufacturing, sale, and use of narcotics.[2] In the United States, the Harrison Narcotics Tax Act of 1914 imposed a special tax on "every person who produces, imports, manufactures, compounds, deals in, dispenses, sells, distributes, or gives away" drugs; in 1919 the Supreme Court interpreted the Act as making the "maintenance" of a drug habit illegal.[3] Britain's criminalization of drug addiction proceeded more slowly, with the Rolleston Committee advocating as late as 1926 for the supervised maintenance of an addict's drug habit, if authorized by a physician.[4]

Because of the late development of drug addiction discourse, the first examples of addicts on the nineteenth-century stage were not hooked on drugs, but alcohol.[5] In temperance melodramas that emphasized the immorality of falling victim to the "demon drink," stage drunkards like Edward Middleton in *The Drunkard; or the Fallen Saved* (1844) and Joe Morgan in *Ten Nights in a Bar-room* (1858) required actors to bypass subtlety and embrace the histrionic, particularly during climactic enactments of delirium tremens. The mid-century stage drunkard and the late-century stage addict shared more surface similarities than compositional anatomy, due to changing theatrical trends as well as variances in how the public regarded alcoholics and drug users. Alcoholic inebriates, presumed to have fostered their own dependencies at the local tavern, faced harsher censure than drug addicts, who were commonly cast as unwitting victims of a legitimate doctor's prescription (what became known in the twentieth century as "iatrogenic addiction").[6] Similarly, in order to fully demonize alcohol, the temperance movement discredited liquor's therapeutic benefits, whereas few could deny the awesome power of a drug like morphine; as an analgesic, sedative, and anti-diarrheal medicine, it could make chronic pain bearable and cholera survivable. Even for physicians cognizant of the dangers of medical narcotics, the wholesale rejection of drugs would have been tantamount to scrapping the most effective weapons in their palliative arsenal. Better to keep the drugs and rehabilitate those who become addicted, some rationalized, than limit or prohibit their use.

The nineteenth-century theatre's first major drug addicts began as literary characters of considerable notoriety. Robert Louis Stevenson's *The Strange Case of Dr. Jekyll and Mr. Hyde* (1886) and Arthur Conan Doyle's *Sherlock Holmes* series (beginning with 1887's *A Study in Scarlet*) captured the imaginations of the English-language reading public. Discounted by the period's critics as sensational "shilling thrillers," both works are now regarded as evocative expressions of *fin-de-siècle* anxieties: the indomitable juggernauts of modernity and technology; the degeneration of humanity and the British Empire through crime, drugs, interracial mixing, vulgarity, and decadence; and the atrophying of Victorian masculinity, among others. The author-endorsed stage versions of *The Strange Case of Dr. Jekyll and Mr. Hyde* and *Sherlock Holmes*, however, are seldom appreciated as medicocultural artifacts of import, nor have Richard Mansfield and William Gillette's embodiments of the title characters been scrutinized as influential articulators of nascent drug addiction discourses. These claims provide the basis for the next two chapters. When he first assumed the dual roles of Henry Jekyll and Edward Hyde, thirty-year-old Richard Mansfield was best known for his work in the light operettas of Gilbert and Sullivan and plays like *A Parisian Romance* and *Prince Karl*.[7] *Dr. Jekyll and Mr. Hyde* became an integral part of his repertoire, and despite later forays into the plays of Shakespeare and Shaw he was unable to shake the conjoined specter of Jekyll and Hyde for the remainder of his career. American playwright, actor, and director William Hooker Gillette built his career on suspenseful Civil War dramas (1886's *Held by the Enemy* and 1895's

Secret Service), English-language adaptations of foreign novels, and his definitive version of *Sherlock Holmes*. To many fans of Conan Doyle's serial stories, Gillette possessed the qualities that most typified Holmes: intelligence, elegance, self-composure, and a touch of eccentricity. That Gillette was an American stung less with time.

Before Sherlock Holmes and Dr. Jekyll stepped (or, in Mr. Hyde's case, skulked) onto the boards of the popular stage, their dramatic interpreters crucially refashioned their two-dimensional sources for the three-dimensional medium. Mansfield enjoined author Thomas Sullivan to pen a stage play of *Dr. Jekyll and Mr. Hyde* within a year of its first publication, intending the dual roles of Jekyll and Hyde for himself. After receiving Stevenson's blessing, Mansfield collaborated with Sullivan on introducing his own unique interpretations to the script. The play first premiered at the Boston Museum theatre on May 9, 1887; five days later it was withdrawn for revisions, with Mansfield appearing in the modified version on September 12 in New York.[8] Other American and British playwrights clamored to adapt *Dr. Jekyll and Mr. Hyde* for the stage, but legal actions by Longmans, Green, & Co., Stevenson's book publishers, halted or delayed several unauthorized adaptations in Britain by claiming copyright infringement. George Grossmith's one-act musical farce *Hide and Seekyll (The Real Case of)*, which portrayed Hide as an alcoholic and Seekyll as a temperate man who wakes each day with a terrible headache, ran in London without challenge.[9] *Sherlock Holmes*'s adaptation was longer in coming, as Conan Doyle himself attempted to write the script before American producer Charles Frohman encouraged Gillette, an actor-playwright with a history of penning hits, to rewrite Conan Doyle's draft. The product was 1899's *Sherlock Holmes; or the Strange Case of Miss Faulkner*, with Conan Doyle and Gillette credited as the play's co-authors. Like Stevenson's *Dr. Jekyll and Mr. Hyde*, Conan Doyle's *Sherlock Holmes* inspired a surfeit of theatrical adaptations, burlesques, and music hall parodies. British actor Charles Brookfield, who in 1893 co-wrote and starred in a musical parody featuring Holmes and Watson called *Under the Clock*, was the first to perform the role of Holmes, and the following year Charles Rogers's "pirated play" *Sherlock Holmes, Private Detective* premiered in Glasgow and ran for ten years. Conan Doyle and Gillette's *Sherlock Holmes*, however, proved the tale's most enduring theatrical adaptation, inspiring its own 1901 parody, Malcolm Watson and Edward Le Serre's deliciously titled *Sheerluck Jones, or Why D'Gillette Him Off*?[10]

For a number of Victorian critics and several modern scholars, the nuanced complexities of Stevenson and Conan Doyle's novellas were lost in translation as playwrights shoehorned the tales into the formulaic molds of melodrama.[11] While this argument carries weight, a far more intriguing story unfolds when the adaptations are recognized for plotting incipient dramaturgies of drug addiction. Part II's chapters work together to situate Gillette and Mansfield's stage addicts within concurrent discourses on drugs, drug use, and the "disease" of addiction. This chapter introduces the primary drug classes of the nineteenth-century pharmacopeia and the medicalization of habitual drug use before detailing the ways Gillette, Mansfield, and their collaborators adapted the novellas' drug narratives for the popular stage. Chapter 4 then endeavors to both reconstruct and decode the actors' approaches to embodying Conan Doyle and Stevenson's notorious users. Typifying Gillette's performance of Sherlock Holmes was a controlled intensity (what the *Illustrated London News* called a "calm self-command [with] lightning alertness") that enabled the detective to navigate treacherous situations with relative ease.[12] This somewhat paradoxical state of restrained vitality extended to the character's onstage drug use, which was normalized in and through Gillette's unforced acting. His performance left no doubt that Holmes, whose precisely measured injections of cocaine enhanced his mental functioning and keen sense of intuition, was the phlegmatic professional habitué of Victorian lore. Dr. Henry Jekyll's deviant addiction, in contrast, devastated his intellectual potential (not to mention his love life) and warped his privileged bourgeois masculinity. Mansfield's acting style, which juxtaposed crowd-pleasing histrionics with more internalized techniques of modern realism, proved the perfect instrument to convey Jekyll's capricious bipolarity.

Though it is perhaps tempting to oversimplify Gillette and Mansfield's performances as expressing irreconcilable pro- and anti-drug viewpoints, the *fin-de-siècle* "drug problem," as it came to be branded, was rarely drawn in black and white. Rather, both stage depictions included moral and medical justifications for the characters' habits, a fitting reflection of the age's evolving constructions of drug dependency. Though I pair Holmes and Jekyll/Hyde together as "addicts," it is also important to distinguish between the characters' illnesses. Holmes avows to Dr. Watson early in the series that he only requires chemical stimulation when not on a case, suggesting his condition might not be drug addiction, but habituation: a psychological or emotional dependence on taking drugs because of their desirable effects, often with little to no lasting physiological health issues or withdrawal symptoms. Still, Watson fears that Holmes, if not already an addict, is dangerously close to becoming one, given that his thrice-daily ritual of cocaine injections repeats for months at a time. There is far less ambiguity in Jekyll's case: he is physiologically and psychologically addicted to his experimental tincture. His deepening tolerance pushes him to strengthen his doses; in Stevenson's text the doctor admits "Once, very early in my career, [the drug] had totally failed me; since then I had been obliged on more than one occasion to double, and once, with infinite risk of death, to treble the amount."[13] I make these distinctions at the outset of Part II for two reasons. First, even as physicians began plotting drug habits along a spectrum of perceived severity, concepts like "habituation," "dependence," "inebriety," "drug mania," "tolerance," and "addiction" were applied rather imprecisely in late nineteenth-century medical and popular discourses. Second, as natural and synthetic drugs became medicalized in the late 1800s and criminalized in the early 1900s, advancing theories and policies regarding recreational, unauthorized, or unmonitored drug use implicated even self-possessed habitués like Holmes.

The nineteenth-century pharmacopeia

In the age of rigid anti-drug legislation and "just say no" rhetoric, it is perhaps difficult to imagine a world in which narcotics were not a priority for public health and law enforcement officials. The few drugs in use in Britain and the United States prior to the Victorian period occupied peripheral spaces in medicine and culture, and discussions of substance addiction focused almost exclusively on the evils of liquor, ale, and wine. Though *cannabis sativa* was cultivated in British colonial territories in the early seventeenth century, hashish had little impact on the mainland until several centuries later. Opiates were easily acquired during the Enlightenment for medical and recreational purposes; many regarded opium smoking as benign of a habit as smoking tobacco. It was in the nineteenth century that the notion of drug dependency became concretized, pharmacology emerged as a discrete scientific field, and literary and artistic depictions of society's stratified "drug cultures" proliferated. Among the triggers of this revolutionary overhaul in thought and practice was a triumvirate of easily obtainable drugs that together created legions of addicts: opiates, inhalants, and cocaine.

The largest class of drugs present in the nineteenth century were the opiates. Harvested from the minuscule capsules of the *papaver somniferum*, raw opium contains twenty-five alkaloids, poisonous and bitter-tasting chemicals that if taken in small doses serve as extremely effective medicaments. Opiates can sedate, alleviate pain, calm muscle spasms, induce euphoric states, and alter mental functioning, whether through a near-prescient mental clarity or what Geoffrey Harding calls "mental clouding."[14] Victorians smoked, ate, and swallowed opiates in a variety of over-the-counter elixirs, some of which were patent medicines marketed to parents for fussy or teething babies. The poppy plant's Indian origins, the Opium Wars, and the prevalence of Chinese-operated opium dens in British and American cities tethered opium supplies to the Orient literally, via trade routes, as well as symbolically (Figure 3.1). A sizable portion of opiate habitués hailed from affluent, cultured upper-class homes; nevertheless, xenophobic prejudices against the Chinese tainted the use of opium in Western cultural imaginings, as did biases against the working poor and unemployed.[15] Despite opium-eating intellectuals like Thomas De Quincey and Samuel Taylor Coleridge reporting flights of creative and spiritual rapture induced by their habits, raw opium's reputation as a drug of the shiftless underclasses remained strong throughout the century.[16]

The discovery of the opium alkaloid morphine revolutionized the treatment of ailments as varied as acute and chronic pain, neurological conditions, and gastrointestinal disorders. The drug, named for the Greek god of dreams, soon became indispensable to Western physicians who used it in private practice, hospitals, birthing rooms, and battlefield infirmaries.[17] Morphine also inspired a substantial change in the reputations of opiate users. By the 1870s, the widespread sale of home hypodermic kits fueled a dangerous but

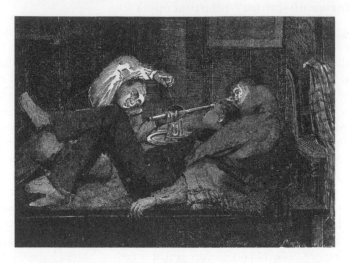

Figure 3.1 "Smoking Opium." *Galliard's Medical Journal* 33, no. 2 (Feb 1882). The National Library of Medicine.

fashionable morphine craze in society's upper echelons. According to Susan Zieger, the "compulsive, clandestine use of new hypodermic technology to inject morphine," sensationally dubbed "morphinomania" in Britain, was perceived as primarily a genteel lady's disease, though men of privilege could also become morphinomaniacs. The shameful nature of drug use was partially eroded by morphine's *au courant* status. In an 1887 issue of *Nineteenth Century*, commentator Seymour Starkey claimed:

> Ladies even, belonging to the most elegant classes of society, go so far as to show their good taste in the jewels which they order to conceal a little syringe and artistically made bottles, which are destined to hold the solution which enchants them! At the theatre, in society, they slip away for a moment, or even watch for a favourable opportunity of pretending to play with these trinkets, while giving themselves an injection of morphia in some part of the body which is exposed, or even hidden from view.[18]

The tincture laudanum, a concoction of opium and alcohol infused with spices like saffron or cinnamon, became a preferred analgesic and soporific for women wishing to alleviate menstrual cramps or soothe colicky infants. A far different social group became associated with the abuse of another opiate, heroin, discovered in 1898. Heralded by physicians as the non-addictive super drug of the *fin de siècle*, heroin was quickly embraced as a street drug, triggering anti-drug backlash and inspiring the cultural icon of the criminalized drug fiend.[19] As its reputation as a just-for-pleasure street drug rose in the early decades of the twentieth century, heroin's use in medical settings waned.

In the mid-1800s, the related chemicals of chloroform, ether, and chloral hydrate joined opiates as popular, habit-forming drugs. Inhalation anesthesia improved surgical procedures in times of peace and war, with sulfuric ether developed in 1846 and chloroform invented one year later. With the patient safely under the spell of these soporifics, surgeons could perform more complicated, lengthy, and delicate operations. Doctors also prescribed them for home use to reduce mild discomfort from ailments like abscessed teeth or migraine headaches. Inhalants took immediate effect and, in the words of one chloroform addict, produced "the delightful sensation of being wafted through an enchanted land into Nirvana."[20] Used as a surgical anesthetic and prescribed frequently to insomniacs and those with neuralgia, physicians thought chloral hydrate produced healthier sleep and pain management than opiates. While chloroform, ether, and chloral hydrate are not addictive in the sense that the user suffers the physiological agonies of withdrawal, their effects are habit-forming nonetheless; the development of tolerances required addicts to inhale larger doses to satisfy their cravings.[21] In perhaps its most egregious misapplication, chloral hydrate was proscribed to alcoholics and morphine habitués to help disrupt their dependencies, only to create a legion of chloral addicts. Sir Benjamin Ward Richardson first warned against habitual use of chloral in 1871. He conceived of chloral not as a feminine or lower-class drug, but one favored by the period's "brainworkers," middle-class men active in professions that taxed the intellect: medicine, law, commerce, clerical work, literature, the arts, and others. While opium addicts could potentially use the drug for years without it impeding their everyday functioning, Richardson and others argued, chloral rendered "its habitués dysfunctional at home and in workplaces."[22] Because even moderate dosage amounts could be fatal, highly poisonous inhalants played a recurrent role in suicides and accidental overdoses. Though some continued to argue that chloral hydrate was non-habit forming, memoirist and opium addict William Rosser Cobbe noted in 1895: "there are some who still persist in the claim that one may take the drug indefinitely without harmful results; in the fact of indisputable testimony that [the United States] is full of chloral habitués."[23]

Physicians first heralded cocaine as a wonder drug possessing the highest level of medicinal benefits and no addictive qualities. The coca leaf, from which the cocaine alkaloid was extracted, was indigenous to South America where it was chewed to strengthen stamina and stave off hunger. Intrepid Western travelers had for centuries returned to their homelands with tales of the South American coca, but the leaf gained little attention until several physicians experimented with the therapeutic benefits of coca following the American Civil War.[24] By that time, medicines were undergoing more stringent laboratory testing, due primarily to growing confidence in empirical research findings (a side effect of medicine's institutional expansion), but perhaps also because of the era's shameful array of prematurely declared "miracle drugs." Though early laboratory studies with the leaf proved inconclusive and disappointing, the work of ophthalmologist Carl Koller and neurologist Sigmund Freud (the latter a habitual cocaine user) dramatically revised coca's reputation. Koller utilized a solution of cocaine to anesthetize the surface of an eye during surgery in 1884; that same year, Freud's "Über Coca" summarized cocaine's therapeutic properties. According to Virginia Berridge and Griffith Edwards, one 1885 issue of the *British Medical Journal* featured sixty-seven separate items on cocaine and its myriad uses (including treating morphine addiction).[25] Unlike the coca leaf, which Westerners disparagingly associated with the indigenous customs of Latin American "savages," cocaine was revered as a thoroughly modern drug with analgesic, stimulant, anesthetic, and anti-depressive properties.[26] Lifelong addict James S. Lee enumerated cocaine's effects in his travel memoir *The Underworld of the East* (1936), proclaiming that the drug "banished" exhaustion, leaving in its place "a marvelous clearness of vision," "a feeling of perfect well being and happiness," and "extreme fertility of the imagination."[27] Cocaine's ability to stimulate mental faculties while reducing fatigue endeared it to the professional classes, including a startling number of medical men and its most famous nineteenth-century habitué, the fictional Sherlock Holmes. However, because the narcotic was relatively inexpensive to acquire, tradesmen and laborers being paid hourly wages also used cocaine to combat exhaustion. The latter group encompassed a growing contingency of black workers, especially in post-Reconstruction America, forging the discriminatory connection between cocaine use and lower-income African Americans that endures today.

Imagining addiction in the late nineteenth century

Drug historian Virginia Berridge places the genesis of "addiction" as a viable, enduring concept in the nineteenth century: "It was then that addiction was either discovered or created."[28] While chronic drug use was certainly ideated in previous centuries, there was far less impetus to define, conceptualize, and treat addiction before the late 1800s. Those in the mainstream shrugged off drug use as a minor nuisance affecting the outer fringes of society: tramps, racialized others, prostitutes, artists, and intellectuals, as H. Wayne Morgan notes, who were "all easily quarantined from society." Such individuals, it was presumed, lacked both the moral courage and the pressures of social responsibility to resist the pleasures of drug use.[29] In this way, early theories of drug addiction echoed common mid-century stereotypes of alcoholism. Soon, however, a culmination of factors gradually reshaped public attitudes toward recreational and therapeutic drug use: the return of American Civil and Crimean War soldiers addicted to analgesics; physician over-prescription; the surge in opiate-laced patent medicines; the invention of the hypodermic needle and home injection kits; and the first attempt to legislatively restrict non-medical opiate use (Britain's 1868 Pharmacy Act). Even as evidence mounted, physicians hesitated to demonize the very drugs that revolutionized patient care, some denying any existence of addictive properties in modern narcotics. Others acknowledged the possibility of substance-based addiction (particularly raw opium) but vouched for the safety of laboratory-manufactured narcotics like morphine, chloral, and cocaine. Still others attempted to compartmentalize addiction by linking it with the user's method of taking drugs. Patients who administered narcotics hypodermically, it was believed, could evade addiction because injections bypassed the digestive system, where bodily cravings were believed to originate—hence the term "opium appetite."[30]

The voices of addicts themselves deepened the drug debate. Beginning with De Quincey's 1821 *Confessions of an English Opium Eater*, the published testimonies of drug users chronicled the physical, behavioral, interpersonal, and financial effects of their habits. Not all addiction narratives condemned chronic drug use, of course. Some addict-authors detailed their lives as functional, socially responsible habitués while others invited readers to vicariously experience being high through vivid tales of drug-fueled euphoria, hallucinations, and spiritual insight. The majority, however, attempted to spark sympathetic responses to the addiction epidemic by assigning blame to cavalier physicians or bad-apple acquaintances. Like advocates of temperance, drug addicts appropriated the metaphor of slavery to explain their physical and mental subjugation: only death, they feared, would release them from their invisible bondage.

Prior to the disease model of addiction, physicians and theorists placed little blame on the chemical substances. Rather, they located deficiencies in the addict's "weak will," or a constitutional shortcoming that increased that person's vulnerability to substance abuse.[31] The ambiguity of the "weak will" made it both tricky to locate anatomically—was it in the nerves? the brain? the blood?—and remarkably easy to condemn. Drug use was variously classed a lower-class compulsion (born of an impoverished lifestyle that drove plebeians to seek escapist pleasures in the form of liquor, opium, and later heroin), a professional-class necessity, or an upper-class consolation. Because the educated and higher born were imagined to be predisposed to nervous conditions, they were thought more likely to require the pacifying effects of sedatives. Nineteenth-century addict William Rosser Cobbe proclaimed that "[Opium] has no part or lot with the ignorant and degraded. Its victims are those who build up thought, who advance material wealth, and give polish to society. Hence the destruction it works is frightful."[32] The habitué's socioeconomic status, therefore, proved a vital, meaning-making component of his illness, one that branded him either a fashionable user or a drug-addled fiend. The era's abundant female addicts inspired theorists to locate the weak will in the constitutions of the "weaker sex," noting that women's finer organizations made them especially susceptible to stimulant abuse. While men gained access to drugs through numerous medical and non-medical channels, female drug-consumers were confined by social mores to frequent physicians' offices and the neighborhood pharmacy, where shelves of mind- and mood-altering consumables promised relief from headaches, insomnia, "female complaints," and the vapors. As Mara L. Keire has argued, in all likelihood, the feminizing of addiction in the late 1800s forestalled stringent narcotics regulations until drug abuse was culturally re-masculinized in the twentieth century by the urban "hustling junkie."[33]

The susceptibility of society's "thinkers" to developing a drug habit was a recurrent Victorian-era trope, one unequivocally reinforced by the fictional excesses of Sherlock Holmes and Dr. Henry Jekyll. Brainworkers in many fields presumably turned to narcotics to invigorate dormant faculties for greater productivity or to dull the effects of mental over-stimulation and fatigue. (Indeed, Dr. Myron G. Schultz extrapolated that Stevenson, an admitted user of opium and hashish, was able to write *The Strange Case of Dr. Jekyll and Mr. Hyde* in six days because of a stimulating cocaine binge, a hypothesis he supported with historical and pharmacological research.)[34] Such high-functioning habitués were of particular interest to Americans, who viewed drug use as an unavoidable byproduct of an ambitious nation of innovators. "This is an inquisitive, an experimenting, and a daring age," one addict wrote in 1876, "an age that has a lively contempt for the constraints and timorous inactivity of ages past. Its quick-thinking and restless humanity are prying into everything. Opium will not pass by untampered with."[35] The separate writings of Americans George M. Beard and Harry Hubbell Kane, a neuroscientist and physician respectively, chronicled the proliferation of overtaxed minds and bodies requiring drugstore palliatives with a strange, reverent pride.[36] Ironically, many brainworking habitués were men of medicine who self-administered cocaine during long hours in the laboratory, operating theatre, or hospital ward. Drug use in the professional classes was thusly conceived of as a necessary evil of modernity, one that individuals engaged in to cope with demanding careers, emotional trials, and the disorienting speed of industrialized urban living. Not surprisingly, this rather conciliatory perspective was met with growing ambivalence as the century progressed, and soon a precursor of the criminalized drug fiend materialized on both sides of the Atlantic, the veritable embodiment of mounting public fears of drug addiction. Terry M. Parssinen sees the 1870 publication of Charles Dickens' unfinished work *The Mystery of Edwin Drood* as symbolically ushering in a new, malignant construction of the drug addict. In Dickens' novel,

> the filthy but harmless opium den described by Victorian reporters was superseded by the depiction of the opium den as a palace of evil. Gone was the image of the opium addict, set forth in De Quincey's *Confessions* and accepted by his contemporaries, as noble self-experimenter. In late Victorian literature, the opium addict was portrayed as a secret degenerate.[37]

In an age when health was equated with prudent self-discipline and decadence with deviancy, the "opium inebriate" posed a direct threat to the wellbeing of the body politic. Lazy and parasitic, he contributed nothing to society, but instead delighted in self-serving overindulgences and diminished inhibitions, leading to erotic and violent behavior.

In the early 1880s, Victorian medical science reformulated compulsive drug use as a classified and treatable disease, thanks in large part to the 1878 English publication of Edward Levinstein's seminal work *Morbid Craving for Morphia*.

Advocates for the disease model of addiction asserted that drugs altered the user's physiology on a cellular level, rewriting the addict as a participant in his affliction rather than its sole creator. Dr. Norman Kerr, a chief English proponent of the disease theory, posited in 1884:

> The moral, social, political, economical and spiritual mischiefs arising from intemperance [are] the result of the operation of natural law, of the physiological and pathological action of an instant narcotic poison on the brain and nervous centres of human beings endowed with a constitutional susceptibility to the action of this class of poisonous agents.[38]

As Kerr's contention indicates, the disease model incorporated some aspects of earlier theories of addiction and jettisoned others. Addicts could still possess "a constitutional susceptibility" to drug dependency, for example, and gender, race, and class remained factors in assessing the addict's deficiencies in self-regulation. Along with another highly stigmatized "condition" of homosexuality, addiction's medicalization generated viewpoints that "were never … scientifically autonomous, [as] their putative objectivity disguised class and moral concerns," offer Berridge and Edwards. "[Addiction] was disease *and* vice," and this hybrid formulation prompted physicians like Oscar Jennings to combine medical therapeutics with the rehabilitation of the addict's weakened will in addiction treatments. Lawrence Driscoll concurs, arguing that while drug addiction's medicalization was "meant to be above morality, sanctioned by science and medical fact, it [could not] avoid redeploying a whole host of values and morals."[39] Among these values was a collective insistence from the medical establishment, sometimes implied and sometimes directly stated, that only addicts with a formidable desire to recover their health (and their self-control) warranted medical interventions. Dr. Leslie Keeley appealed to unhappy addicts by offering a "Gold Cure" for opium habituation: a mail-order remedy that at "ten dollars a pair [of bottles]" would cure even the worse cases of hypodermic morphism.[40]

Nevertheless, addiction's position as a newly pathologized illness shielded addicts from absolute accountability and gave drugs heightened material and metaphorical potency. Not every drug was recognized as negatively impacting the body physiologically, though the entire class of opiates was implicated. As one opium addict admitted in 1881, "I fear in my case, after so long a time, there must be structural disease in the brain, degeneration of tissue, &c., &c., which, even were the cause entirely removed, would still leave *incurable* damage."[41] In acknowledging narcotics' lasting physiological impact, experts became concerned with differentiating true addiction from recreational experimentation and moderate use, as well as shoring up related terminologies. Could a person, for example, regularly use narcotics without building up a biological tolerance that required higher dosages to satiate? Should all drug users— even fully functional habitués with no desire to quit—undergo therapeutic treatments for their own sakes or the sake of society-at-large? Was the word "addict" applicable to both voluntary and compulsive drug users? Similarly, distinguishing "good" drugs from "bad" drugs (and "good" users from "bad" users) continued into the twentieth century. Did synthetically manufactured narcotics and raw forms of addictive substances affect the body in distinctive ways? Should physicians and legislators intervene in drug consumption practices within both medical and recreational contexts, where the identities of addicts were believed to divide along racial, gender, and socioeconomic lines?[42] Such questions engaged medical experts and researchers across the disciplinary divides of neurology, biochemistry, pharmacology, toxicology, and, after the turn of the century, the newly minted field of clinical psychology.

Adapting addiction for the late nineteenth-century popular stage

Gillette loosely based his adaptation of *Sherlock Holmes; or the Strange Case of Miss Faulkner* (itself a reworking of Conan Doyle's failed draft) on three Holmes stories: *A Scandal in Bohemia*, *The Final Problem*, and *A Study in Scarlet*.[43] To helm the plot's criminal conspiracies, Holmes's nemesis Professor Moriarty made the jump from page to stage, as did Holmes's cautious companion, Dr. Watson.[44] In the play, Holmes must disrupt a blackmailing scheme that threatens to jeopardize a European royal's reputation, not to mention the lives of an innocent mother and daughter. Suspense builds through several mini-crescendos before the fourth act's action-packed climax, in which Holmes evades death, captures the criminals, and gets the girl at the atmospheric Stepney Gas Chamber. The characteristics of Britain's beloved sleuth remain much the same in the play. He is an isolated and eccentric gentleman, witty and egotistical but possessing a strong ethical compass. Within him resides an incongruous but appealing mix of scientific intellectualism and aesthetic bohemianism, and though he could not be called an athlete, he is agile in mind and body. Collectively these traits make Holmes a dynamic stage persona, but for Gillette something important was still missing. In the most significant departure from the source material, Gillette incorporated a love interest for Conan Doyle's legendary bachelor. "With a fine disregard for the sensibilities of Holmes purists," write Rosemary Cullen and Don B. Wilmeth, "Gillette cabled to Conan Doyle, 'May I marry Holmes?' Conan Doyle replied that 'you may marry or murder or do what you like with him'."[45] While Holmes's romance with Alice Faulkner rendered the play more palatable to audiences accustomed to cheering onstage lovers, I suspect Gillette was up to more than merely satisfying theatrical conventions, a hunch to which I will return in due course. Most germane to this study is the detective's onstage injection of cocaine occurring in act two, scene two in his rooms at 221B Baker Street. A comparison of this scene with its literary counterpart highlights how Gillette dramaturgically shaped Holmes's drug use.

Conan Doyle's Sherlock Holmes enjoys decidedly catholic extracurricular activities when not on a case. In Holmes's debut story, *A Study in Scarlet* (1887), the detective's new flatmate notes that his habits are "regular"; Holmes spends much of his time in the laboratory, in the dissecting-rooms, and on long walks that often take him through London's less coveted addresses. Writes Watson: "Nothing could exceed his energy when the working fit was upon him; but now and again a reaction would seize him," and Holmes would lounge in a near catatonic state for days at a time. "On these occasions I have noticed such a dreamy, vacant expression in his eyes," offers Watson, "that I might have suspected him of being addicted to the use of some narcotic, had not the temperance and cleanliness of his whole life forbidden such a notion."[46] If Holmes is a born detective, Watson appears to be a psychic. As the doctor comes to discover, the violin, the chemistry set, the tobacco pipe, and the hypodermic syringe serve as the detective's preferred instruments of mental distraction. In the opening paragraph of *The Sign of Four* (1890), Dr. Watson recounts the ritual he has witnessed "three times a day for many months":

> Sherlock Holmes took his bottle from the corner of the mantel-piece, and his hypodermic syringe from its neat morocco case. With his long, white, nervous fingers he adjusted the delicate needle and rolled back his left shirtcuff. For some little time his eyes rested thoughtfully upon the sinewy forearm and wrist, all dotted and scarred with innumerable puncture-marks. Finally, he thrust the sharp point home, pressed down the tiny piston, and sank back into the velvet-lined armchair with a long sigh of satisfaction.[47]

As Joseph McLaughlin notes, despite professing in the very next paragraph to being "irritable at the sight" of Holmes's drug-taking, Watson's conspicuously erotic description suggests a second response to the spectacle: fascination.[48] The doctor's conflicting feelings of revulsion and intrigue at Holmes's injection are a fitting reflection of the Victorians' ambivalent attitudes toward habitual drug use. Gillette's version of Holmes's ritual follows the original quite closely, and yet Watson's interest in Holmes's injection is strictly condemnatory. "*As WATSON sees HOLMES open* [the morocco] *case*," the stage directions read, "*he rises and goes right restlessly and apparently annoyed at what HOLMES is about to do, throwing cigarette on table and sitting again soon.*" Watson watches again as Holmes inserts his needle and presses the piston home with "*an expression of deep anxiety but with effort to restrain himself from speaking.*"[49]

Watson's subsequent interrogation of Holmes reveals more revisions by the playwright. Both renderings of this exchange commence with Watson's question: "Which is it today? Morphine or cocaine?" Intriguingly, the list of possible substances remains unfinished in Gillette's play as Watson asks "Cocaine or morphine, or − " before being interrupted, implying Holmes is both a consumer and an experimenter.[50] "A seven-percent solution" of cocaine is Holmes's answer in both cases, as the detective politely tenders the syringe and phial to Watson. The doctor immediately declines Holmes's offer, though the stage Watson's "Certainly *not!*" (to be spoken "*emphatically*" while rising) is less reflective than the response of Conan Doyle's Watson, whose "brusque" refusal is contextualized: "My constitution has not got over the Afghan campaign yet," he states; "I cannot afford to throw any extra strain upon it." The scenes then diverge substantially with the development of Watson's line of reasoning and Holmes's defense. In the novella, their argument proceeds thusly:

> He smiled at my vehemence. "Perhaps you are right, Watson," he said. "I suppose that its influence is physically a bad one. I find it, however, so transcendently stimulating and clarifying to the mind that its secondary action is a matter of small amount."
>
> "But consider!" I said earnestly. "Count the cost! Your brain may, as you say, be roused and excited, but it is a pathological and morbid process which involves increased tissue-change and may at least leave a permanent weakness. You know, too, what a black reaction comes upon you. Surely the game is hardly worth the candle. Why should you, for a mere passing pleasure, risk the loss of those great powers with which you have been endowed? Remember that I speak not only as one comrade to another but as a medical man to one for whose constitution he is to some extent answerable."
>
> He did not seem offended. On the contrary, he put his fingertips together, and leaned his elbows on the arms of his chair, like one who has a relish for conversation.
>
> "My mind," he said, "rebels at stagnation. Give me problems, give me work, give me the most abstruse cryptogram, or the most intricate analysis, and I am in my own proper atmosphere. I can dispense then with artificial stimulants. But I abhor the dull routine of existence. I crave for mental exaltation. That is why I have chosen my own particular profession, or rather, created it, for I am the only one in the world."

Gillette's version takes another tack:

HOLMES: (*as if surprised*) Oh! I'm sorry! (*Draws hypo and phial back and replaces them on mantel.*)

WATSON: *I* have no wish to break *my* system down before its time!

HOLMES: Quite right, my dear Watson – quite right – But you see, my time has come! (*Throws himself languidly into sofa, leaning back in luxurious enjoyment of the drug.*)

WATSON: (*Goes to table, resting hand on upper corner looking at HOLMES seriously.*) Holmes, for months I have seen you using these deadly drugs – in ever increasing doses. When they once lay hold of you, there is no end! It must go on, and on, and on – until the finish!

HOLMES: (*lying back, dreamily*) So must you go on and on eating your breakfast – until the finish.

WATSON: (*approaching HOLMES*) Breakfast is food! These drugs are poisons – slow but certain. They involve tissue changes of a most serious character.

HOLMES: Just what I want! I'm bored to death with my present tissues and
           am out after a brand new lot!
WATSON: (*going near HOLMES*) Ah, Holmes – I'm trying to save you!
           (*Puts hand on HOLMES' shoulder.*)
HOLMES: (*Earnest an instant; places right hand on WATSON's arm.*) You
           can't do it, old fellow – so don't waste your time.

Later in the scene, Gillette's Holmes echoes Conan Doyle's in professing no
need of cocaine if his mind is properly occupied. Delighting in the surfacing of
a new investigation, Holmes claims: "It saves me any number of doses of those
deadly drugs upon which you occasionally favor me with your medical views!"

Even allowing for the enlivened pacing and liberal use of exclamation marks
as necessary concessions to the popular stage, the theatrical scene is markedly
different from its literary source. Under Conan Doyle's authorship, Holmes
attentively listens to Watson's scientific objections and acknowledges the
habitué's risk for permanent physiological damage. Moreover, his justification
for injecting drugs—intermittent mental torpor for which cocaine is the only
curative—is as thoughtfully articulated as Watson's protestations. With a confidence in his analytical superiority that borders on narcissism, Holmes's suitably Victorian brainworker defense, argues Timothy R. Prchal, suggests that
narcotics are his means not of "escaping but *transcending* the secular realm."[51]
Conan Doyle made Holmes an addict "because he wanted his readers to
view Holmes as an aesthete," contends Martin Booth. "Drug addiction had a
romantic, artistic ring to it. Poets and writers, artists and musicians were, as the
parlance had it, *habitués*, their habits a sign of their uniqueness and intellectual
or even spiritual superiority."[52] Conan Doyle's Watson hopes to appeal to
Holmes's intellectual arrogance by foregrounding the pathological repercussions of drug addiction in his arguments.

In contrast to the careful deliberations of Conan Doyle's characters, Gillette's
scene operates as a somewhat comical *contretemps* on drug dependency, with
the addict himself delivering the punch lines. Holmes is gleefully recalcitrant,
destabilizing each of Watson's arguments while reposing languidly on his sofa.
Because Holmes resists earnestly engaging in a scientific discussion of drug use,
the frustrated Watson grows sanctimonious in his volleys, thereby prioritizing
the secondary prerequisite of addiction qua disease: the addict's moral failing.
With these revisions, Gillette subtly but perceptibly shifts the contested site of
Holmes's disease from his remarkable grey matter to his compromised soul,
a far more effective choice for nineteenth-century audiences accustomed to
melodramas, as well as a more ethically ambiguous foundation upon which to
build his performance of addiction. Closer scrutiny of the detective's behavior
in these two scenes uncovers an intriguing paradox. Whereas Conan Doyle's
Holmes is content to engage in Watson's scientific contemplation of cocaine's
toxicity and the perils of addiction because he views himself as a moderate
user with a genuine need for "artificial stimulants," it is precisely the theatrical
Holmes's jocularity that discloses a latent awareness of his condition's severity.

Such a reading is confirmed in how the drug discussion is concluded in both versions. In Conan Doyle's text, Holmes redirects Watson's attention by transitioning the conversation onto his position as the world's "only unofficial consulting detective," a carrot Watson eagerly bites. Gillette's Holmes, however, explicitly terminates the exchange by professing (cordially but unbendingly) the futility of any attempts of Watson's to save his life. While the former knowingly postpones Watson's pleas for a future date, the latter attempts to resign Watson to his drug use in order to forever silence the doctor on the subject. The release of *The Sign of Four* (1890) and the premiere of *Sherlock Holmes* (1899) straddle cocaine's rapid reappraisal in the 1890s from wonder drug to addictive toxin; it is certainly possible the authors digested and integrated evolving drug discourses when redrafting Holmes's drug use for the stage. Though Gillette's script is perhaps less nuanced than its source material, its dramaturgical changes succeed in deepening and complicating Holmes's drug problem. And yet Holmes seems positively ascetic when compared with Dr. Henry Jekyll.

Over the last twenty years, Victorianists, medical historians, and literary scholars have tendered rich inquiries into *The Strange Case of Dr. Jekyll and Mr. Hyde*'s composition of addiction. Scholars including Adam Colman, Patricia Comitini, Terry D. Cooper, Debbie Harrison, Helle Mathiasen, and Daniel L. Wright illuminate the shadows of Stevenson's addiction narrative, appraising Jekyll as the archetypal Victorian physician-addict and Hyde as his ugly "pharmacological creation."[53] Far fewer studies, however, track Stevenson's addiction narrative as it enters the theatrical realm. With a cyclical storytelling structure, three different narrators, and human transfiguration as a major plot point, Stevenson's novel resists easy theatrical adaptation. Sullivan and Mansfield's 1887 play, the only authorized adaptation of Stevenson's work, was the first of several to impose a linear plot structure on the tale, eliminate its narrative complexities, reduce its allegorical elements, and insert a romantic entanglement for Jekyll. Daniel E. Bandmann's *Dr. Jekyll and Mr. Hyde* (1888), adapted from Mansfield's production and not Stevenson's novella, introduced a collection of dimensionless characters (including several ingénues and a handful of cheerful choir boys) and a midnight stake-out at the vicarage led by an Irish policeman. *Dr. Jekyll and Mr. Hyde, Or a Mis-Spent Life* (1897), written by Luella Forepaugh and George F. Fish for Philadelphia's Forepaugh's Family Theatre and published by Samuel French in 1904, was itself a near-facsimile of Bandmann's melodramatic script.[54] Of the nineteenth-century stage adaptations, Sullivan and Mansfield's largely succeeds in preserving Stevenson's plot and its considerable gothic charm. Moreover, in its staging of Jekyll's ungovernable addiction, the 1887 play ratcheted up the horror for middle-class audiences by gentrifying the doctor, hyper-demonizing his alter ego, and physicalizing the monstrous transformations of Jekyll into Hyde and back again.

Dr. Henry Jekyll satisfies several late-century addiction stereotypes in Stevenson's original text.[55] First, he is a physician-addict, a simultaneously piteous and contemptible figure in the collective Victorian imagination. Second, like Holmes, Stevenson's Jekyll is a reclusive scientific intellectual—one of the addict types easily quarantined from polite society according to pre-disease theories of addiction—whose small coterie of male confidants are similarly asocial, unmarried brainworkers of the professional class.[56] Known to others as charitable men of moderate means, Jekyll and his friends nevertheless eschew London society fêtes and romantic courtships in favor of private dinner parties at their own residences (in effect quarantining themselves). Couple this with Jekyll's compulsion to unleash his dormant wretchedness in the form of Hyde, and "Stevenson represents the bourgeois male in a state of terminal decline," posits Andrew Smith.[57] This terminal decline is manifest not only in Jekyll's drug addiction and his circle's antisocial conduct, but also in Darwinian descriptions of Hyde's simian features and atavistic movements. However, as Smith argues: "the true horror [of Stevenson's novella] is not reflected in Hyde but through the fragile, because empty, world inhabited by the bourgeois professional. In this way the normative becomes demonized."[58] Sullivan's script capsizes Stevenson's world of middle-class degeneration by isolating the deviancy within Jekyll/Hyde alone. Third, Jekyll's irreversible parturition of Hyde suggests narcotics' permanent physiological impact on users, reaffirming the disease theory's cornerstone principle and rendering Jekyll's addiction a pathological illness. The turning point in Jekyll's illness, in which Hyde takes over their shared body without the potion's inducement, authenticates the *fin-de-siècle* fear that the drugs, and not the addicts, possess ultimate control and mastery. "In the historical moment of *The Strange Case*," writes Susan Zieger, "the medical discourse of habituation was combining with the older temperance model to produce a proliferation of terms – Stevenson uses 'malady,' 'madness,' 'cerebral disease,' 'disgrace,' and 'evil' – and a failure to specify Jekyll's 'nameless situation,' situated somewhere between vice and disease."[59] And yet, Jekyll's initial cocksure attitude toward his drug use in the novella suggests that he doubts the substance's physical authority. As Daniel L. Wright contends:

> Jekyll's reaction to Hyde, the emblem of his addiction, is typical; as he proclaims to Utterson, "to put your good heart at rest, I will tell you one thing: the moment I choose, I can be rid of Mr. Hyde" (p. 40). The addict untutored in the pathology of addiction will always so mistakenly suppose that he can regulate the use and effects of his intoxicant. Of course, he cannot – no more than a similar exertion of will can spontaneously heal a compound fracture, reverse the aging process, or eradicate genetic deformity.[60]

Sullivan diverged little from Stevenson's story, but modifications to Jekyll's social milieu as well as his self-perceptions as an addict exploited *fin-de-siècle* fears of a white, middle-class epidemic of addiction.

The play's first act, tellingly titled "Slave and Master," is worth detailing, as the significant dramaturgical changes are all introduced within it.[61] It opens in the tearoom of Sir Danvers Carew's house, the quintessential site of cultured

British socialization, where Sir Danvers (the man Hyde murders), his daughter
Agnes, Mr. Utterson and Dr. Lanyon (Jekyll's closest friends), and Mrs. Lanyon
discuss Henry Jekyll, the "dearest and best man in London," and his unex-
pected absence at dinner.[62] Together they rationalize Jekyll's uncharacteris-
tic breach of etiquette and pale countenance as consequences of the doctor's
excessive work schedule. Jekyll's altered condition is of particular interest to
Agnes, his young fiancée, who is "sure that Harry has something on his mind."
When Jekyll finally enters the scene, his first aside to the audience confirms
Agnes's supposition: "It must not be. I can never marry her, with this hideous
secret, this new danger threatening me at every step. My duty is clear. I must
see her no more."[63] Though he is convivial to Sir Danvers and his guests, Jekyll
drops his sanguine façade once alone with Agnes and confesses himself to be
a man divided:

AGNES: (*Following him*) Are you not Henry Jekyll?
JEKYLL: The philanthropist, the man of science, the distinguished surgeon –
          before the world – yes. How if it were all a lie? If I were like one
          possessed of a fiend – wearing at times another shape, vile, mon-
          strous, hideous beyond belief?
AGNES: (*Hiding her face in hands.*) Oh, be silent.
JEKYLL: Yes, a fiend, without a conscience, and without remorse – invent-
          ing crimes and longing only to commit them.
AGNES: This is horrible. Who accuses you? You are ill and tired. You are
          not yourself.
JEKYLL: That is true. I am but half myself – the other half is –
AGNES: Mine. You have no right to accuse it, falsely.
JEKYLL: You will not believe – if I dared to tell you –
AGNES: You shall tell me nothing.[64]

After reaffirming their love, the couple exits through the garden for some
impromptu stargazing. Agnes soon returns to the tearoom without Jekyll, as
he was called away on an "important case." The next figure to appear in the
garden window is the creeping Edward Hyde, who lasciviously demands of Sir
Danvers: "Call [your daughter] back, I say. I saw her face through the window, and I *like* it." The older gentleman refuses and commands Hyde to leave
his house. "Go?" laughs Hyde. "I. Why, I will make the house mine, the girl
mine if I please." Sir Danvers attempts to physically throw Hyde out, a struggle
ensues, and Hyde "*throttles him*" as the curtain drops.[65]

   If, as Smith suggests, Stevenson's novella normalizes deviancy and degrades
the middle-class male professional who inhabits a "fragile, because empty,
world," Sullivan's play restores the bourgeoisie to their place of sociocultural
dominance. Utterson and Dr. Lanyon, once antisocial bachelors, are rewritten
as respected, benign (and in Lanyon's case, married) members of London society. The playwright also purged Jekyll of his social reclusiveness. He is instead
a popular, philanthropic doctor engaged to the daughter of a military-ranked

aristocrat.[66] Writes Brian A. Rose: "[Sullivan's adaptation] rehabilitates through displaying Jekyll not as an isolated neurotic (Stevenson) but a revered if complicated member of a bourgeois society expected to participate in its usual patterns of quotidian action."[67] Many of Jekyll's ambiguities were also lost in the shift from gothic allegory to stage melodrama. In the novella, the young, pre-addiction Jekyll (in the doctor's own words) masked "a certain impatient gaiety of disposition" beneath a "commonly grave countenance," resulting in a "profound duplicity of life."[68] Jekyll's struggle against wicked impulses explicitly motivated his scientific experimentation, and his bravado during the addiction's early months bespeaks an initial gratification with, and *through*, Edward Hyde. In contrast, the theatrical Jekyll is virtually bereft of evil or arrogant tendencies, and at the play's opening already condemns Hyde as his "hideous secret." Mansfield's admiration for his character is clear in an 1888 interview with the *New York Sun*, in which he describes Jekyll as:

> a dreamer and a visionary. While his every inclination is toward the good, while he himself is inclined toward all that is honorable, pure, and noble, he still recognizes in himself the germs of sin and evil, the desire to satisfy, to let loose a passion, no matter what it may be, and that it is only the restricting force of good, the power of the discriminating conscience, which deters him from indulgence.[69]

According to Rose, in the adapted script "the largely selfish neuroticism of Stevenson's Jekyll becomes the adapted Jekyll's heroic and self-sacrificial search for salvation for mankind from evil."[70] And yet, while Mansfield's Jekyll is a melodramatic hero, his goodness is not as oversimplifying as Rose submits. If we reclassify the play as a play about *fin-de-siècle* notions of drug addiction, then Jekyll's "goodness" (as a philanthropist, fiancé, friend, and male professional) renders his victimization all the more tragically profound. Because Jekyll is a fully entrenched member of the bourgeoisie instead of Stevenson's proverbial black sheep, he draws the threat of a drug addiction epidemic far closer to the nucleus of proper society than the novella permits. Such a shift makes explicit that which Stevenson implies: Jekyll/Hyde's addiction places in jeopardy innocent women (Agnes), children (the young girl Hyde tramples in the street as well as Agnes and Henry's potential offspring), and the upper echelons of the body politic.

Love in the time of narcotics

"Of course a play without a woman in it could have no love," one *Jekyll and Hyde* critic maintained in 1887, "and without love – well, there would be little hope of success on the stage."[71] A fitting assessment of the period's theatrical tastes, and yet I suspect the creation of onstage love interests for Holmes and Jekyll serve a more meaningful function than merely satisfying expectations. Homosexuality and addiction were sister deviances in the

Victorian age, when it was presumed that "the state of craving itself [was] unnatural to a well-regulated nineteenth-century body" and that one craving naturally begot another.[72] If Holmes and Jekyll's drug dependencies are inextricably linked to their analogous rejections of heteronormativity, as is often posited, it is conceivable that the detective (whose lasting romance, many have argued, is with Dr. Watson) and the doctor (whose alter ego can be recast as the embodiment of Jekyll's closeted impulses) are homosexual. By transforming Holmes and Jekyll from resolute bachelors to devoted beaus for the popular stage, Sullivan and Gillette fundamentally stem the homosexual undercurrents flowing within the original novels, thereby safeguarding their heteronormative masculinity and diagnosing Holmes and Jekyll's drug addictions as solitary vices.

For Holmes, Alice Faulkner provides a potential incentive for relinquishing his bohemian lifestyle, including his hypodermic needle that, according to James W. Maertens, has been a "sort of technological fix for [a] loss of connection to the body and the feelings," enabling him "to withdraw ... into his narcissistic shell." [73] He first bristles at Watson's suggestion that a mutual affinity has blossomed between him and Alice: "You mustn't – tempt me – with such a thought! That girl! Youth – exquisite – just beginning her sweet life! – I – seared, drugged, poisoned – almost at the end! No! No! I must cure her!"[74] In the play's final moments, Holmes justifies to Alice his fear of overtaking her purity with his toxicity, but then a long embrace symbolically ushers in a new era in which Holmes is prepared to assume a more productive societal role. For Jekyll, who merited the love and respect of Agnes Carew before becoming a habitué, his addiction is a corrosive, malignant force that derails his domestic agenda. "Then and now," Zieger advances, "narratives about addicts characteristically show them demurring, faking, destroying, or otherwise sabotaging possibilities for heteronormative romantic love and kinship and the bourgeois striving that underwrites them. In conventional wisdom, addiction destroys families."[75] Jekyll's guilt over lying to Agnes generates much of his inner torment, his romanticized suicide marking the character's final attempt to save his woman from his addiction. Agnes's presence also aids in the hyper-demonizing of Hyde as the grotesque avatar of drug addiction.[76] Just as it glorifies Jekyll's goodness, Sullivan's play renders Hyde's evilness even more despicable because of its undisguised carnality and unprompted aggressiveness. The period's medical and popular discourses communicated a shared apprehension that drug users were prone to violent or lewd behavior, as narcotics reputedly lowered inhibitions and liberated the addicts' "lower natures." Hyde's appearance in act one, in which the fiend's spontaneous murder of Sir Danvers Carew interrupts what clearly was the intended rape of Agnes, corroborates late Victorian apprehensions about addict-menaces.[77] The Hyde of Sullivan and Mansfield, attests Irving S. Saposnik, was "a manifestation of Jekyll's lust, a creature of infinite sexual drive who 'unable by reason of his hideous shape to indulge the dreams of his hideous imagination,' proceeds to satisfy his cravings in violence."[78]

In adapting *The Strange Case of Dr. Jekyll and Mr. Hyde* and the *Sherlock Holmes* series for the stage, Mansfield and Gillette steered into, not away from, the characters' illness narratives. That Sullivan and Mansfield's script constructs Jekyll's addiction as a debilitating, unremitting disease seems almost beyond question. Hyde, the "fiend" that Jekyll dares not name to Agnes, first surfaces with the doctor's chemical concoction but soon materializes unbidden, thwarting Jekyll's attempts to master his creation. Conan Doyle's Holmes ostensibly maintains control over his drug habit, and yet readers of 1890's *The Sign of Four* learn from Watson that countless puncture-marks riddle his arm, hardly the sign of an occasional user. By placing Holmes's cocaine injection onstage, Gillette's adaptation obligated the audience, like Watson, to witness this intimate act and then reconcile or dismiss its ambiguities. In dosing himself with the seven-percent solution, was Holmes engaging in a process of physiological regulation or deregulation? As the next chapter suggests, even as drug addiction discourses continued to develop beyond the boundaries of medical science, Gillette's elegant performance of Holmes largely shielded the character from pity or stigmatization.

Gillette was not finished writing Holmes or his drug habit with 1899's *Sherlock Holmes*. His 1905 curtain raiser *The Painful Predicament of Sherlock Holmes* pits Sherlock against Gwendolyn Cobb, a garrulous, frenzied admirer seeking the detective's assistance in freeing her jailed lover.[79] Holmes, who is silent for the entirety of the scene, correctly deduces that Gwendolyn is an escaped lunatic and by passing a handwritten note to his pageboy expedites her capture and recommitment. In *Painful Predicament*'s one-sided dumb show Gillette satirizes Holmes's methodical cerebralism (and perhaps his own subtle depiction of the character). The piece capitalizes on the audience's familiarity with Holmesian objects and habits: a chemistry experiment bubbles over a lamp; Gwendolyn steps on and breaks Holmes's violin; the detective smokes his pipe and surreptitiously examines the woman's handkerchief with a magnifying glass. In the final sequence of the dumb show, Holmes engages in his signature diversion, a cocaine injection. He then retires to the lounge in front of the fire and reclines on the pillows. As the stage falls dark, Holmes's psychotropic reverie begins anew.

Notes

1   Marco-Antoine Crocq, "Historical and Cultural Aspects of Man's Relationship With Addictive Drugs," *Dialogues in Critical Neuroscience* 9, no. 4 (Dec 2007): 355–361.

2   Terry M. Parssinen and Karen Kerner, "Development of the Disease Model of Addiction in Britain, 1870–1926," *Medical History* 24 (1980): 275–296.

3   Ch. 1 of H. R. 6282, Sess. 63 of US Congress (1914).

4   Terry M. Parssinen, *Secret Passions, Secret Remedies: Narcotic Drugs in British Society, 1820–1930* (Philadelphia: Institute for the Study of Human Issues, 1983), 202. The British Parliament passed several Pharmacy and Dangerous Drugs Acts between 1916 and 1925 that defined poisonous drugs and restricted the distribution of narcotics to licensed persons.

5   According to John Frick, the writing and performing of alcoholic characters equipped the temperance movement with an outreach tool capable of influencing a broader swath of the population than literary tracts or pulpit speeches. See Frick's *Theatre, Culture, and Temperance Reform in Nineteenth-Century America* (Cambridge: Cambridge University Press, 2003).

6   See D. F. Musto, "Iatrogenic Addiction: The Problem, its Definition and History," *Bulletin of the New York Academy of Medicine* 61, no. 8 (1985): 694–705.

7   Mansfield was German-born and British-educated, arriving in the United States at age fifteen.

8   Martin A. Danahay and Alex Chisholm, *Jekyll and Hyde Dramatized: The 1887 Richard Mansfield Script and the Evolution of the Story on Stage* (Jefferson, NC: McFarland, 2005), vii.

9   Longmans succeeded in cancelling William Howell Poole's *Jekyll and Hyde* at Croydon's Theatre Royal, and Fred Wright and Thomas Morton Powell's touring production only performed once before it was shut down. Daniel Bandmann attempted to appease Longmans by removing all direct quotations from Stevenson's text. Danahay and Chisholm, *Jekyll and Hyde Dramatized*, vii–x and 133–137.

10   Henry Zecher, *William Gillette: America's Sherlock Holmes* (n.p.: Xlibris Corp., 2011), 287 and 322.

11   See Brian A. Rose's Jekyll and Hyde *Adapted: Dramatizations of Cultural Anxiety* (Westport: Greenwood Press: 1996), 37–77.

12   "The Playhouses," *Illustrated London News*, Sept 14, 1901, quoted in Horst Frenz and Louis Wylie Campbell, *William Gillette on the London Stage*, offprint from *Queen's Quarterly* 52, no. 4 (1945), BRTC.

13   Robert Louis Stevenson, *Dr. Jekyll and Mr. Hyde* (New York: Signet Class, 1980), 113.

14   Geoffrey Harding, *Opiate Addiction, Morality and Medicine: From Moral Illness to Pathological Disease* (New York, St. Martin's Press, 1988), 3.

15   H. Wayne Morgan, *Drugs in America: A Social History, 1800–1980* (New York: Syracuse University Press, 1981), 43. The late nineteenth-century popular press portrayed Chinese-operated opium dens in San Francisco and London as underground lairs of filth and vice, rendering their Anglo frequenters unseemly and disreputable by association.

16   Thomas De Quincey, *Confessions of an English Opium-Eater: Being an Extract from the Life of a Scholar* (n.p.: George Routledge and Sons, 1886). An opium-induced dream inspired Samuel Taylor Coleridge's poem "Kubla Khan" (1797 and published in 1816).

17   Frederick W. A. Serturner, an uneducated assistant of a German druggist, isolated the alkaloid from opium between 1803 and 1806, depending on the source.

18   Susan Zieger, "'How Far am I Responsible?': Women and Morphinomania in Late-Nineteenth-Century Britain," *Victorian Studies* (Autumn 2005): 65–66.

19   H. Wayne Morgan, *Yesterday's Addicts: American Society and Drug Abuse, 1865–1920* (Norman: University of Oklahoma Press, 1974), 28. Though few addicts concerned themselves with pharmacodynamics (the actions of drugs on the human body), Barbara Hodgson offers a clear description of how opiates work once introduced into the system: "[Opium] inhibits pain and produces calm by attaching itself to receptors on certain nerves cells in the brain. These receptors already produce similar but natural narcoticlike substances known as endorphins, sort of homemade pain relievers. So the body, accustomed to its own, albeit not as effective, form of painkiller, recognizes and welcomes the morphine molecules" (*Arms of Morpheus*, 2–3).

20   Anonymous, "The Chloroform Habit as Described by One of Its Victims," *Detroit Lancet*, vol. 8 (1884–1885), 251, reprinted in Morgan, *Yesterday's Addicts*, 147.

21   H. Wayne Morgan, *Drugs in America: A Social History, 1800–1980* (Syracuse: Syracuse University Press, 1981), 13.

22   Richard Davenport-Hines, *The Pursuit of Oblivion: A Global History of Narcotics* (New York: W.W. Norton, 2002), 135.

23   William Rosser Cobbe, *Doctor Judas: A Portrayal of the Opium Habit* (Chicago: S.C. Griggs, 1895), 135.

24   Joseph F. Spillane, *Cocaine: From Medical Marvel to Modern Menace in the United States, 1884–1920* (Baltimore: Johns Hopkins University Press, 2000), 9.

25   Virginia Berridge and Griffith Edwards, *Opium and the People: Opiate Use in Nineteenth-Century England* (New Haven: Yale University Press, 1987), 219 and 221. The actual

isolation of cocaine from the coca leaf occurred in Germany and Peru twenty-five years before Koller's landmark experiments. Spillane, *Cocaine*, 8.

26 Spillane, *Cocaine*, 12.

27 Quoted in *The Drug User: Documents 1840–1960*, eds. John Strausbaugh and Donald Blaise (New York: Blast Books, 1991), 9–10.

28 Virginia Berridge, "Dependence: Historical Concepts and Constructs," in *The Nature of Drug Dependence,* eds. Griffith Edwards and Malcolm Lader (Oxford: Oxford University Press, 1990), 1–18, 2.

29 Morgan, *Yesterday's Addicts*, 5.

30 Barbara Hodgson, *Arms of Morpheus: The Tragic History of Laudanum, Morphine, and Patent Medicines* (Buffalo: Firefly Books, 2001), 82.

31 Recent studies have shown that there indeed can be a genetic predisposition to addiction, but it is chromosomally, not hereditarily determined.

32 Morgan, *Drugs in America*, 43.

33 Mara L. Keire, "Dope Fiends and Degenerates: The Gendering of Addiction in the Early Twentieth Century," *Journal of Social History* 31, no. 4 (Summer 1998): 809–822. Keire acknowledges the influence of David Courtwright's *Dark Paradise: Opiate Addiction in America Before 1940* on her thesis.

34 Myron G. Schultz, "The 'Strange Case' of Robert Louis Stevenson," *Journal of American Medical Association* 216, no. 1 (1971): 90–94.

35 Quoted in Morgan, *Drugs in America*, 45.

36 H.H. Kane, *Drugs That Enslave: The Opium, Chloral, Morphine, and Hashisch* [sic] *Habits* (Philadelphia: Presley Blakiston, 1881).

37 Parssinen, *Secret Passions*, 61.

38 Norman Kerr, quoted in Berridge, "Dependence," 5.

39 Berridge and Edwards, *Opium and the People*, 150 and 155; and Lawrence Driscoll, *Reconsidering Drugs: Mapping Victorian and Modern Drug Discourses* (New York: Palgrave, 2000), 12.

40 Leslie Keeley, *The Morphine User, or From Bondage to Freedom* (Dwight: L. E. Keeley, 1883). See also B. Ball, *The Morphine Habit (morphinomania): With Four Lectures* (New York: Fitzgerald, 1887).

41 Leslie Keeley, "Experiences of Recent Opium Eaters," in *Yesterday's Addicts*, 111–120, 112.

42 In his study of habitual drug use and the professionalization of the medical field, Timothy Hickman takes up some of these questions, arguing that the etymological origins of the word "addiction" suggest its early twentieth century applicability to both "juridical" and "volitional" conditions of drug habituation. He also takes pains to divide the disease theory of drug use and the development of "addiction" as a medicalized term, though I would contend that the introduction of "addiction" into the medical lexicon and the construction of compulsive drug use as an illness requiring medical care overlapped and were conflated in the late nineteenth century. See Hickman's "The Double Meaning of Addiction: Habitual Narcotic Use and the Logic of Professionalizing Medical Authority in the United States, 1900–1920," in *Altering American Consciousness: The History of Alcohol and Drug Use in the United States, 1800–2000,* eds. Sarah W. Tracy and Caroline Jean Acker (Amherst: University of Massachusetts Press, 2004), 182–202.

43 Rosemary Cullen and Don B. Wilmeth, "Introduction," *Plays by William Hooker Gillette* (Cambridge: Cambridge University Press, 1983), 12.

44 While *Sherlock Holmes* possesses many melodramatic traits, the intelligent Professor Moriarty, whose schemes are more opportunistic than truly evil, resists classification as the stereotypical villain. Such deviations from the melodramatic genre have led scholars to characterize the play as originating a new type of play, the detective drama.

45 Cullen and Wilmeth, "Introduction," 12.

46 Arthur Conan Doyle, *A Study in Scarlet*, *The Complete Sherlock Holmes*, Vol. 1 (New York, Barnes and Noble Classics, 2003), 13.

47   Conan Doyle, *The Sign of Four*, in *The Complete Sherlock Holmes*, 99.

48   Joseph McLaughlin, *Writing the Urban Jungle: Reading Empire in London from Conan Doyle to Eliot* (Charlottesville: University of Virginia Press, 2000), 53–55.

49   William Hooker Gillette and Arthur Conan Doyle, *Sherlock Holmes*, in *The Plays of William Hooker Gillette*, ed. Rosemary Cullen and Don B. Wilmeth (Cambridge: Cambridge University Press, 1983), 193–272, 226.

50   All quotations from this exchange appear on pages 99 to 100 (Conan Doyle) and 226 to 227 (Gillette).

51   Timothy R. Prchal, "Secular Guardians of Scared Justice: Fictional Detectives and Asceticism," in *Sherlock Holmes: Victorian Sleuth to Modern Hero*, eds. Charles R. Putney, Joseph A. Cutshall King, and Sally Sugarman (Lanham: Scarecrow, 1996), 157–169, 162.

52   Martin Booth, *The Doctor and the Detective: A Biography of Sir Arthur Conan Doyle* (New York: Thomas Dunne, 2000), 149.

53   Terry D. Cooper, "A Chemically Induced 'Shadow'? Jekyll and Hyde as a Tale of Addiction," *Pastoral Psychology* 49, no. 2 (2000): 121–132, 122. See Patricia Comitini, "The Strange Case of Addiction in Robert Louis Stevenson's *Strange Case of Dr. Jekyll and Mr. Hyde*," *Victorian Review* 38, no. 1 (spring 2012): 113–131; Adam Colman, "The Optative Movement of Dr. Jekyll and Mr. Hyde's Addicts," *Extrapolation* 56, no. 2 (summer 2015): 215–234; Debbie Harrison, "Doctors, Drugs, and Addiction: Professional Integrity in Peril at the Fin de Siecle," *Gothic Studies* 11, no. 2 (Nov 2009): 52–62; Helle Mathiasen, "Dr. Jekyll Impaired," *The American Journal of Medicine* 122, issue 5 (May 2009): 492; and Daniel L. Wright, "'The Prisonhouse of My Disposition': A Study of the Psychology of Addiction in *Dr. Jekyll and Mr. Hyde*," *Studies in the Novel* 26 (1994): 254–267.

54   Sometimes John McKinney is cited as a co-author of Bandmann's script. Bandmann, *Dr. Jekyll and Mr. Hyde*, in *Jekyll and Hyde Dramatized*, 138–163; and Forepaugh and Fish, *Dr. Jekyll and Mr. Hyde, Or a Mis-Spent Life* (New York: Samuel French, 1904).

55   According to Thomas L. Reed, Jr., twentieth-century scholarship on Stevenson's *Jekyll and Hyde* largely discards Jekyll's illness of addiction, opting instead to emphasize the book's allegorical and metaphorical themes, particularly the threats of degeneration, homosexuality, and technology to Victorian bourgeois masculinity. At the commencement of his study on *Jekyll and Hyde* and alcoholism, Reed states: "We'll do well to begin by establishing the clear but under-appreciated fact that Henry Jekyll is an addict." However, at the turn of the millennium, a renewed interest in Jekyll's addiction is registered in a spate of studies. In addition to those listed in Note 53, see Reed's *The Transforming Draught: Jekyll and Hyde, Robert Louis Stevenson and the Victorian Alcohol Debate* (Jefferson, NC: McFarland, 2006); Andrew Smith's *Victorian Demons: Medicine, Masculinity and the Gothic at the fin-de-siècle* (Manchester: Manchester University Press, 2004); and Susan Zieger's *Inventing the Addict: Drugs, Race, and Sexuality in Nineteenth-Century British and American Literature* (Amherst: University of Massachusetts Press, 2008).

56   My contentions regarding Jekyll's reclusiveness and his asocial circle of friends conform to the scholarly consensus reached during the last two decades. Though earlier scholars including Irving Saposnik pointed to Utterson's ethical benevolence and Enfield and Utterson's weekly walks together as proof that theirs was a compassionate and socially visible group, most now agree that the novella's featured men were socially exclusive and largely self-involved.

57   Smith, *Victorian Demons*, 37.

58   Ibid., 7.

59   Zieger, *Inventing the Addict*, 186–187.

60   Wright, "Psychology of Addiction," 255.

61   Of the four acts' names, "Slave and Master," "Hide and Seek," "Two of the Same," and "The Last Night," only the final act's name is taken from Stevenson's chapter titles. The rest were of Sullivan's invention.

62   T. R. Sullivan, *Dr. Jekyll and Mr. Hyde* in *Jekyll and Hyde Dramatized*, eds. Martin A. Danahay and Alex Chisholm (Jefferson: McFarland, 2005), 47–79, 48.

63 Ibid., 48–51.
64 Ibid., 53. It is important to note the repetition of the label "fiend" in this exchange, as the feared early twentieth-century drug addict was regularly referred to as the "drug fiend."
65 Ibid., 57.
66 In Sullivan's play, Carew is addressed as "General Sir," a title that is absent in Stevenson's work. Its addition suggests Sullivan was elevating Carew's status in order to heighten Jekyll's by association, as well as make Carew's murder by Hyde an even more heinous offense.
67 Rose, Jekyll and Hyde *Adapted,* 56.
68 Stevenson, *Jekyll and Hyde,* 103–104.
69 "Mansfield vs. Stevenson: New and Interesting Conceptions of Dr. Jekyll and Mr. Hyde," *New York Sun,* Jan 1, 1888.
70 Rose, Jekyll and Hyde *Adapted,* 23 and 40.
71 "The Passing Show," unidentified newspaper, May 7, 1887, HTC.
72 Zieger, *Inventing the Addict,* 155 and 170.
73 James W. Maertens, "Masculine Power and the Ideal Reasoner: Sherlock Holmes, Technician-Hero," in *Sherlock Holmes: Victorian Sleuth to Modern Hero,* 296–322, 319 and 331.
74 Gillette, *Sherlock Holmes,* 265.
75 Zieger, *Inventing the Addict,* 162.
76 Sullivan's play defines evil as "those forces that act toward the dissolution of the familial bonds, the disintegration of social discourse and the abnegation of recognized means of controlling disruptions to established codes of social behavior" (Rose, Jekyll and Hyde *Adapted,* 70).
77 "Mansfield vs. Stevenson: New and Interesting Conceptions of Dr. Jekyll and Mr. Hyde," *New York Sun,* Jan 1, 1888.
78 Irving S. Saposnik, "The Anatomy of *Dr. Jekyll and Mr. Hyde," Studies in English Literature, 1500–1900* 11, no. 4 (Autumn 1971): 715–731, 715n1. Saposnik is quoting Mansfield's notes that are housed at the Huntington Library.
79 William Hooker Gillette, *The Painful Predicament of Sherlock Holmes* (Chicago: Ben Abramson, 1955).

Bibliography

Ball, B. *The Morphine Habit (Morphinomania): With Four Lectures.* New York: Fitzgerald, 1887.

Bandmann, Daniel E. "*Dr. Jekyll and Mr. Hyde.*" In *Jekyll and Hyde Dramatized,* edited by Martin A. Danahay and Alexander Chisholm, 138–163. Jefferson: McFarland, 2005.

Berridge, Virginia. "Dependence: Historical Concepts and Constructs." In *The Nature of Drug Dependence,* edited by Griffith Edwards and Malcolm Lader, 1–18. Oxford: Oxford University Press, 1990.

Berridge, Virginia. "The Origins of the English Drug 'Scene', 1890–1930." *Medical History* 32 (1988): 51–64.

Berridge, Virginia and Griffith Edwards. *Opium and the People: Opiate Use in Nineteenth-Century England.* New Haven: Yale University Press, 1987.

Booth, Martin. *The Doctor and the Detective: A Biography of Sir Arthur Conan Doyle.* New York: Thomas Dunne Books, 2000.

Cobbe, William Rosser. *Doctor Judas: A Portrayal of the Opium Habit.* Chicago: S.C. Griggs, 1895.

Colman, Adam. "The Optative Movement of Dr. Jekyll and Mr. Hyde's Addicts." *Extrapolation* 56, no. 2 (summer 2015): 215–234.

Comitini, Patricia. "The Strange Case of Addiction in Robert Louis Stevenson's *Strange Case of Dr. Jekyll and Mr. Hyde.*" *Victorian Review* 38, no. 1 (spring 2012): 113–131.

Conan Doyle, Arthur. *A Study in Scarlet, The Complete Sherlock Holmes*, Vol. 1. New York: Barnes and Noble Classics, 2003.

Conti, Meredith. "Ungentlemanly Habits: The Dramaturgy of Drug Addiction in *Fin-de-Siecle* Theatrical Adaptations of the Sherlock Holmes Stories and The Strange Case of Dr. Jekyll and Mr. Hyde." In *Victorian Medicine and Popular Culture*, edited by Louise Penner and Tabitha Sparks, 109–124. London: Routledge, 2015.

Cooper, Terry D. "A Chemically Induced 'Shadow'? Jekyll and Hyde as a Tale of Addiction." *Pastoral Psychology* 49, no. 2 (2000): 121–132.

Crocq, Marco-Antoine. "Historical and Cultural Aspects of Man's Relationship With Addictive Drugs." *Dialogues in Critical Neuroscience* 9, no. 4 (Dec 2007): 355–361.

Cullen, Rosemary and Don B. Wilmeth, eds. *Plays by William Hooker Gillette*. Cambridge: Cambridge University Press, 1983.

Danahay, Martin A. and Alex Chisholm, eds. *Jekyll and Hyde Dramatized: The 1887 Richard Mansfield Script and the Evolution of the Story on Stage*. Jefferson: McFarland, 2005.

Davenport-Hines, Richard. *The Pursuit of Oblivion: A Global History of Narcotics*. New York: W.W. Norton & Co., 2002.

De Quincey, Thomas. *Confessions of an English Opium-Eater: Being an Extract from the Life of a Scholar*. n.p.: George Routledge and Sons, 1886.

Driscoll, Lawrence. *Reconsidering Drugs: Mapping Victorian and Modern Drug Discourses*. New York: Palgrave, 2000.

Forepaugh, Luella and George F. Fish. *Dr. Jekyll and Mr. Hyde, Or a Mis-Spent Life*. New York: Samuel French, 1904.

Frick, John. *Theatre, Culture, and Temperance Reform in Nineteenth-Century America*. Cambridge: Cambridge University Press, 2003.

Gillette, William Hooker. *The Painful Predicament of Sherlock Holmes*. Chicago: Ben Abramson, 1955.

Gillette, William Hooker and Arthur Conan Doyle. *Sherlock Holmes*. In *The Plays of William Hooker Gillette*, edited by Martin A. Danahay and Alexander Chisholm, 193–272. Jefferson: McFarland, 2005.

Harding, Geoffrey. *Opiate Addiction, Morality and Medicine: From Moral Illness to Pathological Disease*. New York, St. Martin's Press, 1988.

Harrison, Debbie. "Doctors, Drugs, and Addiction: Professional Integrity in Peril at the Fin de Siecle." *Gothic Studies* 11, no. 2 (Nov 2009): 52–62.

Hickman, Timothy. "The Double Meaning of Addiction: Habitual Narcotic Use and the Logic of Professionalizing Medical Authority in the United States, 1900-1920." In *Altering American Consciousness: The History of Alcohol and Drug Use in the United States, 1800–2000*, edited by Sarah W. Tracy and Caroline Jean Acker, 182–202. Amherst: University of Massachusetts Press, 2004.

Hodgson, Barbara. *In the Arms of Morpheus: The Tragic History of Laudanum, Morphine, and Patent Medicines*. Buffalo: Firefly Books, 2001.

Kane, H.H. *Drugs That Enslave: The Opium, Chloral, Morphine, and Hashisch Habits*. Philadelphia: Presley Blakiston, 1881.

Keeley, Leslie. *The Morphine User, or From Bondage to Freedom*. Dwight: L. E. Keeley, 1883.

Keire, Mara L. "Dope Fiends and Degenerates: The Gendering of Addiction in the Early Twentieth Century." *Journal of Social History* 31, no. 4 (Summer 1998): 809–822.

Maertens, James W. "Masculine Power and the Ideal Reasoner: Sherlock Holmes, Technician-Hero." In *Sherlock Holmes: Victorian Sleuth to Modern Hero*, edited by Charles R. Putney, Joseph A. Cutshall King, and Sally Sugarman, 296–322. Lanham: Scarecrow, 1996.

Mathiasen, Helle. "Dr. Jekyll Impaired." *The American Journal of Medicine* 122, issue 5 (May 2009): 492.

McLaughlin, Joseph. *Writing the Urban Jungle: Reading Empire in London from Doyle to Eliot.* Charlottesville: University Press of Virginia, 2000.

Morgan, H. Wayne. *Drugs in America: A Social History, 1800–1980.* New York: Syracuse University Press, 1981.

Morgan, H. Wayne. *Yesterday's Addicts: American Society and Drug Abuse, 1865–1920.* Norman: University of Oklahoma Press, 1974.

Musto, D. F. "Iatrogenic Addiction: The Problem, its Definition and History." *Bulletin of the New York Academy of Medicine* 61, no. 8 (1985): 694–705.

Parssinen, Terry M. *Secret Passions, Secret Remedies: Narcotic Drugs in British Society, 1820–1930.* Philadelphia: Institute for the Study of Human Issues, 1983.

Parssinen, Terry M. and Karen Kerner. "Development of the Disease Model of Addiction in Britain, 1870–1926." *Medical History* 24 (1980): 275–296.

Prchal, Timothy R. "Secular Guardians of Scared Justice: Fictional Detectives and Asceticism." In *Sherlock Holmes: Victorian Sleuth to Modern Hero*, edited by Charles Putney, Joseph A. Cutshall King, and Sally Sugarman, 157–169. Lanham: Scarecrow, 1996.

Putney, Charles R., Joseph A. Cutshall King, and Sally Sugarman, eds. *Sherlock Holmes: Victorian Sleuth to Modern Hero.* Lanham: Scarecrow, 1996.

Reed, Jr., Thomas L. *The Transforming Draught: Jekyll and Hyde, Robert Louis Stevenson and the Victorian Alcohol Debate.* Jefferson: McFarland, 2006.

Rose, Brian A. Jekyll and Hyde *Adapted: Dramatizations of Cultural Anxiety.* Westport: Greenwood Press: 1996.

Saposnik, Irving S. "The Anatomy of *Dr. Jekyll and Mr. Hyde.*" *Studies in English Literature, 1500–1900* 11, no. 4 (Autumn 1971): 715–731.

Schultz, Myron G. "The 'Strange Case' of Robert Louis Stevenson." *Journal of American Medical Association* 216, no. 1 (1971): 90–94.

Smith, Andrew. *Victorian Demons: Medicine, Masculinity, and the Gothic at the Fin-de-Siècle.* Manchester: Manchester University Press, 2004.

Spillane, Joseph F. *Cocaine: From Medical Marvel to Modern Menace in the United States, 1884–1920.* Baltimore: John Hopkins University Press, 2000.

Stevenson, Robert Louis. *The Strange Case of Dr. Jekyll and Mr. Hyde.* New York: Signet Class, 1980.

Strausbaugh, John and Donald Blaise, eds. *The Drug User: Documents 1840–1960.* New York: Blast Books, 1991.

Sullivan, T. R. *Dr. Jekyll and Mr. Hyde.* In *Jekyll and Hyde Dramatized*, edited by Martin A. Danahay and Alex Chisholm, 47–79.

Wright, Daniel L. "'The Prisonhouse of My Disposition': A Study of the Psychology of Addiction in *Dr. Jekyll and Mr. Hyde.*" *Studies in the Novel* 26 (1994): 254–267.

Zecher, Henry. *William Gillette: America's Sherlock Holmes.* n.p.: Xlibris Corp., 2011.

Zieger, Susan. "'How Far am I Responsible?' Women and Morphinomania in Late-Nineteenth-Century Britain." *Victorian Studies* 48, no. 1 (Autumn 2005): 59–81.

Zieger, Susan. *Inventing the Addict: Drugs, Race, and Sexuality in Nineteenth-Century British and American Literature.* Amherst: University of Massachusetts Press, 2008.

4 Master, martyr, monster
The addict archetypes of William Hooker Gillette and Richard Mansfield

The tenant of 221B Baker Street stands behind a table wearing a silk smoking gown.[1] Holding the tip of a hypodermic needle to his wrist, William Gillette's Sherlock Holmes applies pressure to the syringe's plunger. In the left side of the image sits Dr. Watson, observing the proceedings with unconcealed revulsion. Unmoved by—or, more to the point, inattentive to—his companion's objections, Holmes appears placid and self-possessed: the very picture of an elegant, controlled Victorian drug habitué. No analogous image exists of Richard Mansfield's Dr. Henry Jekyll ingesting his enslaving elixir of red liquid and white powder, and yet the famous double-exposure photograph by Van der Weyde of the actor as Jekyll and Hyde affords a striking portrait of drug-induced biformity (Figures 4.1 and 4.2). Dressed in a double-breasted frock coat with erect posture, coiffed hair, and an open comportment, the doctor's appearance bears all the archetypal markers of privileged bourgeois masculinity. The angst inscribed on Jekyll's face, however, contradicts his body's studied ease. With the specter of Mr. Hyde (both the incarnation of Jekyll's inescapable cravings and the fractured self that results from surrendering) crouching villainously behind him, the doctor raises his eyes and right arm both to the heavens, gestures signifying not only Jekyll's inherent moral virtue, as Irving Saposnik suggests, but also his guilt, powerlessness, and spiritual supplication.[2]

In suggesting that relationships and even identities must splinter to accommodate an addict's habit, both photographs make visible the divisive nature of compulsive drug consumption. The images also document two compositions of theatricalized drug abuse that together delineated an optics of performed addiction for the popular stage, optics that permitted the juxtaposition and interplay of drug addiction theories circulating at the *fin de siècle*. What follows moves away from the textual and dramaturgical and toward the embodied and performative, analyzing how Gillette and Mansfield manifested the varied symptomatologies of drug abuse in 1899's *Sherlock Holmes* and 1887's *Dr. Jekyll and Mr. Hyde*. If Gillette, as the elegant, understated, and tranquil Holmes, forged a performance of controlled habituation, then Mansfield's embodiment of immoderate addiction as Jekyll/Hyde was one of immoderate mimesis.

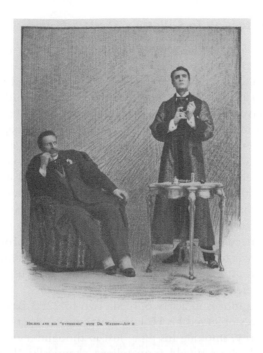

Holmes and his "Hypodermic" with Dr. Watson—Act II

Figure 4.1 "William Gillette as Sherlock Holmes as produced at the Garrick Theatre, New York" (New York: R.H. Russell, 1900). HTC Clippings 14 Gillette Programs. Harvard Theatre Collection, Houghton Library, Harvard University.

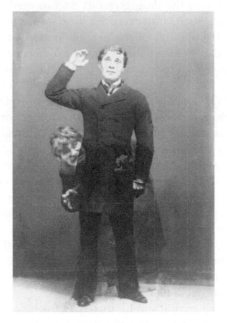

Figure 4.2 "Richard Mansfield as Dr. Jekyll and Mr. Hyde." Library of Congress.

Dosing and detecting in Gillette's *Sherlock Holmes*

In 1904's *The Adventure of the Missing Three-Quarter*, Arthur Conan Doyle put an end to Holmes's drug habit. "For years," Watson declared in the story, "I gradually weaned him from that drug mania which had threatened once to check his remarkable career. Now I knew that under ordinary conditions he no longer craved for this artificial stimulus; but I was well aware that the fiend was not dead, but sleeping."[3] This gradual weaning began in the 1890s when, as experts progressively acknowledged the dangers of cocaine consumption, Conan Doyle downplayed Holmes's drug usage and heightened Watson's rhetoric of abstinence. Watson's declaration that the "fiend was not dead, but sleeping" proves that, as Martin Booth writes, "Conan Doyle was ahead of his time, aware that drug addiction was rarely overcome and could only be suppressed, not extinguished."[4] The serialized Holmes may have relinquished his hypodermic needle and seven-percent solution, but throughout William Gillette's thirty-year tenure as the authoritative Sherlock Holmes, his detective retained his most exceptional flaw, hypodermic drug use, to the apparent pleasure and gratification of audiences.

Sherlock Holmes moves in act two, scene two to 221B Baker Street, where Gillette's audiences observed his Holmes lounging on floor cushions with his violin laying nearby, smoking his pipe, lost in thought: a composition of the signature ennui Holmes would soon relieve chemically. Then, the onstage injection. Just as in Conan Doyle's *The Sign of Four*, Holmes's lethargy deepened as the cocaine solution entered his bloodstream, a somewhat peculiar physiological response to the drug given its documented effects. The opiates sedated, not cocaine. Soon, however, the drug's stimulating effects vitalized Gillette's Holmes. By the end of the act, Holmes's outwitting of Moriarty assured audiences that cocaine sharpened the detective's intellect without blunting his judgment. "From lassitude and light irony to vibrant nerves and an alert pistol was the direction in which [Gillette] chose to lead his action," remarked *Chicago Tribune*'s Charles Collins of Holmes's transformation.[5] Holmes's behavior never grew agitated, choleric, or lewd while under the influence of cocaine, as *fin-de-siècle* critics of habitual drug use warned. Theatregoers found little to dislike about the brilliant and debonair Holmes: "[Gillette] presents a man of fine and dominant intellect, intense feeling, perfectly controlled, vigilant sagacity, implacable purpose, cold, imperturbable demeanor, muscular physique, and polished, elegant manner."[6] With such a litany of sterling qualities, it is no wonder Gillette's Holmes possessed—or at least believed he possessed—absolute control over his drug habit. Still, in a 1937 retrospective on Gillette's Holmes, John Mason Brown conceived of Holmes's cocaine use as the hero-detective's Achilles heel: "He is a superman, joined to the lesser race of men only by the slim ties of his one weakness, his call to Watson for the needle."[7]

Though Holmes's injection and his subsequent debate with Watson occupy no more than two minutes of the play's running time, the detective is, in effect, high for the entirety of act two. Lest spectators forget Holmes's impaired state, his inability to read a letter later in the act serves as a reminder: "Read it, Watson, there's a good fellow – my eyes – (*with a motion across eyes; half smile*) You know – cocaine."[8] But is "impaired" even an appropriate descriptor? As the script, reviews, and publicity stills of the production suggest, Gillette signified Holmes's doped condition through a brief bout of languidness and lingering blurred vision. In all other observable ways, the detective's faculties, including his legendary powers of deduction, remained unhampered by the drug. "When Holmes carefully measures his 7 percent solution," Joseph McLaughlin maintains, "he subordinates the substance to his will and pleasure."[9] As Alan Dale of the *New York Journal and Advertiser* wrote of Gillette's performance:

> [Sherlock Holmes] was not only keen-witted, but he was amazingly non-chalant, apparently lethargic, able to see through at least half a dozen stone walls, and a better mind reader than anybody not addicted to the secret sciences. Perhaps he was quite too wonderful for implicit admiration.[10]

A hyper-functional addict whose body betrayed only minimal signs of drug dependence, Gillette's Holmes seemed almost an antiquated figure in 1899, when increasingly drug-literate Europeans and Americans viewed cocainism as disease and vice. The mythic Holmesian habitué grew only rarer in the 1910s and 1920s, as the criminalized drug fiend eclipsed other addict archetypes in popular culture.

Gillette affiliated Holmes's drug use with bohemian aestheticism even more directly than Conan Doyle's writings. The serialized stories introduced all the building blocks of Holmes's bohemianism at some point (pipe-smoking in elegant lounging robes, meditating on floor cushions, violin-playing, and of course drug-taking), but Gillette compressed all of these activities into the space of one theatrical scene, creating an explicit and integrative portrait of *fin-de-siècle* aestheticism. As Pasquale Accardo writes in his study of medical iconography in *Sherlock Holmes*:

> with William Gillette's stage performances an exaggerated Bohemianism became the rule for later representations of Holmes in the media … His almost ridiculous attire accented certain Byronic strains in Holmes's character and served to link the antisocial scientific detective to the antisocial artist and aesthete – the dandy.[11]

But, cautions James W. Maertens:

> [Holmes's] bohemianism signals not so much that he is a poet but that he is not a conformist or a company man. He defies officialdom in all its guises … If there is something Byronic in Holmes, it is his tendency to melancholia, which he treats with cocaine.[12]

Accardo and Maertens's use of "Byronic" in separate writings suggests several things about Holmes's drug use. First, it is conceivable that Holmes suffered from chronic depression, or at least from a melancholic predisposition he managed two ways: by solving crimes and by self-medicating. Second, Gillette's performance of bohemian aestheticism—including his habitual drug use—discourages more simplistic readings of Holmes as a no-nonsense sleuth guided only by objectivity and pragmatism. Conan Doyle's Holmes, Douglas Small argues, is a non-addicted polymath whose identity as a rational, dispassionate brainworker fully encased his habit. "The pleasures of the drug are not what he desires, but only a stopgap for the mental exertion of detection," writes Small of the literary Holmes. "Holmes is indifferent to his body so long as his mind is energised; his use of cocaine is contextualised so that it indicates the extent to which Holmes prefers the life of the mind over a bodily or emotional one."[13] The Holmes of Gillette's imagination, however, was a realist and a dreamer. It was the balancing of the right and left sides of his brain, the commingling of intuition and logic, that made Gillette's Holmes an elite detective, not to mention a compelling stage protagonist. Critic Amy Leslie, upon seeing *Sherlock Holmes*, regarded Gillette as "so exotic and elegant that his detective is the very orchid of his kind."[14]

This Byronic orchid of a man, however extraordinary, made injecting cocaine appear almost prosaic, in large part due to Gillette's acting style. The actor played Holmes for over half of his six-decade career and for good reason; the role capitalized on Gillette's natural magnetism, perspicacity, and restraint. For Gillette, actors were not Diderotian *tabula rasas* waiting for a playwright's inscription to give them life. Rather, he attested, "[Personality] is the most singularly important factor for infusing the Life-Illusion into modern stage creations that is known to man."[15] He suffused his characters with aspects of himself, regarding the notion of actors "disappearing" into their roles as both inane and impossible. "Many proclaim him as the most finished and polished actor of the day, the acme of realism," mused the critic at Hartford's *Courant*, "others say he simply acts William Gillette in any part he may have to play. Perhaps the mean of these two extremes is nearest the truth."[16] If Gillette lacked the versatility of some of his contemporaries, he owned his limits, adopting a repertoire of somewhat homogeneous characters that showcased his particular gifts as a performer: subtlety, intensity, poise, intelligence, and a trace of vulnerability. The actor's methods proved instrumental in normalizing Holmes' onstage drug use. "He was natural in the finest sense, the truest sense," turn-of-the-century playwright Edwin Milton Royle praised, "not with the monotonous, inaudible, colorless naturalism of some of our contemporary performers, but with all the vivid, colorful variety and zest of the life we actually live, the life around us and within us."[17] In his most admired roles, including Holmes and Dumont/Thorne in the spy drama *Secret Service*, Gillette's effortlessness as an actor helped render the plays' spectacular circumstances more plausible and palatable for audiences weary of melodramatic posturing and vocal bombast. As Norman Hapgood observed in 1901, Gillette's acting was "cold, yet producing feeling in the observer; apparently natural and disdainful of the theatrical, yet alert, active, and deeply theatrical every second."[18] What most distanced Gillette's naturalism from the performative Zolaism embraced by some of his contemporaries was the actor's refusal to depict man at his most coarse or disgraceful. Even Holmes's hypodermic drug use offered little temptation for Gillette to plumb the lower depths of human behavior.

Economy governed Gillette's work. The actor could famously hold audiences with lengthy silences or convey an emotion with a glance, relying on minute physiological responses to fill characters with what he called the "Breath of life."[19] His body often mimicked a compressed coil: motionless, but full of tension and poised to spring. "His acting is indeed a paradox," Montrose Moses once remarked, "for it is the acme of nervous ease."[20] Gillette's angular face and lithe figure, so strikingly similar to Doyle's descriptions and Sidney Paget's illustrations of the detective, externalized Holmes's drug habit without sacrificing the character's status as a man of self-discipline. Registering the physiological effects of habitual drug use were the actor's hands—which languorously gestured in the moments prior to and following Holmes's cocaine injection but acquired a subtle, tremulous quality in the play's later acts—and his eyes, which were "half-lidded, almost sleepy eyes intelligently observant; watchful, at times wavering eyes with little variety of expression."[21] The subtlety with which Gillette recalibrated Holmes's symptomatology from drug withdrawal to that of drug satiation marked the character as both a high-functioning habitué and one unlikely to desire or independently pursue sobriety.

Regarded retrospectively, Gillette's thirty-year run as the enigmatic detective seems to spell unqualified success, but early critics of *Sherlock Holmes* were not universally adulatory. Following a copyright performance at London's Lyceum Theatre, the play premiered in 1899 at New York's Garrick Theatre to largely favorable reviews. Though a number of reviews chided Gillette for the play's love story, critics commended his "untheatrical" tack in embodying "this fantastic, imaginative, and at the same time potently human conception."[22] After crossing the Atlantic and garnering solid reviews in Liverpool ("a most realistic Sherlock Holmes," declared the *Era*, and "perfectly magnetic"), Gillette opened *Sherlock Holmes* on September 9, 1901 at the Lyceum to a mixed reception.[23] Those with seats distant from the stage audibly complained of not being able to hear Gillette, and Gillette's physical restraint displeased some Lyceum spectators who perhaps had grown accustomed to the resident company's more pictorial style (à la their recently retired actor-manager Henry Irving). The scrutiny of Gillette's Holmes was made all the more intense because of the beloved character's English roots. "Surely no playhouse is large enough to hold that colossal figure?" scoffed *The Times*:

> Print has the advantage of always leaving a margin for the imagination. Now Dr. Doyle and Mr. Gillette between them have cut away that margin. They give us our Sherlock not as he was, a composite photograph, a serious of kaleidoscopic patterns, a splendid image, but a definite individual with a very rococo dressing-gown and a not very audible voice.[24]

British audiences, like those in America, remained skeptical about Holmes's affections for Alice Faulkner but concluded that Gillette's icy portrayal of Holmes-in-love at least tempered the damage wrought by the love plot. Gillette cut a striking figure as Holmes, reviewers acknowledged, and some regarded the actor's understated approach to the character as the production's saving grace, "lift[ing the play] altogether out of the ruck of melodrama." For the *Tatler*, Gillette's subtle style "is most useful as a corrective to our own bawling methods in melodrama which the unhappy provincial playgoer has to listen to week after week."[25] In a notable endorsement of Gillette's naturalistic acting, the outspoken champion of modernism and founder of London's Independent Theatre Society, J. T. Grein, proposed (using a suitably scientific metaphor) that: "The performance will confirm Mr. Gillette's reputation as an actor of great resources, but I fear that at best his fame as an artist will remain unimpaired by his thankless experiment."[26]

Holmes' cocaine habit, once perceived only in the imaginations of Conan Doyle's readers, became an embodied ritual in Gillette's *Sherlock Holmes*, an intimate avocation within the world of Holmesian literature rendered spectacular within the world of the theatre. But contextualized by Gillette's patented "calm intensity," Holmes's drug use rarely registered to British or American critics as the injurious disease against which Watson inveighed; rather, most respondents allude to the detective's injections with what can best be described as boys-will-be-boys rhetoric. Holmes, after all, was an elegant Victorian brainworker with delicate nerves whose deductive powers improved with cocaine. Moreover, as we will see at the end of this chapter, "drug habitué" was but one in a list of characteristics used to describe Gillette's Holmes and therefore never overshadowed his perceived self-mastery. For the *Washington Post* reviewer, Sherlock Holmes was a "cocaine-soaked, hard, cold, reasoning, and self-possessed man."[27] If Gillette's debonair detective-aesthete enjoyed thrice-daily injections with no more ill effects than blurred vision and a bout of lethargy, Richard Mansfield's Jekyll destroyed his career, love life, and selfhood with his first swallow of red liquid and white powder.

"His failure is a disease": Virtue and vice in Mansfield's *Dr. Jekyll and Mr. Hyde*

As actors and public figures, Mansfield and Gillette acquired reputations of nearly oppositional tenor. Both on and offstage, Gillette's cordial professionalism endeared him to collaborators, fans, and the press, while Mansfield was by many accounts a charismatic but temperamental autocrat. Although scholars credit both men with participating in or originating transitional acting forms that bridged mid-century melodramatic techniques with psychological realism, Gillette and Mansfield were very different performers. Gillette's aforementioned skills lay in intensely detailed, technical naturalism, while Mansfield painted psychological states with evocative but broad brushstrokes. This approach proved effective in farcical or melodramatic fare, but left Mansfield ill-equipped to flesh out the weightier characters, as Garff B. Wilson has noted:

> [Mansfield] could grasp and project the simple, violent, baser emotions which are characteristic of melodrama … [but] discriminating viewers felt that, with few exceptions, he could not touch either the depths or the heights of great tragic emotion and though he often simulated these emotions there was no "informing soul" behind the simulation.[28]

Still, even Mansfield's detractors acknowledged his dynamic magnetism as a performer. While Mansfield could not boast a chameleon-esque versatility, his portrayals benefitted from the uncommon plasticity of his face and body. He exercised similar control over his voice, modulating it into a buoyant lilt for Beau Brummell or a sonorous baritone for Henry V, though some found his elocutionary efforts intrusive. Short of stature and square-jawed, Mansfield lacked the matinee-idol looks of Gillette and was reportedly sensitive about his appearance. His approach to character creation, too, markedly diverged from Gillette's. Note Mansfield's *Jekyll and Hyde*-esque description of how, through the actor's artistry and diligence, character eventually displaces player:

> [T]he actor, the poet actor, sees and creates in the air before him the being he delineates; he makes him, he builds him during the day, in the long hours of the night; the character gradually takes being; he is the actor's genius; the slave of the ring, who comes when he calls him, stands beside him, and envelops him in his ghostly arms; the actor's personality disappears; he is the character.[29]

Mansfield's public image bore a strong resemblance to his dual role of addiction. Like the famous photograph that superimposed Mansfield's Hyde upon his Jekyll, critical assessments of even a single performance seemed to address two distinctive Mansfields: sensitive genius and sensational hack.[30] The actor's offstage reputation was no less bifurcated. Overbearing and mercurially tempered, the actor periodically made the gossip pages thanks to fits of anger in public places, some resulting in damaged property, injured waiters, and frightened housekeepers. Reporting on one such outburst in "Mr. Mansfield in a Rage: Great Actor Got Real Mad While in Sioux City," an anonymous author playfully proclaimed: "The Mansfieldian temper was tried to the uttermost, the excoriating eloquence of the Mansfieldian tongue was hardly equal to the test, and the Mansfieldian irascibility was given a refreshing exhibition."[31] Friends and fans of the actor, however, testified to Mansfield's gentle nature, and the actor himself attempted to counteract his poor public image with a series of interviews in which a jovial Mansfield ruminated on his career while engaging in tranquil activities like sailing. The actor, it would seem, had much in common with Jekyll and Hyde: a veneer of congeniality, restraint, and charm masked the irascible and impulsive dictator within, an ambition for personal aggrandizement "tempered by a sense of conscientious duty to his public."[32] As noted by Mansfield friend and biographer William Winter, the actor's collaborators regarded him "sometimes as affable and kind, sometimes as unreasonable, tyrannical, and offensive. That testimony, both ways, is authentic."[33] Admirers and detractors alike admitted Mansfield was the best actor to bring *Dr. Jekyll and Mr. Hyde* to the stage, citing his total (and somewhat dangerous) immersion into the role of Edward Hyde as proof of his suitability. Newspapers printed tales of Mansfield-as-Hyde trampling backstage crewmembers as he rushed to the stage, and of forceful onstage chokeholds in the fatal act one meeting of Hyde and Carew that left the victim lightheaded. In such cases, the press proved uncharacteristically generous to the actor, absolving him of any willful wrongdoing because, as *The Post* rationalized in a retrospective on the dual role, "He is said to have lived so deeply the part of Mr. Hyde."[34]

Reviewers of the play's initial run (and the Mansfield revivals that followed) centralized Jekyll's immoderate drug use and Hyde's narcoticized hedonism in their appraisals of the piece, even if some found the subject too pronounced or distasteful. "The modern stage does not require a dose of hideous stories nor does it demand the dramatization of dreams caused by painful indigestion or a course of opiates," carped London's *Daily Telegraph* in its coverage.[35] Critics routinely dissected Mansfield's Jekyll/Hyde and analyzed each component part, mirroring the common bifurcation of states-of-being (sober and high, pain and pleasure) applied by addict-authors throughout the 1800s. With a few exceptions, theatregoers celebrated Mansfield's fiendish Hyde but considered the actor's softened, guilt-ridden Dr. Jekyll an ineffective deviation from Stevenson's work. Of his electrifying transformations, in which the actor changed from Jekyll to Hyde or Hyde to Jekyll, Mansfield received nearly unanimous commendation.

Mansfield reshaped Jekyll into a more sympathetic, ennobled scientist than Stevenson's creation, a character with an elaborate addiction narrative. To do so, the actor first lessened Jekyll's moral culpability in his own addiction by replacing the original character's egotism and intellectual opportunism with an altruistic (if misapplied) inquisitiveness. No longer Stevenson's self-absorbed physician, Mansfield's Jekyll fancied himself a sacrificial lamb on the altar of scientific progress: "And I, who have toiled for man am doomed to eternal wretchedness," he laments in act one before collapsing into a chair. "Ah, Heaven help me, Heaven help me!"[36] While Gillette's Holmes participated willfully in his addiction without measurable contrition, Mansfield wrapped his reluctant drug inebriate in a mantle of shame, echoing many of the period's addiction narratives. This metaphorical self-flagellation began immediately upon his first entrance and extended throughout the play's acts, rather than developing gradually. By staging the destruction of character's meaningful relationships and his immaculate bourgeois façade through his intemperate drug use, Mansfield also heightened the individual and communal stakes of Jekyll's addiction. Finally, the actor's enfeebled Jekyll externalized for audiences the mental and physiological impacts of chemical addiction.

These changes to Jekyll's character gratified some observers and perturbed others. The *Illustrated Sporting and Dramatic News* seemed to wholly grasp

Mansfield's interpretation of Stevenson's character, particularly the actor's more tragic construction of Jekyll's illness. Protesting the novella's depiction of a cheerful Jekyll who "holds out to his friends the hand that has killed their friends," the critic claimed, Mansfield ... evolves a nobler, subtler, and more logical conception ... [Jekyll] could not be jolly – he is crushed by remorse for the crimes he has committed as Hyde; he is in despair at the inexorable fate that binds him to his baser part and renders his resistance to the noxious drug weaker and weaker.[37] The *London Times* applauded Mansfield's "humanizing Jekyll, making him hate Hyde, and suffer mentally from his knowledge of Hyde's villainies," even going so far as to say "Mr. Stevenson ought to be much obliged to Mr. Mansfield for not only making his story profitable on the stage, but for giving to the character of Jekyll something like consistency."[38] And the *Chicago Record-Herald* tendered its approval of Mansfield's Jekyll by way of a backhanded compliment: "Genius would not be required to make Hyde a creepy figure; but to give him larger significance by enforcing the woe of Jekyll and by keeping poignantly before the spectator the sense of Jekyll's consciousness of his doom – this does require feeling and prowess of the first order."[39]

Far more reviews, however, critiqued Jekyll's anemic flatness, particularly in comparison with his forceful Hyde. The *Athenaeum* proclaimed the character "too lackadaisical," the *Boston Evening Transcript* "too inveterately gloomy."[40] The *London Letter* claimed that English audiences and reviewers "unanimously voted [it] a jerky, spiritless, and utterly commonplace impersonation ... His Jekyll is absurd and magnifies all his old faults."[41] Mansfield's virtuous and melancholic doctor "too palpably carried about with him" the horrible knowledge of his alter ego's wrongdoings, lamented *The Boston Post*.[42] Just as 1880s addicts inspired both sympathy (as sufferers of a diagnosable disease) and censure (as co-architects of their disease), Mansfield's Jekyll, a protagonist-addict directly responsible for his own downfall, troubled critics. The *Boston Evening Transcript* articulated this moral ambivalence:

> Hyde is Jekyll's malady, and our abhorrence of the disease is lessened by our pity for the sufferer, for, in this case, disease and sufferer are one. Then, too, as the disease is essentially shameful, and, to a certain extent, voluntarily incurred, our sympathy with and pity for Jekyll is not quite free from a dash of contempt.

Here the *Transcript* collapses person and pathology into one indivisible identity, at once pathetic and culpable. The review then compares Mansfield's Jekyll with a similarly divisive figure, the drunkard: "You may tell us [the alcoholic's] failing is a disease, and convince our understanding that it is so; but in our heart of heart we do not quite respect him, even in his sober days."[43] Such assessments of Jekyll tallied with the *fin-de-siècle* construction of the compulsive drug user as both physically and morally ill.

In 1888, Mansfield gave several interviews justifying his controversial interpretation, insisting that Jekyll's righteousness was vital to the theatrical dynamism and duality of Jekyll/Hyde. Hyde's indulgence of Jekyll's inner demons, the actor reasoned, purged all evil from the doctor, leaving only goodness. It was only natural, then, that Jekyll felt horror and remorse for his actions as Hyde and could not be the "jovial … dinner party giving" Jekyll of Stevenson's imagination. Mansfield guaranteed the originality of his Jekyll with characteristic conceit, telling London's *The Star* that other actors playing the dual role "can all find Hyde in Mr. Stevenson's book, but my Jekyll they cannot find, for he is not there," presumably a swipe at Daniel Bandmann's rival portrayal.[44] In answering critics who disapproved of the gentler, more vulnerable Jekyll of Mansfield's imagination, the actor explained: "Now, rightly or wrongly, I have a theory that all that is good in a man's character – his affection for others, his love of truth and mercy, his self-sacrifice, patience, and other virtues – all come to him from his mother; and so I make Jekyll somewhat effeminate, that is to say, gentle in his manner and passionate and self-sacrificing in his love."[45] While his hedonistic Hyde validated *fin-de-siècle* fears of the addict-menace, the effeminate comportment of Mansfield's Jekyll confirmed a parallel construction of male drug addicts as weak willed, overly sensitive aesthetes, for as Mara L. Keire affirms, "[A]ddiction made men less manly."[46] With Agnes at his side, Mansfield's Jekyll was explicitly heterosexual, and yet the character's fragility gestured toward addiction's medicocultural linkages to feminine sensibility and homosexuality.

Mansfield's Jekyll was sallow-skinned, rheumy-eyed, upright but slightly sway-backed in posture, and somewhat conservative in movement in the play's early acts. His longer black hair, which several critics labeled inappropriate for the character's profession, was parted on the side and curled, permitting Mansfield to shift from Jekyll to Hyde by way of a rapid tousle. As Jekyll's condition worsened, the actor's posture bowed and his arm movements grew tremulous. "The terrific strain upon a once powerful system begins to tell, and he finds himself generally less and less able to withstand, both physically and mentally, the encroachment of evil," wrote Mansfield. "He is bowed down with remorse at the thought of the monster he has conjured up betwixt himself and the beautiful woman to whom he is engaged … Worse is added to worse."[47] Jekyll's "terrific strain" mimicked the drug addict's characteristic symptomatology, as enumerated in Levinstein's *Morbid Craving for Morphia*: pale and slack skin, dull and unfocused eyes, trembling hands, and involuntary muscular twitches. Of those addicts suffering from "abstinence from morphia," known now as withdrawal, Levinstein reported: "They are overcome by a feeling of uneasiness and restlessness; the feeling of self-consciousness and self-possession is gone, and is replaced by extreme despondency … Some of the patients will be found walking about in deep despair, hoping to find an opportunity of freeing themselves for ever from their wretched condition."[48] Compare Levinstein's record of acute drug withdrawal with the *Pall Mall Budget's* description of Mansfield's final scene as Jekyll: "Imagine him locked up in his laboratory … pacing to and fro in mortal agony. The drug, which was once so potent in effecting convenient transformations, cannot be procured in its native purity, and with its purity its potentiality has gone … So great is Jekyll's agony that he writhes in unutterable torments."[49] Without his tincture, the active components of which replicated those of opium-infused laudanum, Mansfield's Jekyll suffered the effects of abstinence in full view of the audience, a somatic spectacle of performed withdrawal.

Mythically the cause of fainting spectators and post-theatre nightmares, Mansfield's savage Hyde became an attraction for thrill-seeking theatregoers. That the novella's Mr. Utterson describes Hyde as giving "the impression of deformity without any nameable malformation" seemed inconsequential to Mansfield's interpretation of the role.[50] Indeed, the actor himself argued that translating Hyde from page to stage required heightening his corporeal abnormalities: "The form shrinks to fit the spirit, which remains," he stated of his conception, "and the form and features accommodate themselves to the likeness of the being within."[51] With the increased stigmatization of habitual drug use in the 1880s and 1890s, medical and popular presses itemized or illustrated addiction's disfiguring scars, among them an emaciated frame, infected puncture wounds, and glassy, dilated eyes. Cast in this light, the theatrical Hyde's misshapenness signaled not just the character's depravity, but the symptomatic markings of the addict's self-mutilation. Reviewers attended assiduously to Hyde's non-normative corporeality. Widely refusing to acknowledge Mansfield's creation as anthropomorphous, critics instead labeled him as a "gnome," "dwarf," "bogy," "demon," "monster," or "imp," as in the *Pall Mall Gazette*'s invitation to readers to "imagine a crouching imp of stunted stature, misshapen and crook-backed, halting in his gait, a mass of towzled [*sic*] black locks covering his forehead, his eyes glowing like coals, without teeth, and varying his raucous bass tones with hisses and gasps."[52] Mansfield's primitive posture, irregular gait, and what the *Athenaeum* described as "ape-like agility" served as weighty signifiers of atavistic savagery and retrograding degeneration, given the cultural prominence of Darwinian and Spencerian theories of human evolution.[53] Others saw in Hyde's spontaneous ferocity, straining hands, and talon-like fingers the makings of a "hellish hawk"; in his serpentine undulations the motions of a "reptile," "crocodile," or "cobra"; and in his "mouth with its leering bestiality," feral crouch, and sharp eyes the body and face of a cat.[54] Hyde's voice—grating, croaking, raspy—also marked his creation as subhuman, as did the character's legendary hiss.

Audiences and critics alike hailed his creature a triumph. Mansfield's muscular volatility, which many felt he squandered in his milquetoast rendition of Jekyll, gave life to Hyde. "Mr. Mansfield's reserves of nervous force and of vocal volume and intensity (to say nothing of his knowledge of the lust, hatred, and fury that the human heart can generate), are wonderfully shown in this performance," proclaimed a New York reviewer; the *London Letter* concurred, maintaining Mansfield's Hyde "is full of weird power and ferocity, and proves that Mansfield has (as I have often said in the past) great capabilities for character acting. His Hyde is simply a revelation."[55] William Winter applauded the actor's "horrible animal vigor," and "tremendous power" in creating a "carnal monster of unqualified evil."[56] If we consider Mansfield's production of *Dr. Jekyll and Mr. Hyde* as "*The Drama of the Drug*," as one critic sardonically advised, then the actor's deformed Hyde reified the coexisting biological and moralistic factors for drug dependence permitted by the late-century disease model of addiction, as well as the powerful authority of the disease itself. "[I]n spite of a crouching gait suggestive of physical weakness," one Boston critic remarked, "the spirit of sin was stamped so mightily upon him that he suggested brute strength that could well conquer whatever it attacked."[57] Echoing the marketing strategies for spectacular and "monstrous" bodies exhibited in dime museums, side shows, and lecture halls, a moralistic illness narrative enfreaked the character of Hyde. As the material outgrowth of Jekyll's addiction and an expression of his/its amoral appetites, the aggregate traits, gestures, and locomotions of Hyde's non-normative form externalized the disease within.

It was precisely Mansfield's material transformations that most encapsulated Dr. Jekyll's struggle to maintain control over his addiction. Just as in Stevenson's original text, Sullivan's script initially disaffiliates Jekyll from Hyde by concealing his first transformation offstage and introducing both identities to the audience separately. Jekyll is, in both his literary and theatrical renderings, a closeted addict laboring to compartmentalize and insulate his habit. Soon, however, several onstage transformations expose Jekyll's illness, compelling the audience to witness explicit and embellished spectacles of drug-taking. Whether Mansfield utilized special makeup, wigs, prosthetics, or mechanical apparatuses in his nightly metamorphoses became a disputed matter in the press; likely it was a combination of physical manipulations, quick-change artistry, and lighting effects (Jekyll was lit from above, Hyde from below).[58] The importance of these scenes, however, lay not in their illusionary merits. Hyde's transfiguration into Jekyll, detailed here by *The Daily Telegraph*, translated for the stage an addict's passage from withdrawal to satiation:

> The fiend grovels and begs for the priceless drug … At last Lanyon yields, and the deformed, shapeless, withered Hyde sinks in a heap on the floor, feverishly mixing the drug by the light of the winter fire, the red glow falling upon his towsled hair and revolting features. There is a pause but of an instant, when to the surprise and admiration of everybody, there arises, without screens, or gauzes, or traps, or anything, from the groveling, ill-dressed jabbery mass on the ground, the well-knit frame, the well-dressed body, and the pale, calm, clear-eyed face of the renewed Jekyll.[59]

The transformations, as part of Mansfield's larger composition of addiction, manifested the documented consequences of habitual drug-taking (exhilaration; loss of control; the transfiguring of body and identity; the relieving of withdrawal symptoms) and returning to sobriety (feelings of guilt and shame; memory loss; increased cravings and physical discomfort; the reemergence, perhaps, of the pre-consumption identity).

Mansfield's performance of addiction impelled commentators to explicitly compare or correlate his Jekyll/Hyde with other stage inebriates, including but not limited to Daniel Bandmann's competing portrayal of the dual roles, which

London critics summarily panned as a "wearisome" and ridiculous "harlequin-ade."[60] A closer counterpart of Mansfield's portrayal was Charles Warner's Jean Coupeau, the lead character of Charles Reade's social drama *Drink* (1879). Indeed, at the time of Mansfield's *Dr. Jekyll and Mr. Hyde*, Warner's career-making portrayal of Coupeau was the most acclaimed performance of addiction to date. *Drink*, a dramatization of Émile Zola's 1877 novel *L'Assommoir*, follows the descent of Coupeau, a once amiable mechanic and devoted family man, into the lowest depths of alcoholism. Though he is "cured" of his cravings by a stint in a hospital ward and pledges sobriety for the sake of his wife and daughter, his illness enslaves him again after the play's villainess swaps the claret he is ordered to drink with brandy. Coupeau strains to resist his old temptation before draining the bottle. Overtaken by a brutal assault of delirium tremens, replete with hallucinations, ravings, and paroxysmal seizures, Copeau succumbs to his disease.

Like Mansfield's *Dr. Jekyll and Mr. Hyde*, *Drink* profited almost solely from Warner's illness role, and the two performances often inspired direct comparisons. Warner's depiction "of a man crazed with drink and in the throes of delirium tremens can only be compared with Mansfield's impersonation of Mr. Hyde," asserted one critic, while another labeled it "a more minute, graphic, and terrible study of character than any which Sir Henry Irving ever gave; it makes Richard Mansfield's dual creation of Dr. Jekyll and Mr. Hyde seem like a babe in arms."[61] It is telling that out of the nearly twenty reviews on Warner's Coupeau, only one mentioned the role's affiliation to mid-century stage alcoholics like W. H. Smith's Edward Middleton. Rather, the repeated linkage of Warner's and Mansfield's inebriates implies that critics considered both only distantly related to the agonies of the melodramatic drunkard. Operating within the Zolaist milieu of *Drink*, Warner reconstituted the performance of alcoholism by infusing it with naturalistic details (or what one reviewer labeled "photographic acting") while Mansfield, whose performance of drug addiction (and particularly Hyde) pivoted on and articulated itself through somatic expressivity, professed on countless occasions that his approach to Jekyll/Hyde was first and foremost a study in psychology.[62] The discrepancy between Mansfield's reputedly lofty aims in embodying Jekyll/Hyde and the performance's popular reception vexed the actor greatly. According to Franklyn Fyles:

> He read Stevenson's tale with keen appreciation of its astonishing psychology ... He longed for a purely intellectual exploit; to distinguish himself by exposing what took place inside of the amiable Dr. Jekyll in his shifts of soul to the cruel Mr. Hyde and back again; and he did that explicitly enough to be seen clearly by all who looked for it; but far more impressive to the multitude than the mental transitions was the transformation of palpable matter.[63]

American and British critics judged the merits of Mansfield's *Dr. Jekyll and Mr. Hyde* similarly: the script itself was formulaic and uninspiring, but the actor's protean efforts in the dual roles impressed critics and frightened susceptible theatregoers. London critics were more vociferous in their critiques of Mansfield's sympathetic Jekyll, whose "wavy gestures and transpontine flourishes" in act one, "beloved no doubt in America," left *The Daily Telegraph* unmoved; Mansfield's Dr. Jekyll was "a mixture of a smug young shopwalker and an aesthetic curate, who wishes to be well with the ladies," mused *The Pall Mall Gazette*. Still, despite largely analogous reviews printed in Boston, New York, and London labeling Mansfield's *tour de force* a "must see," his engagement at the Lyceum Theatre failed to sell enough tickets to recuperate tour and production costs. Perhaps the critics' cynicism dissuaded London theatregoers from attending, or perhaps the well-publicized rivalry with Bandmann tarnished Mansfield's reputation in the eyes of the public. However, it is likely the timing of Mansfield's Lyceum residency factored into ticket sales. Just three days after Mansfield's production premiered on August 4, 1888, the stabbed body of prostitute Martha Tabram was found in the East London neighborhood of Whitechapel. Three weeks later, Whitechapel police discovered the first in a series of brutally mutilated corpses of women, instigating citywide panic and the manhunt for the soon-to-be-christened Jack the Ripper. Journalists and theatregoers quickly linked the diabolical Hyde of Stevenson's imagination and Mansfield's representation to the Whitechapel murders; the timing seemed just too coincidental to some of the Lyceum's bourgeois theatregoers, though Whitechapel residents, accustomed to witnessing violence and sexual assaults against women on a more regular basis, were doubtless skeptical of the correlation.[64] Some commentators wondered if Ripper had sat among Mansfield's spectators, finding inspiration in the macabre tale; others recommended that the police study Mansfield's Hyde so as to better understand Ripper's mind; still others deduced that the murderer must be living a double life similar to Jekyll and Hyde. Of particular interest were Mansfield's seamless transformations from gentleman to fiend and Hyde's misogynistic savagery, both suspected to be Ripper *modi operandi*. One night before the famous double murder of Elizabeth Stride and Catherine Eddowes, *Dr. Jekyll and Mr. Hyde* closed, its final night having been advertised for two weeks and not the result of public pressure, as newspapers speculated.

In a remarkable piece of theatre history, the City of London Police received a tip urging them to consider Mansfield a suspect in the Ripper case. "I have A great likeing for acters," the concerned citizen wrote in the October 5th letter, "So that I should be the Last to think because A man take a dretfull Part he is therefore Bad but when I went to see Mr Mansfield Take the Part of Dr Jekel & Mr Hyde I felt at once that he was the Man Wanted & I have not been able to get this Feeling out of my Head."[65] Despite the citizen's urging that the actor be under surveillance, Mansfield was quickly ruled out as a legitimate suspect. Mansfield's association with the Ripper case moves beyond the anecdotal when reconceived as an extra-theatrical outgrowth of the Jekyll/Hyde illness narrative. The character of Dr. Jekyll contributed much to the sensational icon of the mad doctor, which emerged in the 1880s "from pre-existing anxieties relating to the conduct of medicine in general and journalistic anxieties about middle-class men in particular," as the Ripper's penchant for surgically dissecting corpses situated the medical man in "a sinister light."[66] In both Stevenson's text and Sullivan's script, the doctor's "madness" is triggered and accelerated by psychotropic drugs; so too is the entirety of Hyde and his spectrum of malignant acts, including sexual aggressiveness and murder. Medicine, madness, and violence (sexual or otherwise) are thus triangulated in the dual role of Jekyll/Hyde, a synergetic formula for criminal evildoing that found resonance in the Whitechapel case.

The anatomy of a *fin-de-siècle* addict

Before leaving Holmes and Jekyll to their chemical devices, it is important to acknowledge the one challenge shared by those theorizing and treating addiction in the nineteenth century: how to judge addiction's intangible effects on an individual's selfhood and public identity. The physical markers of addiction (puncture wounds, chapped lips) may have been easy to spot, but the internal consequences were extremely varied and difficult to decipher, particularly given the relative newness of drug addiction discourse. Contemplating the links between addiction and identity in the works of novelist and opium addict William Burroughs, Janet Farrell Brodie and Marc Redfield offer:

> [A]ddiction destroys identity not by attacking it from the outside, but by usurping the origin or identity of identity itself. This is the predicament Ronell calls 'Being-on-drugs.' There is no natural identity. Yet there is also no god to set its guarantee on an originary moment of artifice, a 'constructedness' that could guarantee the identity of identity.[67]

While I disagree that addicts are not in possession of a "natural identity," the concept of identity usurpation is instructive. Many addicts struggled with how to define themselves as drug users publicly or privately, trying on various roles (victim, slave, demon, thrill-seeker, experimenter, innocent) until one or several fit, effectively bisecting their lifelines into *B.D.* and *A.D.* (Before Drugs and After Drugs). The words of one opium addict reflect such a dividedness: "Once, I was a prosperous, respected man; now I have lost property, health, character, money, *everything*. I expect to die a pauper and in debt, and leave to my family nothing but the heavy cloud that hangs over my name."[68] Much of what separates the theatricalized addictions of Sherlock Holmes and Henry Jekyll is dependent upon their ability to integrate their illnesses with their pre-addiction identities. While Holmes's dependency seems an organic and indivisible part of his identity (to the extent that his pre-addiction identity is both unimaginable and unimportant), Jekyll's very core rebels at incorporating addiction into the "good doctor's" identity, thereby spawning an intra-identity whose dominant trait *is* addiction: Hyde. And yet as a "Being-on-drugs" Jekyll persists as an unstable entity, his selfhood constantly under threat of usurpation.

As a hyper-functional addict, Gillette's Holmes represented a faction of habitués who reported leading conventional lives despite decades of using drugs, seamlessly incorporating their habits into their existences and identities. Gillette strengthened Holmes's position as the performative surrogate for society's durable addicts by integrating the detective's public pursuits and private pleasures. Though Holmes professes to have no need of cocaine while investigating a case, he injects cocaine directly before discussing with Watson his ongoing, *fourteen-month* pursuit of Professor Moriarty, a case that "is now rapidly approaching a singularly diverting climax," Holmes pronounces.[69] His productiveness as a systematic drug user—particularly in balancing his habituation with the demands of his perilous career—enhanced the character's singularity. Reviews persistently interwove Holmes's drug use with his detective work, such as Amy Leslie's report that the play was "resurrected from the chronicles of [Doyle's] fascinating *dopey sleuth*, a hitherto unveiled episode in that irresistible gentleman's *pipe-and-needle career* of noticing things."[70] Because Holmes's addiction is already present at both his literary and theatrical introductions, it is a fully constitutive component of his selfhood, posing no mutating or destabilizing threat to a pre-addiction identity. Gillette's "adventurous cocaine victim," it would seem, wore his drug habit with the same nonchalant ease that he did his deerskin hat.[71] If Holmes's identity effortlessly *subsumed* his habituation, addiction forcefully destabilized and *consumed* Jekyll's identity. And yet, through Jekyll's sympathetic asides and discussions of the "good doctor" by other characters, the specter of his pre-addiction identity lingered over the drama's action as if wanting to be reunited with its master. The public persona Jekyll contrived to preserve his bourgeois standing, then, is both a shadow figure of what he once was and a decoy to distract from what he has become. Straining to conceal his shame, Mansfield's Jekyll deviated from the novella's more unapologetic drug experimenter and strengthened the role's kinship to the reluctant addicts given prominence in disease theory discourse.

But if the actor's Jekyll epitomized the diseased addict of the late Victorian imagination, what do we make of his Hyde? He was, above all else, the result of a degenerative fracturing of Jekyll's pre-addiction identity through the transfiguring force of drugs. As such, Hyde is defined by his corruption of Jekyll's prized normativity. For Thomas Reed, Hyde can be understood as "the altered state of being in which Jekyll feels comfortable indulging his morally troublesome appetites," an assertion surely applicable to Mansfield's portrayal.[72] Brian Rose conceives of Mansfield's Hyde as a monstrous receptacle for Victorian society's most stigmatized, socially corrosive behaviors: Hyde drinks, murders, leers at women, and walks disreputable neighborhoods under the glow of gaslight.[73] Despite Edward Hyde's legitimate status as a gentleman (which is, of course, reliant upon Jekyll's professional ranking), in both Stevenson and Mansfield's renderings he possesses no sense of bourgeois propriety unless prompted by other similarly classed men of superior ethics. In Mansfield's performance, Hyde's instinctual behavior and comportment align him with the stereotypical lower-class brute of Victorian myth, particularly his ill-fitting clothing, affinity for drink, stooped posture, habitual incivility, and blatant disrespect for women. Even his private lodgings, which stage renderings of the 1887 premiere production show as appointed with the chic furnishings of a prosperous bachelor, are located in Soho, London's entertainment district of theatres, music halls, brothels, and gambling dens, not of desirable middle-class residences.[74] Whereas Mansfield presented Jekyll's diseased condition as the result of audacious scientific experimentation, Hyde's behavior flows conversely. As a spontaneous "Being-on-drugs" (for there is no Hyde before the red liquid and white powder), Mansfield's monster represented the dangers posed to genteel society by the deviant drug use of a corruptible lower class. The novella's Mr. Hyde is both of Dr. Jekyll and apart from Dr. Jekyll. Mansfield's embodied Hyde—who walked "alone," operated without Jekyll's express directives, and barely resembled his host—transposed and intensified Stevenson's dystopic premise.

I propose that Mansfield's Hyde is best appreciated as a personification: Hyde-as-addiction. In this strategy, Hyde's malignity corresponds to both the adverse qualities of addictive narcotics and the disease that results from their habitual consumption, a disease of immeasurable leverage and unpredictability. According to Stacey Margolis, the *fin-de-siècle* term "addiction" encompassed two forms of desire: the desire ascribed to the victim and the desire ascribed to the drug itself. Because the disease theory of addiction endowed drugs with the potential to permanently modify the habitué's psychophysical and biochemical health, many writers warned that the repentant addict's desire for sobriety was often no match for a more powerful competing force: the desire of the narcotic itself to enslave its human host. As Margolis argues, this proposition bore hallmarks of the characteristic personification of alcohol (the "demon" drink) by temperance reformers:

> Indeed, according to a common description of inebriety, alcohol, once ingested, does not evoke a monstrous desire in the drinker so much as replace the individual agent with its own monstrous agency … From this perspective, the problem with the addict is not that he desires too much or too freely, but that he stops desiring altogether. Since the user is actually replaced by the drug, addiction here is constituted not by the self that wants the drug, but the drug that wants itself.[75]

Just as liquor retained the dehumanizing pronoun *it* even in its personified form, several critics referred to Mansfield's character as an *it*, a creature bereft of humanizing masculinity. By act four, when "Hyde has become the master of Jekyll," the desires of the drug/addiction (Hyde) are no longer containable by the hostile addict (Jekyll).[76] Such an interpretation helps to justify Mansfield's predominantly physical portrayal of Hyde, for Hyde-as-addiction's "evil" must be materially determined, not mentally or emotionally. In this way, Mansfield's ape-like Hyde is the proverbial monkey on Jekyll's back.

Traditionally dismissed as crowd-pleasing, superficial fare, Gillette's Sherlock Homes and Mansfield's Jekyll and Hyde warrant increased critical attention as the groundbreaking embodiments of nineteenth-century drug addicts. Gillette exemplified the quintessential bourgeois "brainworker" of Conan Doyle's creation, an isolated intellectual whose cocaine habit staved off mental stagnation and melancholy. Yet by deepening the moral complexities of drug habituation in the playscript and downplaying cocainism's biological and psychological effects in performance, Gillette located Holmes's "moderate" drug use in ambiguous terrain. Mansfield's Jekyll, in contrast, was hooked on drugs from his first voyage into Hyde's world. That the phials of liquid and powder possessed addictive properties was irrefutable in Sullivan's adaptation; otherwise, the actor's righteous physician would have destroyed the remaining stores of the drug, and Hyde with them. Unlike the novella's Jekyll, whose egocentric ambition and reclusiveness partially insulated society against the horrors of Hyde, Mansfield's reincorporation of Jekyll into polite society elevated the stakes of drug addiction to the level of a public threat, a change that substantiated *fin-de-siècle* fears of a societal drug epidemic. The Edward Hyde of Mansfield's invention appeared even more diabolical and diseased than Stevenson's, the chemical monster to Jekyll's human martyr. *Sherlock Holmes* and *Dr. Jekyll and Mr. Hyde* anchored the actors' repertoires for the remainder of their careers, and both Gillette's Holmes and Mansfield's Jekyll/Hyde contributed to a germinal optics of performed addiction only partly indebted to prior methods of staging alcoholism.[77] Commonalities in where the actors located the physical effects of their characters' drug habituation—in the gestures of nervous fingers, in dreamy or unfocused glances, in postural shifts—partially bridged the stylistic and tonal chasms between their representations.

By the 1910s and 1920s, scientific and legislative measures in the United States and Britain recolored the gray areas of the *fin-de-siècle* drug problem in black and white, pathologizing and criminalizing even controlled habitués like Holmes and repentant addicts like Jekyll. Reflective of this gradual revision, Progressive Era—and to a lesser extent Edwardian—addiction plays delimited the spectrum of stage addicts to the most slovenly, villainous, or victimized. Clyde Fitch's *The City* (1909), Eugene O'Neill's *The Web* (1913), and Pendleton King's *Cocaine* (1917), for example, depicted drug addicts as blackmailers, suicidal lovers, abusers, and murderers, though none of these dramas feature onstage drug use. A xenophobic subgenre of plays emerging at the turn of the century led audiences inside dimly lit opium dens, where male and female addicts fed their habits and racialized (often Chinese) purveyors drugged white women in order to kidnap and sell them, associating drug use with prostitution, white slavery, poverty, and immigrant criminality. British playwright Frederick Lonsdale's *The Fake* (1924) even presented a case for justifiable homicide of an abusive drug and alcohol inebriate by means of a lethal overdose.[78] Just as Victorian medicine's shifting and inconclusive theories on drug use set the stage for protagonist-addicts like Holmes and Jekyll (the sympathetic half of the Jekyll/Hyde dyad), the aggressive legislative policies and stigmatizing medical practices of the early twentieth century encouraged antagonist-addicts to flourish in popular culture. Mansfield's Hyde, therefore, proved a harbinger of things to come. Unrefined, lustful, and raging, Hyde operated as a performative blueprint for the next century's archetypal addict, the criminalized "drug fiend": corrupted, diseased, barely human, and beyond repair.

Notes

1 This stage picture was lampooned in one of the many theatrical parodies of *Sherlock Holmes* entitled *Sheerluck Holmes*. In an illustration of the skit featuring actors Montgomery and Stone as Holmes and Watson ("Quick, Watson, The Needle!"), Holmes, with eyes bulging beneath his deerskin hat, wields a gigantic hypodermic needle of at least a foot's length. Unidentified newspaper clipping, Sherlock Holmes clippings file, HTC.

2 Irving S. Saposnik, "The Anatomy of *Dr. Jekyll and Mr. Hyde*," *Studies in English Literature, 1500–1900* 11, no. 4 (Autumn 1971): 715–731.

3 Arthur Conan Doyle, *The Adventure of the Missing Three-Quarter*, in *The Return of Sherlock Holmes* (New York: P.F. Collier & Son, 1905), 291–381.

4 Martin Booth, *The Doctor and the Detective: A Biography of Sir Arthur Conan Doyle* (New York: Thomas Dunne Books, 2000), 151.

5 Charles Collins, "The Stage: Sherlock Holmes," *Chicago Tribune*, Feb 26, 1930, "The Players' Collection" portfolio, William Gillette, BRTC.

6 Unidentified New York newspaper clipping, Clippings File, Sherlock Holmes, BRTC.

7 "Sherlock Holmes as Played by William Gillette: A. Conan Doyle's Master Sleuth as Mr. Gillette Acted the Character and Made It His," *New York Post*, May 1, 1937, William Gillette Clippings File, BRTC.

8 William Hooker Gillette and Arthur Conan Doyle, *Sherlock Holmes*, in *The Plays of William Hooker Gillette*, ed. Rosemary Cullen and Don B. Wilmeth (Cambridge: Cambridge University Press, 1983), 193–272, 230.

9 Joseph McLaughlin, *Writing the Urban Jungle: Reading Empire in London from Doyle to Eliot* (Charlottesville: University Press of Virginia, 2000), 59.

10 Alan Dale, *New York Journal and Advertiser*, Nov 7, 1899, Sherlock Holmes Clippings File, BRTC.

11 Pasquale Accardo, *Diagnosis and Detection: The Medical Iconography of Sherlock Holmes* (Rutherford: Fairleigh Dickinson University Press, 1987), 88.

12 James W. Maertens, "Masculine Power and the Ideal Reasoner: Sherlock Holmes, Technician-Hero," in *Sherlock Holmes: Victorian Sleuth to Modern Hero*, eds. Charles R. Putney, Joseph A. Cutshall King, and Sally Sugarman (Lanham: Scarecrow, 1996), 308.

13 Douglas Small, "Sherlock Holmes and Cocaine: A 7% Solution for Modern Professionalism," *English-Language Literature in Transition, 1880–1920* 58, no. 3 (2015): 341–364, 347.

14 Amy Leslie, "Gillette is a Sleuth: Brilliant Builder of Comedies Invents Exciting Melodrama for Sherlock Holmes," unnamed newspaper, Dec 5, 1900, Sherlock Holmes Clippings File, HTC.

15 William Gillette, *The Illusion of the First Time in Acting*, intro. George Arliss (New York: Dramatic Museum of Columbia University, 1915), 45.

16 Quoted in Doris E. Cook, *Sherlock Holmes and Much More; or some of the facts about William Gillette* (Hartford: The Connecticut Historical Society, 1970), 55, BRTC.

17 "Gillette was Pioneer in 'Natural,'" *New York Times*, Dec 17, 1929, scrapbook on William Gillette's farewell tour, BRTC.

18 Norman Hapgood, *The Stage in America, 1897–1900*, v. 1 (New York: Macmillan, 1901), 69.

19 Gillette, *Illusion of the First Time*, 38.

20 Montrose J. Moses, "William Gillette Says Farewell: A Veteran of Three Generations of the American Theatre," reprinted from *Theatre Guild Magazine* (Jan 1930), William Gillette Clippings File, BRTC.

21 Unidentified newspaper clipping, BRTC.

22 Roland Burke Hennessy, "New Plays in New York," *Broadway Magazine* 4, no. 4 (Jan 1900), 254; and Lewis C. Strang, *Famous Actors of the Day in America* (1900), 92, quoted in Zecher, *William Gillette*, 301.

23 "Sherlock Holmes," *The Era*, Sept 7, 1901.

24 "Lyceum Theatre," *The Times* (London), Sept 10, 1901.

25 "Mr. William Gillette as Sherlock Holmes," *Candid Friend*, Sept 14, 1901; and "Sherlock Holmes at the Lyceum Theatre," *The Tatler*, Sept 18, 1901.

26 J.T. Grein, *Dramatic Criticism*, v. 3 (Greening and Co., 1902), 257–260, quoted in Zecher, *William Gillette*, 321.

27 "At the Theaters, William Gillette as 'Sherlock Holmes' at the New National," *Washington Post*, Nov 20, 1900.

28 Garff B. Wilson, "Richard Mansfield: Actor of the Transition," *Educational Theatre Journal* 14, no. 1 (March 1962): 38–43, 40–41.

29 Richard Mansfield, "Man and the Actor," *Atlantic Monthly* (May 1906).

30 For biographical information, acting descriptions, and personality sketches of Mansfield, see Clayton Hamilton, "Richard Mansfield: The Man," *The North American Review* (Jan 1908): 60–69; Eaward Wagenknecht, "Richard Mansfield: Portrait of an Actor," *The Sewanee Review* 38, no. 2 (1930): 150–160; Wilson, "Richard Mansfield"; Paul Wilstach, *Richard Mansfield, the Man and the Actor* (London: Chapman & Hall, 1908); and William Winter, *Life and Art of Richard Mansfield*, vols. 1 and 2 (New York: Yard and Co., 1910).

31 Unidentified newspaper clipping, Richard Mansfield Clippings File, BRTC.

32 Wagenknecht, "Richard Mansfield," 152. See also James O'Donnell Bennett, "Richard Mansfield," *Munsey's Magazine* (March 1907), Richard Mansfield Clippings File, BRTC.

33 Winter, *Life and Art*, I, 331–332.

34 "The Biggest Hits of the Old Days: The Most Popular Plays and Musical Comedies of the American Stage, No. 86 – Richard Mansfield as Dr. Jekyll and Mr. Hyde," *The Post*, Dec 20, 1933, Jekyll and Hyde Clippings File, HTC.

35 *Daily Telegraph*, reprinted in unidentified American newspaper clipping, Jekyll and Hyde Clippings File, HTC.

36 Sullivan, *Dr. Jekyll and Mr. Hyde*, in *Jekyll and Hyde Dramatized*, 53.

37 *Illustrated Sporting and Dramatic News*, July 28, 1888, BRTC.

38 Unidentified review, *Boston Home Journal* reprinted from the *London Times*, Aug 1888, Clippings File, Jekyll and Hyde, HTC. William Winter avowed that: "Mr. Mansfield rises to a nobler height than [the acting of Hyde] – for he is able[,] in concurrent and associate impersonation of Dr. Jekyll, to interblend the angel with the demon, and thus to command a lasting victory, such as his baleful image of the hellish Hyde could never, separately, achieve … [He presents] the image of a man who is convulsed, lacerated, and ultimately destroyed by a terrific and fatal struggle within the theatre of his own soul and body." William Winter, "Richard Mansfield as Dr. Jekyll and Mr. Hyde," *New York Tribune*, Sept 13, 1887, Jekyll and Hyde Clippings File, HTC.

39 James O'Donnell Bennett, "Music and the Drama," *Chicago Record-Herald*, Nov 29, 1903, Fred G. Ross Scrapbooks, vol. 1, BRTC.

40 "Mansfield and Bandmann," *Athenaeum* reprinted in *Boston Post*, Aug 22, 1888, Jekyll and Hyde Clippings File, HTC; and "Dr. Jekyll and Mr. Hyde," *Boston Evening Transcript*, May 10, 1887, Jekyll and Hyde Clippings File, HTC.

41 *London Letter*, Aug 9, 1888, reprinted in *New York Mirror*, Aug 25, 1888, Jekyll and Hyde Clippings File, HTC. For the *Pall Mall Budget*, "[I]t is difficult to understand how an actor who is possessed of such abilities as Mr. Mansfield should show us a Jekyll who is a mixture of a smug young shop-walker and an aesthetic curate, who wishes to be well

with the ladies." "The Nightmare at the Lyceum," *Pall Mall Budget*, Aug 9, 1888, Jekyll and Hyde Clippings File, BRTC.

42 *The Boston Post*, May 10, 1887, Jekyll and Hyde Clippings File, HTC.
43 "Dr. Jekyll and Mr. Hyde," *Boston Evening Transcript*, May 10, 1887, Jekyll and Hyde Clippings File, HTC.
44 "The Real Dr. Jekyll and Mr. Hyde, An Interview with Mr. Richard Mansfield," *Pall Mall Gazette*, July 24, 1888; and "A Chat with Richard Mansfield," *The Star*, July 27, 1888, reprinted in *Jekyll and Hyde Dramatized*, 105.
45 "The Real Dr. Jekyll and Mr. Hyde," *Pall Mall Gazette*, July 24, 1888.
46 Mara L. Keire, "Dope Fiends and Degenerates: The Gendering of Addiction in the Early Twentieth Century," *Journal of Social History* 31, no. 4 (Summer 1998): 809–822, 812.
47 "Mansfield vs. Stevenson: New and Interesting Conceptions of Dr. Jekyll and Mr. Hyde," *New York Sun*, Jan 1, 1888.
48 Eduard Levinstein, *Morbid Craving for Morphia* (London: Smith, Elder: 1878), 11–14 and 16.
49 "The Nightmare at the Lyceum," *Pall Mall Budget*, Aug 9, 1888.
50 Stevenson, *Jekyll and Hyde*, 52.
51 "Mansfield vs. Stevenson," *New York Sun*, Jan 1, 1888.
52 "The Nightmare at the Lyceum," *Pall Mall Gazette*, Aug 7, 1888. Describing for their readers the bizarre character and physicality of Mansfield's Mr. Hyde, critics tapped a wide array of notable literary and theatrical figures. In a rash of contemporary reviews, the actor's Hyde was pronounced "an intensified murderous Quilp" with "a Uriah Heep bearing," "a monster more mis-shapen than Caliban; more demonical than Quasimodo; more ghastly than Hugo's '*homme qui rit*,'" "[akin to] the Frankensteins and Vampires and all their uncanny brood," "the compound of Quilp and Caliban," "as ghastly a mixture of Quilp, Quasimodo, and the 'Man Cat' of the old Victorian Theatre as can be imagined," "a sickening compound of greedy Ghoul, of hideous Leprechaun, and dream-haunted Jabberwock," and perhaps my favorite, "[possessing] the manners of Quilp and the methods of the demon lobster." Such clearly exaggerated references encourage readers to imagine Mansfield's creation as a demon of the highest caliber: monstrous, deformed, paranormal, and profoundly malevolent. Unidentified newspaper clipping, Mar. 22, 1906, Clippings File, Jekyll and Hyde, HTC; unidentified Boston newspaper, May 14, 1887, HTC; *Piccadilly*, Aug 9, 1888, 120, BRTC; "Lyceum Theatre," *The Daily Telegraph*, Aug 6, 1888, reprinted in *Jekyll and Hyde Dramatized*, 123; "The Nightmare at the Lyceum," *Pall Mall Budget*, Aug 9, 1888, BRTC; "Dr. Jekyll and Mr. Hyde," unknown newspaper, Sept 22, 1888, HTC; "Lyceum Theatre," *The Daily Telegraph*, Aug 6, 1888, reprinted in *Jekyll and Hyde Dramatized*, 123; and *The Illustrated Sporting and Dramatic News*, Aug 18, 1888, 695, BRTC.
53 "Mansfield and Bandmann," *Athenaeum* reprinted in *Boston Post*, Aug 22, 1888, Jekyll and Hyde Clippings File, HTC.
54 "Mansfield and Bandmann: Condemning the Rival Version of Dr. Jekyll and Mr. Hyde," Labouchere's *London Letter*, reprinted in *Kansas City Star*, Aug 13, 1888, Jekyll and Hyde Clippings File, HTC; and William Winter, "Richard Mansfield as Dr. Jekyll and Mr. Hyde," *New York Tribune*, Sept 13, 1887.
55 "Mansfield as Jekyll and Hyde, New Amsterdam Theatre," unidentified newspaper clipping, Mar 22, 1906, HTC; and *London Letter*, Aug 9, 1888, reprinted in *New York Mirror*, Aug 25, 1888.
56 William Winter, "Richard Mansfield as Dr. Jekyll and Mr. Hyde," *New York Tribune*, Sept 13, 1887, Jekyll and Hyde Clippings File, HTC.
57 "The Theatre," unidentified newspaper clipping, April 15, 1888, Jekyll and Hyde Clippings File, HTC; and unidentified Boston newspaper clipping, Jekyll and Hyde Clippings File, HTC.
58 Martin A. Dahanay and Alex Chisholm point out that Mansfield himself would have bristled at being called a "quick-change artist" in *Dr. Jekyll and Mr. Hyde*, as he considered himself a serious theatre artist and not a street performer *Jekyll and Hyde Dramatized*, 32.

59 "Lyceum Theatre," *The Daily Telegraph*, Aug 6, 1888, reprinted in *Jekyll and Hyde Dramatized*, 124.
60 "Opera Comique Theatre," *Daily Telegraph*, Aug 7, 1888; and "Plays and Players," *Sunday Times*, Aug 12, 1888. Reprints of Bandmann reviews appear in Danahay and Chisholm's *Jekyll and Hyde Dramatized*, 163–166.
61 "Zola Parodied," unidentified newspaper clipping, Drink Clippings File, BRTC and unidentified newspaper clipping, Drink Clippings File, BRTC.
62 "Mr. Charles Warner in 'Drink,' The Academy," unidentified newspaper clipping, Drink Clippings File, BRTC.
63 Franklyn Fyles, "What Was Mansfield's Influence on the American Drama?," *American Review of Reviews* (Oct 1907), 430, Scrapbook, Bibbee, BRTC.
64 Alan Sharp, "The Strange Case of Dr. Jekyll and Saucy Jacky," *The Ripperologist*, no. 5 (2004), reprinted in *Casebook: Jack the Ripper*, Stephen P. Ryder, ed. www.casebook.org.
65 M.P., "Letter to City of London Police, naming Mansfield as Murderer," Oct 5, 1888, reprinted in *Jekyll and Hyde Dramatized*, 180. I have retained the original letter's spelling and punctuation.
66 Smith, *Victorian Demons*, 7.
67 Brodie and Redfield, "Introduction," in *High Anxieties: Cultural Studies in Addiction* (Berkeley: University of California Press, 2002), 9.
68 Keeley, "Experiences," in *Yesterday's Addicts*, H. Wayne Morgan (Norman: University of Oklahoma Press, 1974): 112.
69 Gillette and Conan Doyle, *Sherlock Holmes*, 227 (act two, scene two).
70 Leslie, "Gillette is a Sleuth," Dec 5, 1900.
71 Unidentified New York newspaper clipping of Garrick Theatre production, Sherlock Holmes Clippings File, BRTC.
72 Reed, *The Transforming Draught*, 9.
73 Rose, Jekyll and Hyde *Adapted*, 39.
74 Reprints of the production's stage renderings can be found in C. Alex Pinkston, Jr.'s "The Stage Premiere of Dr. Jekyll and Mr. Hyde," *Nineteenth-Century Theatre and Film* 14, no. 1–2 (1986): 21–44, 30.
75 Stacey Margolis, "Addiction and the Ends of Desire," in *High Anxieties*, 21–22.
76 "The Nightmare at the Lyceum," *Pall Mall Budget*, Aug 9, 1888.
77 Gillette played Holmes until age 79 and Mansfield last embodied Jekyll/Hyde six months before his death in 1907.
78 Clyde Fitch, *The City* (Boston: Little, Brown, and Co., 1915); Eugene O'Neill, *The Web*, in *Ten "Lost" Plays* (New York: Dover Publications, 1995), 49–70; Pendleton King, *Cocaine*, in *The Provincetown Plays*, eds. George Cram Cook and Frank Shay (Cincinnati: Stewart Kidd Company, 1921), 71–94; Frederick Lonsdale, *The Fake: A Play in Three Acts* (New York: Samuel French, 1926). The opium den plays *The Bowery After Dark*, *From Broadway to the Bowery*, *From Rags to Riches*, and *The Queen of Chinatown* are discussed in J. Chris Westgate's *Staging the Slums, Slumming the Stage: Class, Poverty, Ethnicity, and Sexuality in American Theatre, 1890–1916* (New York: Palgrave Macmillan, 2014). See also Max Shulman, "The American Pipe Dream: Drug Addiction on Stage, 1890–1940" (PhD diss., Tufts University, 2016).

Bibliography

Accardo, Pasquale. *Diagnosis and Detection: The Medical Iconography of Sherlock Holmes*. Rutherford: Fairleigh Dickinson University Press, 1987.
Booth, Martin. *The Doctor and the Detective: A Biography of Sir Arthur Conan Doyle*. New York: Thomas Dunne Books, 2000.
Brodie, Janet Farrell and Marc Redfield, eds. *High Anxieties: Cultural Studies in Addiction*. Berkeley: University of California Press, 2002.

Conan Doyle, Arthur. *The Adventure of the Missing Three-Quarter.* In *The Return of Sherlock Holmes,* 291–381. New York: P.F. Collier & Son, 1905.

Danahay, Martin A. and Alex Chisholm, eds. *Jekyll and Hyde Dramatized: The 1887 Richard Mansfield Script and the Evolution of the Story on Stage.* Jefferson: McFarland, 2005.

Fitch, Clyde. *The City.* Boston: Little, Brown, and Co., 1915.

Gillette, William. *The Illusion of the First Time in Acting.* Introduction by George Arliss. New York: Dramatic Museum of Columbia University, 1915.

Gillette, William Hooker and Arthur Conan Doyle. *Sherlock Holmes.* In *The Plays of William Hooker Gillette,* edited by Rosemary Cullen and Don B. Wilmeth, 193–272. Cambridge: Cambridge University Press, 1983.

Hapgood, Norman. *The Stage in America, 1897–1900.* v. 1. New York: Macmillan, 1901.

Keire, Mara L. "Dope Fiends and Degenerates: The Gendering of Addiction in the Early Twentieth Century." *Journal of Social History* 31, no. 4 (Summer 1998): 809–822.

King, Pendleton. *Cocaine.* In *The Provincetown Plays,* edited by George Cram Cook and Frank Shay, 71–94. Cincinnati: Stewart Kidd Company, 1921.

Levinstein, Eduard. *Morbid Craving for Morphia.* London: Smith, Elder: 1878.

Lonsdale, Frederick. *The Fake: A Play in Three Acts.* New York: Samuel French, 1926.

Maertens, James W. "Masculine Power and the Ideal Reasoner: Sherlock Holmes, Technician-Hero." In *Sherlock Holmes: Victorian Sleuth to Modern Hero,* edited by Charles Putney, Joseph A. Cutshall King, and Sally Sugarman, 296–322. Lanham: Scarecrow, 1996.

Margolis, Stacey. "Addiction and the Ends of Desire." In Brodie and Redfield, *High Anxieties,* 19–37.

McLaughlin, Joseph. *Writing the Urban Jungle: Reading Empire in London from Doyle to Eliot* Charlottesville: University Press of Virginia, 2000.

Morgan, H. Wayne. *Yesterday's Addicts: American Society and Drug Abuse, 1865–1920.* Norman: University of Oklahoma Press, 1974.

O'Neill, Eugene. *The Web.* In *Ten "Lost" Plays,* 49–70. New York: Dover Publications, 1995.

Pinkston, Jr., C. Alex. "The Stage Premiere of *Dr. Jekyll and Mr. Hyde.*" *Nineteenth-Century Theatre and Film* 14, no. 1-2 (1986): 21–44.

Reed, Jr., Thomas L. *The Transforming Draught:* Jekyll and Hyde, *Robert Louis Stevenson and the Victorian Alcohol Debate.* Jefferson: McFarland, 2006.

Rose, Brian A. Jekyll and Hyde *Adapted: Dramatizations of Cultural Anxiety.* Westport: Greenwood Press: 1996.

Saposnik, Irving S. "The Anatomy of *Dr. Jekyll and Mr. Hyde.*" *Studies in English Literature, 1500-1900* 11, no. 4 (Autumn 1971): 715–731.

Shulman, Max. "The American Pipe Dream: Drug Addiction on Stage, 1890–1940." PhD dissertation. Tufts University, 2016.

Small, Douglas. "Sherlock Holmes and Cocaine: A 7% Solution for Modern Professionalism," *English-Language Literature in Transition, 1880–1920* 58, no. 3 (2015): 341–364.

Westgate, J. Chris. *Staging the Slums, Slumming the Stage: Class, Poverty, Ethnicity, and Sexuality in American Theatre, 1890–1916.* New York: Palgrave Macmillan, 2014.

Wilson, Garff B. "Richard Mansfield: Actor of the Transition." *Educational Theatre Journal* 14, no. 1 (March 1962): 38–43.

Wilstach, Paul. *Richard Mansfield, the Man and the Actor.* London: Chapman & Hall, 1908.

Winter, William. *Life and Art of Richard Mansfield.* Vols. 1 and 2. New York: Yard and Co., 1910.

Part III
Performing mental illness

5 The madwoman in the theatre

Normalizing the disordered female mind in Ellen Terry's Lyceum repertoire

In September of 1895, London's *The Era* published a short piece entitled "The Rose Norreys Fund."[1] "Miss Rose Norreys, early on Tuesday morning, Aug. 20th, was found in Upper George-street, Marylebone, quite delirious" the item begins sensationally. Miss Norreys, the reader soon discovers, was taken first to a workhouse and then "removed" six days later to Colney Hatch, a prominent London psychiatric hospital (or, to use Victorian parlance, lunatic asylum). As for the reason for Miss Norreys' extended detainment, *The Era* reports that "she suffers chiefly from the delusion that she is persecuted." While Rose Norreys' name is now quite unknown to us, in the late 1880s and early 1890s, she was hailed by critics as a rising star of the London stage, proficient in classical works and comedies but perhaps best-suited to the period's modern social dramas and melodramas. As the piece's title indicates, *The Era* has reputedly altruistic purposes in divulging Norreys' troubles: the actress will soon be released from Colney Hatch because of her improved mental state, and, as the newspaper declares, "a long period of rest and seclusion in the country is urgently needed; but this will, of course cost money." The paper announces the creation of a subscription fund to help support Norreys during her recovery, printing the names of subscribers as well as their pledged donations. Another more extensive article on Norreys' condition appearing in the same issue speculates on the toll the acting profession takes on its most gifted delegates, arguing that "the born actor or actress is, like all artists, keenly impressionable. Hard and severe nervous strain, acting on an organization of this kind, is often too great for the brain to bear."[2] But, the article remarks, actors and actresses respond differently to this overtaxation: "the man seeks solace where it may easiest be found," it pronounces, "while the woman's mind, 'like sweet bells jangled out of tune and harsh,' yields to the strain, and weakens under it." Of Norreys, *The Era* proclaims:

> We cannot restore to the unhappy lady the plentitude of her reason. That is too much to hope for. But we can give the wavering intellect a chance of recovering its balance; we can, at least, spare the poor weak mind the additional visitation of actual distress.

Evident in *The Era*'s reporting are the intermingled desires to diagnose, infantilize, and romanticize Norreys and her condition. As for the root causes of her breakdown, *The Era* is transparent in its hypothesis: Norreys was a stage actor, and she was a woman.

Unwieldy and imprecise, the nineteenth-century category of mental illness encompassed purportedly functional disorders like hysteria, hypochondriasis, and neurasthenia and permanent conditions like insanity and senile dementia. Prior to the mid-1700s, "lunatics"—largely regarded as bearable, if not irksome, members of the populace—were cared for within communities or committed to private madhouses run by non-medical custodians, their disorders regarded as deviant social conditions rather than physiological or psychological illnesses. Soon, however, British society grew intolerant of the mentally ill in public spaces. Georgian and early Victorian asylums operated as repositories for behavioral outcasts, less dedicated to rehabilitating the inmates than to containing their aberrant conduct, often through abusive measures. Such establishments often served as terminal residences of the most incurable cases of insanity, particularly for inmates of meager or no income; citizens suffering from hysteria or hypochondriasis, particularly those of bourgeois or upper-class pedigree, were likely nursed through their illness at home.

The ways in which the mentally ill were viewed, diagnosed, and treated in England changed markedly over the nineteenth century for a number of reasons, chief among them legislative reforms (including the Lunacy and County Asylum Acts of 1845), the "moral management" approach to patient care and rehabilitation pioneered at William Tuke's York Retreat, and Victorian medical science's reappraisal of mental illness as a variable but nevertheless definable set of medically treatable conditions.[3] To bring mental disorders under the direct purview of their profession, doctors attempted to strengthen links between mental illness and anatomical and physiological deficiencies, while loosening the ties that historically bound mental disorders to metaphysical, spiritual, or even demonic agents. The positivist turn compelled scientists of diverse disciplines—neurology, gynecology, biochemistry, evolutionary psychology, nosology, and pathology—to find perceptible somatic markers of "mental disease": a tumorous uterus, perhaps, or an insufficiency of cerebrospinal fluid. Even so, diseases of the mind remained moral for many Victorian alienists in that indulging in excesses (alcohol, masturbation, or overwork, as well as epic passions like grief and lovesickness) seemed to actuate psychological breaks. In the 1870s and 1880s, French neurologist Jean-Martin Charcot's work at Paris's Salpêtrière Hospital, in which he used hypnosis as a means of both inducing and relieving hysterical symptoms, bolstered a hitherto tenuous link between mind and body in Western understandings of mental illness. Soon Sigmund Freud and Josef Breuer's psychoanalytic approach recalibrated the fields of psychology and psychiatry, and through their work, the newly identified unconscious mind became a fortress to be unlocked by a vigilant and empathetic therapist.

According to Andrew Scull, studies on mental illness often misrepresent its Western history in one of two dichotomous ways. First are the metanarratives of medicine's progress toward benevolent care for the insane. Sympathetic Enlightenment physicians and Victorian alienists, these histories contend, rescued the mentally ill from shaming and abusive techniques (including iron restraints, water cures, isolation, bleeding, and brute force) designed to stem objectionable behaviors, adopting instead Tuke's moral management model of patient care.[4] These chronicles normally climax at the introduction of Freud's psychoanalysis, which de-popularized the use of physical therapies in cases of mental illness and instead advocated the "talking cure" as a means of identifying catalytic past traumas. Such metanarratives offer uncomplicated, "Great Man" histories that disregard conflicting patient experiences, not to mention any negative social, political, and scientific fallout from the *fin de siècle*'s psychiatric revolution. And yet, Scull cautions, the counterarguments advanced by esteemed critics Michel Foucault and Thomas Szasz, in which the moralistic, evangelical-based lunacy reform of the nineteenth century and the expanding asylum system that accompanied it are condemned as even more abasing and repressive to the mentally ill than ostensibly crueler strategies, are similarly fraught. Certainly, critics are right to challenge overly commendatory depictions of lunacy reform and simplified histories of modern psychiatry, and Foucault's "medical gaze" succinctly articulates how the patient's subjective appreciation of his illness was displaced by the supposedly objective (or objectifying) evaluations conducted by medical professionals. However, it is hard to ignore that Victorian-era advances did improve the general welfare of at least some of those institutionalized in Britain and the United States.

For both Scull and historian Janet Oppenheim, the considerable changes to the categorization, diagnosis, and treatment of mental illness in the nineteenth century cannot be reduced as either "humane" or "inhumane"; indeed, in Scull's words, this evolution was "fundamentally ambiguous." While much recommended the mid-century moral treatment as gentler in design than earlier correctional approaches, it was also "a mechanism for inducing conformity" operating on the "tactful manipulation" of patient by doctor.[5] Like the bacteriological revolution and drug addiction's medicalization, the complex (and often interrupted) conversions from mentalist to physicalist theories of mental illness—and back again with the birth of psychoanalysis—found reflection in British and American theatres, where by the early 1900s, playwrights and actors shifted both the locus and symptoms of mental illness inward.

The intimate relationship of psychology and theatre entered a new stage in the late 1800s. Charcot's *théâtre d'hystérie* captivated audiences in Paris. Hamlet, Oedipus, and Rebecca West all spent well-documented time on Sigmund Freud's couch, and playwrights like Émile Zola, Arthur Wing Pinero, and James A. Herne penned dramatic meditations on human psychology for subscription and popular audiences. And at 21 Wellington Street in London's bustling Strand district, the Lyceum Theatre, under the management

of actor Henry Irving, staged a host of gendered mental disorders for a fascinated theatregoing public. From Shakespearean revivals to intricately plotted
melodramas, Irving's Lyceum appealed to middle-class patrons of varied tastes
but comparable pocketbooks. During his tenure (1878–1899), the company
adopted a "picturesque" or "pictorial" style of theatre-making that married
theatrical realism (both in acting and design) with elaborate *mise en scènes* and
the comprehensive physicalization of characters' inner thoughts and emotions,
an ideal aesthetic for exploring the performative nature of neurotic and psychotic states. While portrayals of the mentally ill were certainly not exclusive
to the Lyceum, Irving's fascination with the human mind transformed his
theatre, when money and time permitted, of course, into a sort of laboratory
in which configurations of mental illness were tested and generated through
performance. Irving was not alone in his experiments, however. The stage
hysterics and madwomen created by Ellen Terry, Irving's co-star, dovetailed
with the increasingly feminized notions of insanity circulating in Victorian
Britain and were among the most photographed and illustrated of her roles.
By locating these chapters at the Lyceum and not at an intimate subscription
house specializing in naturalism, I aim to challenge the problematic prioritiza-
tion of the "New Drama" in studies of mental illness on the late nineteenth-
century stage. Indeed, Henry Irving and Ellen Terry's somatically expressive
renderings of hysteria, mania, melancholia, and madness entranced audiences
for twenty years before significant changes to modern psychiatry and acting
methods gradually outpaced the Lyceum's approach to staging mental illness.

Determining exactly which psychogenic disorders inspired Irving and
Terry's performances of mentally ill characters is an inexact science. Both
actors often blended symptoms from multiple discrete pathologies or warped
an illness's characteristic trajectory in order to heighten its theatrical affectiv-
ity. Their methods are perhaps unsurprising given the imprecision with which
Victorian medical professionals diagnosed and treated mental illnesses.[6] My
labeling of performances as enactments of specific disorders, therefore, is more
conjectural than concrete, a reflection of the actors' earnest but inexplicit portrayals of neuroses or psychoses. What is not hypothetical, however, is that
Irving and Terry constructed their performances of mental illness as expressions
of gendered psychological suffering. Though recent histories of Victorian asylum care have usefully foregrounded the patient's socioeconomic status as the
primary shaper of his treatment (both social and medical), the so-called "mind
disorders" had long been gendered. Together, the patient's biological sex and
cultural notions of gender distinguished male and female mental illnesses, and
such distinctions grew even more crucial as psychiatry became a legitimate
branch of institutionalized medicine.[7] In the mid-1800s, the public face of
insanity morphed from the raging, combative male to the emotionally vulnerable but sexually aggressive female, and the relationship between the male
physician and female patient became an iconic emblem of Victorian medicine.[8]
As I suggest in the following chapters, Terry's characters, all the more genuine
and womanly for having gone mad, naturalized feminine mental illness and

contained its impact to the domestic realm. Conversely, Irving's embodiments represented masculine madness as an aberrant and often effeminate state-of-being, tragic in its design and sweeping in its socio-political consequence. Perceptions of male and female mental illness in the nineteenth century's last decades diverged significantly enough to call for different methodological approaches to analyzing Terry and Irving's illness roles. In this chapter, I will introduce the etiologies, symptomatologies, and treatments of female hysteria and insanity before detailing Terry's portrayals of Ophelia, Lady Macbeth, and Lucy Ashton. In the next, I will "diagnose" Irving's Mathias, Hamlet, and King Lear with three discrete mental disorders that became masculinized, either implicitly or explicitly, in Victorian medicocultural discourses.

"A mind diseased" in Ellen Terry's Lyceum repertoire

"I have engaged Ellen Terry – not a bad start – eh?" Henry Irving wrote to a friend after the actor visited Terry's lodgings at Longridge Road, London. At this meeting, during which "formalities disintegrated" after Irving's beloved dog defecated on Terry's rug, the actress agreed to serve as the Lyceum's leading lady at "40 guineas a week and half the takings from a benefit performance."[9] By the time she became a contractual player at the Lyceum, Terry was already an actress of some acclaim, but her partnership with Irving catapulted her into the stratosphere of national celebrity where she remained until her death as Dame Ellen Terry, Order of the British Empire, in 1928. Terry was born in 1847 to parents Ben and Sarah, the fifth of eleven children (several of whom died in infancy). The Terry siblings, including successful stage performers Kate, Florence, Marion, and Fred, received their initial actor training from their parents, who were provincial traveling players. The adolescent Terry performed in Bristol and at London's Royalty, Princess, and Haymarket theatres until one week before her seventeenth birthday, when she married the much older artist George Frederic Watts. All three of Terry's marriages were short-lived; an illegitimate affair with famed architect E. W. Godwin that resulted in two children, Edith and Edwin Gordon Craig, suspended her career from 1867 to 1874.[10] Terry performed with the Lyceum company from 1878 to 1902, the longest and most successful professional engagement in her sixty-nine-year acting career, with seven American tours expanding her circle of admirers.[11] A speculated romance between the king and queen of the Lyceum stage was confirmed much later by Terry. Irving denied all such rumors. Both before and during Terry's time at the Lyceum, the actress excelled in portraying comic and romantic roles in plays by Edward Bulwer-Lytton, J. M. Barrie, George Bernard Shaw, and of course, Shakespeare. Such roles showcased Terry's warmth, intelligence, and mirthful spirit, but also a contrapuntal sensuality. Whether meant derogatorily or adoringly, the word "charm" appeared time and again alongside the actress's name in newspaper reviews, journals, and souvenir postcards. Terry, an independent and financially secure woman who actively supported women's suffrage in the 1910s, regarded the term as insulting and diminutive.

Perhaps because of her "charms," critics often overlooked Terry's sharp intelligence as well as the weaknesses in her acting: a deficiency of tragic power, a propensity for forgetting lines, and debilitating opening-night nervousness. Indeed, in 1898, Charles Hiatt wrote:

> Ellen Terry's buoyancy, her all-pervading gracefulness, the charm of her singular voice, in which laughter and tears seem to be in everlasting chase, the innate femininity of all she attempts, do in fact to some extent disarm cold and searching criticism.[12]

Terry researched her roles assiduously and filled notebooks and script margins with insights, questions, line readings, and blocking notations. Like Rose Norreys and many actresses of their time, Terry's mental health was often the subject of targeted scrutiny, and she herself admitted to several bouts of nervous exhaustion provoked by her profession. "The actress is evidently a woman of extreme nervous sensibility," the *New York Herald* declared upon Terry's arrival in America in 1883, "with an organization so highly strung that in the words of a friend yesterday, 'she always has her heart in her mouth.'"[13] Critics found Terry's presence, voice, and temperament inadequate for portraying tragic roles, but she was supremely adept at expressing the "weaker" emotion of pathos, a gift that served her well in the Lyceum's repertoire. Terry's was a pre-Raphaelite appearance—abundant golden hair, wide and expressive mouth, piercing eyes framed with heavy brows, graceful carriage, and thin figure—that endeared her to audiences and rendered her an icon of late nineteenth-century aestheticism. Operating as a performative surrogate for the period's mentally ill women, the alluring and sympathetic Terry normalized hysteria and insanity as organic, feminine states-of-being; indeed, as embodied by Terry, the hysteric and the madwoman simultaneously suffered within and were liberated by their conditions, dovetailing compellingly with gendered constructions of mental illness circulating throughout the Victorian period.

Given the social constraints regulating British and American women in the late 1800s, it is unsurprising that mental illness categories and treatments were reductively gendered, with the elusive pathology *hysteria* (now fraught with semantic, historiographical, and theoretical landmines) and the even more indeterminate state-of-being, *madness*, serving as the primary diagnoses for female sufferers.[14] In recent years, historians have challenged hysteria's reputation as a female affliction. Michael S. Micale, for example, relies upon Charcot's work with male hysterics of all classes, temperaments, and occupations in the 1870s and 1880s to de-feminize the hysterical condition. Still, Charcot's own photographic evidence of hysterical attacks in the 1870s overwhelmingly featured female patients in highly sexualized attitudes, what Micale concedes were "some of the most gender-stereotyped images in nineteenth-century science."[15] Similarly, despite Charcot's efforts to convince the scientific community of the abundance of male hysterics in modern France, he endorsed Pierre Briquet's estimated ratio of male hysteric to female as one to twenty.[16] And in *On the Pathology and Treatment of Hysteria* (1853),

Robert Brudenell Carter asserted that men and women both developed hysteria from the extreme repression of "sexual passions," but because men possessed the "facilities" to gratify their urges, they escaped hysteria in higher numbers than women.[17] Historians similarly challenge hysteria's authenticity as a distinctive pathological illness, defining it rather as a mythic construction or a nebulous, catch-all diagnosis with little scientific specificity. But no matter: for the vast majority of Victorian Britons, hysteria was a real illness that disproportionally impacted women.[18] In what follows, I treat hysteria as a female affliction of genuine force.

The hysteric and the madwoman

Over its lengthy history, hysteria's etiologies have run the gamut from erotic urges and masturbation, to miscarriages, to overindulgence in foods rich in animal fats.[19] As Elisabeth Bronfen offers in *The Knotted Subject: Hysteria and Its Discontents*, hysteria was an "infamously resilient somatic illness without organic lesions," flexible enough to endure several millennia.[20] In its earliest etymological construction, hysteria was the product of reproductive idleness. The uterus, lacking purpose, drifted from its anatomical home, triggering the manifestation of hysterical symptoms. Though Victorian physicians widely ridiculed the notion of a "wandering womb," they time and again reasserted hysteria's linkage with a woman's reproductive system and lifecycles (puberty, menses, pregnancy, postpartum, lactation, and menopause), finding support in the burgeoning medical specialty of gynecology. Female sexuality proved a thorny issue in the nineteenth century: society celebrated procreation as the ultimate endowment of womanhood but feared and scorned female sexual arousal, inspiring the medical community to pathologize both women's erotic urges and their deliberate suppression of such desires. Mid-century gynecologists warned that even the most natural of life events for biological females provoked madness, including childbirth (puerperal insanity) and menopause (climacteric insanity). "In short," writes Roy Porter, "the female reproductive system was so precariously poised that almost any irregularity, whether excitation or repression, was sure to provoke hysteriform disorders ... This prognosis (uterine disturbances lead to hysterical conditions that precipitate insanity proper) became standard to nineteenth-century medicine."[21] Victorian psychiatry bolstered the uterine theory of hysteria by claiming that fluctuations in the overall health of the reproductive system impacted the patient's cerebral fibers. Gynecology and psychiatry, the "twin pillars supporting the rehabilitation of uterine theories of hysteria," also amplified the occurrence of hysterectomies and, less prominently, clitorectomies in Victorian England.[22] So firmly entrenched was the uterine theory of female madness that physicians often disregarded the importance of their patients' lived experiences in diagnosing mental disturbances. "Expressions of unhappiness, low self-esteem, helplessness, anxiety, and fear were not connected to the realities of women's lives," Elaine Showalter writes, "while expressions of sexual desire, anger, and aggression were taken as morbid deviations from the normal female personality."[23] In this way, emotional responses to childbirth, child-loss, marital strife, the pressures of entering the masculine public sphere, or any number of other common life events for the nineteenth-century woman, became pathologized and hystericized. The clinical use of vibrators to alleviate depression, hysteria, and anxiety through induced "paroxysms," or in contemporary terms, orgasms, operates as a curious coda to what was a deeply inimical chapter in women's history.

While the Victorian age played host to revised uterine theories of hysteria, it also accommodated theories attributing the illness to neurological defects or a shortage of nerve force. To be sure, early Victorians valued sensitivity in both sexes, so long as it remained delicate and not debilitating. In the 1850s, the concept of "muscular Christianity," a fusion of robustness and righteous morality, curbed the appeal of the emotional male prized by the Romantics. To later Victorians, a nervous sensibility suggested both effeminacy and impairment; men who experienced nervous breakdowns were deemed shamefully deficient in the masculine traits of purpose, ambition, and self-regulation. "Want of *nerve* betrayed effeminacy," Porter notes; "want of *nerves*, by contrast, exposed plebian dullness."[24] Human beings were equipped with a limited supply of nerve force, argued alienists and physicians, and each gender preserved or depleted its stores differently. Whereas professional men could induce clinical anxiety through overwork, physicians believed a woman's very physiology, devoted as it was to supporting reproductive processes, made the depletion of her nerve force a constant risk.[25]

Soon evolutionary scientists and social reformers hybridized reproductive and neurological theories of female hysteria in an all-out assault on the ambitious New Woman. In 1871's *The Descent of Man*, Charles Darwin argued that men and women possessed opposing traits because of evolutionary processes of natural and sexual selection. Man was given physical strength and intelligence so as to survive, defend his mate, and produce offspring. Because she would be taken care of by man, woman was endowed with an entirely different set of characteristics, save her capacity for procreation. Among woman's innate faculties, according to Victorian physician T. S. Clouston, "were the cheerfulness, vivacity, and powers of endurance that made women capable 'not only of bearing her own share of ills, but helping to bear those of others.'"[26] Herbert Spencer's *Study of Sociology* (1872–1873) further posited that the female brain stopped maturing at an earlier age than the man's so that the body could devote its energies to vitalizing the woman's most important assets: her reproductive organs.[27] This component of evolutionary thought carried with it significant implications for women living at the *fin de siècle*, when fears of social degeneration, race suicide, and female autonomy escalated. Just as middle-class women began to enter male-dominated professions, politics, and educational systems, reports of female nervous disorders skyrocketed. Darwin, Spencer, and their Victorian followers urged that women protect the delicate biological balance designed for them by nature, for if a female should overtax her intellect by entering into the public sphere or pursuing higher education, she would exhaust her nerve force and impair her reproductive organs, leading inevitably to hysteria or insanity.[28] Such assertions justified social and political policies designed to kept women subordinate. Not surprisingly, S. Weir Mitchell's infamous rest cure for the female neurotic confined the patient entirely to her bed, prescribed frequent, fatty meals, and prohibited intellectual stimulation in the hopes of restoring her biological balance and re-containing her within the domestic sphere. To gender matters further, Darwinian psychiatrists agreed that once a mind disorder materialized, it could be passed from mothers to their future daughters, potentially producing familial lines of mentally ill women. Thus, genetics joined physiology as a widely acknowledged root cause of the female maladies.

Whiteness colored the portrait of Victorian-era hysteria. Women of color rarely received the diagnosis, both because female patients with direct access to physicians were often white and middle-class, and because the medicalized concept of "race" erected biological, physiological, and intellectual barriers between white Euro-Americans and people of color. Physiognomists and phrenologists, for example, compared European facial features and cranial measurements with those of African and Native American descent in order to argue that anatomical differences in racialized bodies generated inequalities in their intellectual and emotional processes. The fusion of hysteria with fragile nerves and reproductive health disorders further disassociated women of color from the disease, as medical science—and Victorian society in general—theorized that only white women possessed the delicate sensibilities to develop nervous conditions and that women of color seldom suffered from reproductive infirmities or barrenness. "Native" women, scientists argued, were equipped with robust reproductive organs of animal-like efficiency, allowing them to conceive and birth offspring often and without considerable pain. In short, the Victorians viewed women of color as too biologically and emotionally primitive to become hysterics.

Female hysteria was known for its unpredictable somatic manifestations that, due to their sheer variety, prompted many physicians to over-diagnose the condition and others to doubt its very existence. Hysterics reported involuntary twitches, spasms, seizures, and convulsions; catatonic spells and fainting; extreme emotional states from ecstasy to depression; throat constrictions; abdominal, chest, and genital pains; severe anxiety; and abnormal breathing patterns, among others. Hysterics' reputation for duplicitous and sexual behavior rendered them one of the least sympathetic patient groups of the period.[29] The hysteric was, to her critics, a cunning dissembler and attention-starved exhibitionist who shared much in common with the professional actor. In *Unmaking Mimesis: Essays on Feminism and Theatre*, Elin Diamond alerts us to the "similar repertory of signs" used by the hysteric and the nineteenth-century melodramatic actor: "the facial grimace, eye-rolling, teeth gnashing, heavy sighs, fainting, shrieking, shivering, choking. '*Hysterical laughter*' is a frequent stage direction, usually an indication of despair and abandonment, also a symptom of guilt."[30] Charcot's live scientific demonstrations at the Salpêtrière exploited hysteria's distinctive theatricality. As a neurologist, Charcot sought material evidence that hysterics shared a *tare nerveuse*, or a hereditary weakness of the nervous system. A "great psychical shaking up" (*le grand ébranlement psychique*), he theorized, induced the hysterical condition in those constitutionally vulnerable to the disorder.[31] To his consternation, numerous postmortem autopsies failed to reveal organic lesions or anatomical abnormalities, but his experiments with hypnosis nevertheless fueled Charcot's conviction that hysterical symptoms were genuine and could be treated with inhalants, baths, electricity, the application of magnets and metals, and even "ovarian compressors."[32]

Charcot's observations of his most famous patient, Augustine, prompted him to codify the hysterical attack into four distinct stages. Such attacks began with the "epileptoid phase or 'tonic rigidity.'" This was followed by the *grands mouvements* or clonic spasms in which the hysteric's body performed "circus-like acrobatics" (*le clownisme*). In the third phase, the hysteric would rapidly cycle through the *attitudes passionnelles*, or physical representations of love, fear, loathing, and other emotional states. For Augustine, these *attitudes* included "seduction, supplication, erotic pleasure, ecstasy and mockery," often accompanied by vivid visual and aural hallucinations. The final stage was categorized by "tears and laughter, both of which Charcot saw as a release before the patient comes back to herself."[33] Charcot's four-part hysterical attack was a highly performative, seemingly collaborative exhibition of illness forged by director and actress, though it is important to situate this "collaboration" within the lopsided power dynamics at the heart of Charcot's demonstrations: medical men gazed on, physically manipulated, and induced (often involuntary) behaviors in their sexualized female patients (Figure 5.1). With a simultaneously theatrical and orgastic climactic structure, the attack's emotional reversals, overt eroticism, and reliance on somatic expressiveness intimately tied it to femininity.[34]

Even in the most extreme cases, a hysteric had the potential to recover, but her condition could also deepen, leading to clinical insanity. Alienists tasked with differentiating between the hysteric and the madwoman depended upon notions of temporality and cognizance. Unlike the hysteric, who experienced spells of lucidity and normal functioning and remained at least partially cognizant of her illness, the madwoman's condition was defined by its totality and constancy. Similarly, while a hysteric had the potential for partial or complete rehabilitation, a madwoman was often the recipient of basic maintenance. Though hysteria and insanity produced similar behavioral phenomena, including catatonia, hallucinations, spontaneous laughter, and eroticism, insanity presented (or was thought to present) a slightly different set of expressions. Within the medicocultural iconography of madness, Jane E. Kromm notes:

> there are gestures of hair-pulling, and hair dressed with straw *à la folle*, which have long been associated with the female stereotype of madness. Traits from traditional male stereotypes newly gendered female include the fists clenched with straw, upraised arms of distress or exaltation, and haranguelike gesticulations.[35]

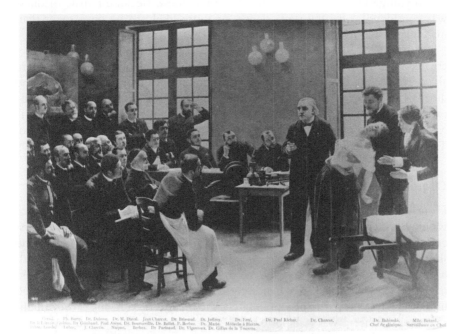

Figure 5.1 Leçon clinique à la Salpêtrière, Pierre-André Brouillet, 1887. The National Library of Medicine.

Rhythmical rocking or swaying, incomprehensible mutterings, and repetitive tasks like shredding cloth or picking hairs all signaled permanent mental degeneration. Clear in this embodied lexicon of madness is the juxtaposition of actions that are contained, isolating, or introspective with those that are exhibitionist and histrionic.

Hysterics and madwomen engaged in behavior that transgressed the restrictive boundaries of Victorian womanhood, but can we interpret such behaviors as socially subversive weapons of resistance? On this question scholars disagree. For Phyllis Chesler, socially and sexually repressed women used "going mad" as a way of reclaiming their bodily autonomy, while for Roy Porter, the "incapacitating symptoms" of hysteria reified "the sufferer's actual social condition" and not some utopic converse of nineteenth-century social strictures.[36] Warning that this binary traps the female patient in a "double-bind of victim or rebel" within a dictatorial, misogynistic institution of Victorian medicine, Jane Wood notes that there were patients in real distress or pain who actively participated in their recoveries as well as compassionate doctors dedicated to understanding mental illness and restoring its sufferers to health.[37] Female madness as a construction of the collective Victorian imagination was a true paradox. Conceived of as irrational beings in possession of ever-changing bodies, women were organically unstable and therefore more apt to plunge into the deep chasm of mental illness. Because female madness was considered a natural state, it was far more likely to be permanent than male madness.

The discursive bodies inscribed by science and literature, aesthetic bodies created by art and fashion, and performative bodies gazed upon in the theatre all contributed to the medicocultural configurations of mental illness operating during the Victorian period. For nearly a quarter of a century, Terry's high-profile hysterical and mad roles at the Lyceum, all white gentlewomen of delicate nerves, contributed to this multimodal synthesis of female mental illness. The first of these was Ophelia.

Ophelia, 1878

From the beginning of *Hamlet* rehearsals Terry struggled to find her place within Irving's uncompromising system of producing theatre. At the first company reading, Irving performed all of the parts except Ophelia, which he skipped entirely. According to Terry, Irving never rehearsed his scenes with his new leading actress, opting instead to stage crowd scenes, supervise orchestra practices, and check gas lighting effects. Terry's apprehension mounted until, ten days before the play premiered, she finally asked Irving if they might rehearse together. "We shall be all right!" he responded, "but we are not going to run the risk of being bottled up by a gas man or fiddler."[38] Terry, it would seem, was on her own.

She first visited an asylum, hoping to observe "authentic" feminine madness in all its contradictory glory. "Like all Ophelias before (and after) me, I went to the madhouse to study wits astray," Terry related in her 1908 memoir *Story of My Life*. This preparatory ritual had grown so commonplace by 1878 that asylum superintendents regularly opened their institutions' doors to actresses preparing for mad roles. "It seems to be supposed," Hanwell Asylum superintendent John Conolly stated:

> That it is an easy task to play the part of a crazy girl, and that it is chiefly composed of singing and prettiness. The habitual courtesy, the partial rudeness of mental disorder, are things to be witnessed … An actress, ambitious of something beyond cold imitation, might find the contemplation of such cases a not unprofitable study.[39]

In describing her fieldwork, Terry admitted to being dissatisfied with the majority of the madhouse's specimens:

> I was disheartened at first. There was no beauty, no nature, no pity in most of the lunatics. Strange as it may sound, they were too *theatrical* to teach me anything. Then, just as I was going away, I noticed a young girl gazing at the wall. I went between her and the wall to see her face. It was quite vacant, but the body expressed that she was waiting, waiting. Suddenly she

threw up her hands and sped across the room like a swallow. I never forget it. She was very thin, very pathetic, very young, and the movement was as poignant as it was beautiful.[40]

Terry concluded from her experience "that the actor must imagine first and observe afterwards"; still, it is probable that the little swallow's pathetic beauty, temporal variations, and flight across the asylum floor influenced her Ophelia.

In performance, Terry's Ophelia conformed to the traditional aesthetics of feminine madness. Cognizant of the importance of evocative costuming and hairdressing, or what she called the "art and archaeology" of dress, Terry appeared first the devoted and winsome ingénue in neatly tailored gowns, wavy hair tamed by pins.[41] After Polonius's death, she re-entered as the despondent but alluring madwoman, her draped white gown and nest of tangled hair adhering to the paradigmatic Victorian iconography of "wits astray." Far less conventional, however, was the actor's initial pronouncement to her Lyceum collaborators that Ophelia would not wear white in the mad scene. As Terry recounted it, "[Irving] had heard that I intended to wear black in the mad scene, and he intended me to wear white. When he first mentioned the subject, I had no idea that there would be any opposition." After confirming that Terry had had a black dress made for the mad scene:

> Henry did not wag an eyelid.
> "I see. In mourning for her father."
> "No, not exactly that. I think *red* was the mourning color of the period. But black seems to me *right* – like the character, like the situation."

At that moment production advisor Walter Lacy appeared, and Irving requested that Terry repeat her costume choices to his advisor:

> Rather surprised, but still unsuspecting, I told Lacy all over again. Pink in the first scene, yellow in the second, black –
> You should have seen Lacy's face at the word "black." He was going to burst out, but Henry stopped him. He was more diplomatic than that!
> "They generally wear *white*, don't they?"
> "I believe so," I answered, "but black is more interesting." ...
> And then they dropped the subject for the day. It was clever of him!
> The next day Lacy came up to me:
> "You didn't really mean that you are going to wear black in the mad scene?"
> "Yes I did. Why not?"
> "*Why not!* My God! Madam, there must be only one black figure in this play, and that's Hamlet!"
> I did feel a fool. What a blundering donkey I had been not to see it before![42]

Here the men's somewhat condescending dismissal of Terry's creative impulses replicates the institutional and personal policing of female mental patients and their symptomatic behaviors by male alienists, physicians, and asylum superintendents. In both cases (not to mention that of the fictional Ophelia), authoritative males regulated and endorsed a narrow range of expressions for the women under their care. Terry later articulated what she was unable to justify to Irving and Lacy: "I could have gone mad much more comfortably in black."[43] Given that Victorians considered insanity a more naturalized state for women than men, Terry's use of the word "comfortable" here is provocative indeed.

Terry's instinct to abandon the character's quintessential iconography for clothes more befitting Ophelia's mental state implies she viewed Ophelia as an illness role in need of more comprehensive signaling. For Terry, the color of black, which seemed "*right* – like the character, like the situation," could have represented Ophelia's internalized desolation, a psychic and spiritual void created by the loss of her father and the rapid onset of insanity. In wishing to wear black instead of virginal white, Terry allied her Ophelia with that of early nineteenth-century actress Harriet Smithson. While performing to great acclaim with Charles Kemble at Paris's Odéon in 1827, Smithson (later Berlioz) used a black cloth as Ophelia's prop during the mad scene. Two drawings by French artists immortalized Smithson's mad Ophelia: Louis Boulanger and Achille Jacques Jean-Marie Devéria's *Hamlet, Acte IV, scene 5* (1827) and Eugène Delacroix's *Le Chant d'Ophèlie (Act IV. Sc. 5)* (1834). Delacroix's work, art historian Kimberly Rhodes notes, prioritizes Smithson's gestural expressivity in depicting Ophelia kneeling down to lay the sable fabric on the ground as she sings "le chant d'Ophèlie." In Devéria's and Boulanger's lithograph, Ophelia dances distractedly as Claudius, Laertes, and two other men look on with concern, the mourning cloth lying inert on the floor before her. She gazes down at it, knee-length dark hair spilling over her shoulder, her empire-waisted gown of standard white outlining a curvaceous silhouette. Smithson's was a suitably emotional Ophelia for the Romantic age, interweaving grief, madness, and sensuality through her manipulation of a simple black cloth. "Smithson relied on her gestural and miming powers to create a more persuasive and affecting mad Ophelia," offers Rhodes. "By doing so, she located Ophelia's madness in her actions and visage rather than in her voice and words."[44] Both prints were widely distributed in France and England, and while it is impossible to know whether Terry came across these sketches, it is probable she knew of Smithson's emblematic black cloth.

Terry did not like Ophelia and she did not like herself as Ophelia, or so she claimed in *Four Lectures on Shakespeare*, posthumously published in 1932. "[Ophelia's] brain, her soul and her body are all pathetically weak," Terry remarked of "Shakespeare's only timid heroine"; the character's main point of interest was her "incipient insanity," an indication to audiences that "from the first there is something queer about her" and that her father's murder was the "shock" that prompted her latent mental condition to activate. "Ophelia is really mad, not merely metaphorically mad – with grief," declared the actress.[45] As noted by biographer Nina Auerbach, Terry's critique of Ophelia seems out-of-place in a volume of lectures "brim[ming] with generous affection even for pathetic heroines," though Terry also asserted that Ophelia's mad scene moves audiences more than all of Shakespeare's "sane" scenes.[46] Terry's lack of deference to a character so beloved by audiences is clear in her account of playing *Hamlet* in Chicago, a city whose citizens were "a rough, murderous, sand-bagging crew":

> I ran on to the stage in the mad scene, and never have I felt such sympathy! This frail wraith, this poor demented thing, could hold them in the hollow of her hand … It was splendid! "How long can I hold them?" I thought: "For ever!" Then I laughed. That was the best Ophelia laugh of my life.[47]

Though Terry herself regarded Ophelia as "pathetically weak" in body, brain, and soul, her performance also conceded the possibility that the character's mental instability, already present at the play's opening, was the result of years of radical self-denial within and acquiescence to a patriarchal system. In this interpretation, then, Ophelia's madness—however pathetic, aesthetic, and pit-ied by the tragedy's male witnesses—served as an unconventional expression of insurrectionist female autonomy. While scholars have since condemned the theory of female madness-as-rebellion, first identified by Phyllis Chesler, Sandra Gilbert, and Susan Gubar, as illusory and injurious to feminism, theories of female psychology in Victorian Britain left ample room for both interpreta-tions of Terry's Ophelia.[48]

Reviews of the Lyceum's *Hamlet* suggest that Terry offered glimpses of Ophelia's "incipient insanity" long before the mad scene. Although her Ophelia remained winsome and docile, obedient to father, king, and betrothed, she was perhaps not the uncomplicated and buoyant heroine audiences had come to expect in the play's earlier acts. In Terry's design, Ophelia's mental fragility was intertwined inextricably with her femininity and, by extension, her appeal. "Miss Terry's Ophelia was a delicious and exquisite creation," the *Baltimore Day* reported during one of Lyceum's American tours:

> Her grief and madness have idealized her, and Miss Terry imbues the char-acter with so much spirituality that we forget all else … The conflict of emotions which swept over her heart was reflected in every lineament of her face, and in her tear-stained eyes, and the mad scene, with its snatches of plaintive song, its fitful gleams of reason and protracted outbursts of grief, was marked by great power and originally [sic].[49]

Unlike other performers who portrayed Ophelia as naturally comfortable in or conditioned to her subservient role, Terry's Ophelia was visibly uneasy in her tenuous sanity; madness was her natural, unencumbered state. "And if … her 'sweet bells were jangled out of tune,' they were never harsh, and their muffled music but gave, perhaps, the more appropriate voice to her piteous sorrow, and more piteous mirth," wrote the reviewer at *Punch*. "Mr. Irving's Hamlet ... we knew already. Ellen Terry's Ophelia we did not know. *That* is the revelation for which we have to thank the new management of the Lyceum."[50] Ophelia's madness, then, was not the result of an abrupt flip from sanity to insanity at her father's death, but the hastened advance of an expected outcome; for Terry, grief served as the catalyst of Ophelia's psychotic break, not its genesis.

Perhaps inspired by her madhouse observations and the Lyceum's pictorial approach to theatre-making, in act four's mad scene, Terry exteriorized Ophelia's mental state by way of unsettled movements, rapid shifts in facial expression, unprovoked mood changes, and spontaneous laughter, one of the key indicators of female lunacy in the Victorian age. "The triumph of [Terry's] impersonation was in the mad scene," claimed the *Boston Traveller*,

> in which her sudden changes of mood, from the pathetic to the hilarious, when the notes of her sad songs, were drowned in a moment in shouts of hysterical laughter, were admirably accomplished. Her scenes of insanity are wonderful in their variety, their unconventionality, their fine commentary on the text, their thrilling pathos.[51]

Though critics described Terry's performance of madness as realistic, it is far more likely that her pre-Raphaelite maiden was "picturesquely pathetic rather than horrifyingly real," as twentieth-century Irving biographer Alan Hughes posits. "A sordidly realistic portrayal of Ophelia mad, if well played, can temporarily turn an audience against Hamlet. Terry depicted a mind 'so shattered as to be beyond hope or help,' but she took care to exclude the squalid and painful."[52] Notable in Hughes's remarks is the implication, one befitting a privileged Victorian physician, that Ophelia's madness is only consequential if and when it affects Hamlet. Nevertheless, what emerges from countless reviews of Terry's Ophelia is a critical narrative that both fetishizes and naturalizes female mental illness. "The semblance of insanity was marvelously shown [in the mad scene]," offered *Dramatic Notes*, "and would have been, even, painful, but that the purity, charm, and grace of Miss Terry's Ophelia."[53] Terry's Ophelia appeared most beautiful, winning, organic, and secure when she was unshackled by her madness. Such an approach suggests that Ophelia's pathetic (*not* tragic) end in the water's depths transpired not because she was mentally ill, but because she breeched the fortifications of the domestic, private realm, where she had been monitored and contained.

Photographs and audio recordings offer clues to Terry's performance. Ophelia's voice, as articulated by Terry, was recorded for posterity in 1911 in America, along with the actress's renderings of four other Shakespearean heroines. It is a mellifluous voice, with rolling "r's" and lilting cadences signaling Ophelia's youthful femininity. As interpreted by Michael Booth, "the madness and the singing seem too refined and prettified to be dramatically convincing to the modern ear, but it is interesting to note the prolongation of the sounds of pain and grief ... a mournful wail pregnant with sorrow."[54] As for Ophelia's form and comportment, three Window & Grove photographic portraits suggest how Terry embodied the role. The first shows the actress in a dress with a clinging bodice, high neckline, and pearl-embellished sleeves and neckline, a set of letters held aloft in her left hand, indicating the nunnery scene. Though her mouth and jaw are relaxed, Terry's eyebrows are furrowed with concern, her eyes directed straight at the camera. Of Terry's three-quarter length pose, Kimberly Rhodes writes: "Her body tilts to the left [of the frame], leaving the viewer with an unsteady feeling analogous to 'Ophelia's' state of mind."[55] Even before madness, Terry's Ophelia appears vulnerable, anxious, and fragile: the outward expression of a weak nervous system. In another photograph, Terry stands in the mad Ophelia's ermine-lined white gown, hair slightly disheveled, and clutches a bouquet of flowers and herbs, the "remembrances" Ophelia distributes to her brother (Figure 5.2). Despite the camera's tighter frame, her gaze is conspicuously distant, perhaps even vacant, and directed slightly off to her left. The final of the three photographs is a close-up portrait of the insane Ophelia, and a study in feminine madness's physiognomy: parted mouth, knitted brow, wide eyes staring with an agonized expression at the viewer, her hands fussing at the ends of her hair (Figure 5.3). Terry's Ophelia appears as a wounded animal peering fearfully at her human captor, her beauty both distorted and enhanced by her manifest suffering. "Taken together," argues Rhodes, "the three of the Window & Grove images form a triptych of

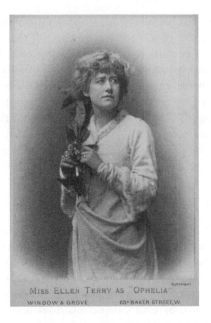

MISS ELLEN TERRY AS "OPHELIA"

WINDOW & GROVE   63ª BAKER STREET, W.

Figure 5.2 Miss Ellen Terry as "Ophelia," Window & Grove photograph. Courtesy of Folger Shakespeare Library.

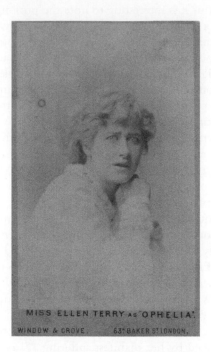

Figure 5.3 Miss Ellen Terry as "Ophelia," Window & Grove photograph. Courtesy of Folger Shakespeare Library.

madness that moves the viewer from consideration of body to mind and forges links between the two."[56] It was in the full throes of her illness, just when Terry's Ophelia became resolutely pathologized, that she also appeared most vital, natural, and womanly: "Miss Terry's Ophelia is an exquisite piece of acting," hailed one enamored reviewer, "marked by the highest beauty of form, and touched by grace so pathetically suggestive that even before the sadness of its tragedy arrives it moves the spirit of the spectator to tears. Its girlish grace is most winning."[57] In a process of mutual authentication, the feminine softness of Terry's Ophelia naturalized her madness, just as her madness reaffirmed and heightened the character's muliebrity.

Lady Macbeth, 1888

John Singer Sargent's *Ellen Terry as Lady Macbeth* (1889) is a stunning, full-length painting of the actress in the character's famous green iridescent beetle-wing gown, red hair in two enormous plaits that reach her knees, holding a golden crown over her head. It is a portrait of fierce, almost obsessive ambition, not to mention a vivid expression of Terry's pictorial aestheticism. Unlike the series of Ophelia photographs, Sargent's depiction does not—by most accounts—accurately capture Terry's performance of the notorious accomplice. Terry's Lady Macbeth was no unmerciful, Machiavellian assassin like Sarah Siddons's or, to a lesser extent, Hannah Pritchard's; she rejected wholesale the traditional methods of playing the Scottish queen. Her resolutely feminine Lady Macbeth was driven mad not by her symbolic masculinization and murderous deeds, but by her womanly devotion to satisfying her husband's greatest ambitions. As such, Terry's Lady Macbeth replicated the mental degeneration that conservatives warned would befall Victorian women, should they challenge conventional gender roles.

In an 1843 essay in the *Westminster Review*, Siddons (the most popular Lady Macbeth of the century) described the character as a "'fair, feminine, nay, perhaps, even fragile' woman, 'captivating in feminine loveliness,' whose power sprang from 'a charm of such potency as to fascinate the mind of a hero so dauntless, a character so amiable, so honourable as Macbeth.'"[58] Despite this, and perhaps due to Siddons's classical acting techniques and imposing height, the ruthless Lady Macbeth she depicted onstage barely resembled the weak woman composed by her imagination. While Ellen Terry was without the tragic power of Siddons, she had feminine grace in abundance. It was Terry, therefore, who, in one of her most polarizing performances, brought a fair and fragile Lady Macbeth to life for audiences. In a letter to William Winter, the actress wrote: "Everyone seems to think Mrs. McB is a Monstrousness & I can only see that she's a woman – a mistaken woman – & weak – not a Dove – of course not – but first of all a wife."[59] Terry's own writings on Lady Macbeth unquestionably depict her as a hysteric. A "delicate little creature," Lady Macbeth is "'a woman of the highest nervous organization, with a passionate intensity of purpose' … [She] was no monster, but a 'womanly woman' who is 'a woman in everything … her strength is all nervous force; her ambition is all for her husband.'"[60] Though Lady Macbeth assists in the murders that place her husband on the throne, her incantatory command to unearthly spirits fail to "unsex" her (1.5.31), leaving her gentle body, soul, and mind intact. According to Booth, "Because [Terry's Lady Macbeth] was so feminine her nature was frail, and it collapsed under the weight of guilt, remorse, and Macbeth's estrangement."[61] Terry's writings on Lady Macbeth do not directly cite the childless character's disclosure "I have given suck, and know/How tender 'tis to love the babe that milks me"(1.7.55-6), lines that suggest she had once birthed a child. Nevertheless, the actress's nurturing Lady Macbeth would seem to sanction the period's routine yoking of female hysteria and insanity to perinatal and postnatal processes, as well as to child loss, trauma, and even excessive stores of breast milk.

By Terry's explicit design (and in an unintentional parody of the stresses of being a domesticated hostess), Lady Macbeth's madness had its origins in the banquet scene. During that "'damned party,'" Terry revealed, "'her [un?] mistakable softening of the brain occurs – she turns quite gentle – and so we are prepared for the last scene's madness and death.'"[62] However, from the outset the seeds of hysteria were present. Crucial to Terry's construction of Lady Macbeth's illness was her fainting in act two, scene three, which actresses commonly played as an improvised attempt to deflect attention from Macbeth. Lady Macbeth's fainting, a key manifestation of hysteria according to the period's experts, was "*Just* like a woman," Terry wrote in the margins of her script. Terry performed it as an authentic articulation of post-traumatic stress following Duncan's murder (and relief that the Macbeths' lies withstood scrutiny). Lady Macbeth's fainting was "unquestionably genuine," argues McDonald of Terry's treatment:

> [It is] very much a physical collapse foreshadowing the internal pressures of the sleepwalking scene. And Terry finds a plausible psychological motive for the action, as her marginal notes reveal: "Strung up, past pitch, she gives in at the end of his speech when she finds he is safely through his story, and *then she faints, really*." No feigned collapse here.[63]

In Terry's embodiment, the character's gentle beauty, neurotic tendencies, and sexualized behavior closely resemble the prerequisites for acquiring the female malady. Labeled "nervous," "finely strung," and "sensitive" by the *Pall Mall Gazette*, Terry's Lady Macbeth boasted a potent sensuality, much like *les femmes hystériques* on display in Charcot's clinic. A select number of critics heralded the decidedly un-fiendish "New Lady Macbeth" as a revelation; others commended Terry for her gutsy departure from dramatic protocol but still voiced their preference for other actresses' portrayals.[64] After all, as *The People*'s critic noted, because audiences were accustomed to (and seemingly preferred) a forceful, overbearing Lady Macbeth, in the Lyceum's *Macbeth* "it was impossible not to recognize that, alike in mental will and its physical expression, the woman, despite her dominating words, was the weaker vessel."[65] And *The World*'s January 2, 1889 review claimed that though Terry's performance was not of Shakespeare's Lady Macbeth, the Bard would have written the character just as Terry envisioned her had he been acquainted with the actress.[66]

Macbeth was a controversial but commercial win for the Lyceum. Terry wrote in her diary "I am a success, which amazes me," though she did acknowledge "some people hate me in it."[67] In reality, a good many critics took umbrage at Terry's Lady Macbeth. Perhaps, hazarded some, Terry's softer interpretation was the only one she could have constructed, given her limitations as a tragic actress. Hers was not *the* Lady Macbeth, wrote the *Graphic*, precisely because she flaunted her womanliness even while committing terrible acts: "Incitements to treason and barbarous murder sit ill upon a woman who is all love and caresses."[68] *Sporting and Dramatic News*'s critique recognized Lady Macbeth's hysterical affliction as both inborn and situational:

> Must she not be something more and deeper and worse than the too affectionate wife *who loses her sense of morality* in her eagerness to serve her husband's ambition, who *hysterically* becomes his accessory after he has

murdered his royal guest, and who later on shows a *touching distress* under
the dismal memories which haunt her in her dreams?[69]

This concisely traces Lady Macbeth's descent into insanity in period-appropriate
terms: a loss of morality via a failed attempt to "unsex" herself (i.e., rejecting
her normative femininity) leading to her banquet scene hysteria and eventual
madness ("a touching distress"). This woman of love and caresses was all too
passionate for some reviewers accustomed to Lady Macbeth as ice queen or masculinized virago. The critic from the *Star* reported:

> The great fact about Miss Terry's Lady Macbeth is its sex ... It is redolent,
> pungent with the *odeur de femme*. Look how she rushes into her husband's
> arms, clinging, kissing, coaxing, and even her taunts, when his resolution
> begins to wane, are sugared with a loving smile.[70]

But while a majority of reviewers lamented Terry's choices, her overtly feminized performance of Lady Macbeth (played, as the *Times* alleged, with "an
energy of character that [is] more hysterical than real") located it squarely
within the period's discourse on gendered mental illnesses.[71] Cursed with a
woman's delicate nerves, Lady Macbeth provoked her own descent into madness by meddling in her husband's hyper-masculine affairs: politics, murder,
ambition, and power.

Just as Ophelia has her mad scenes, Lady Macbeth has her sleepwalking
scene. While the simple act of sleepwalking is not, in reality, symptomatic of
madness, Lady Macbeth's "softened brain" (as Terry labeled it) prohibited her
peaceful slumber. "Sleep is a passive, feminine state," reminds Lisa Appignanesi
in *Mad, Bad and Sad: Women and the Mind Doctors*. "But increasingly it is clear
that activity takes place within it. That activity ... is distinctly other, altered,
and seems to share not a little with the hallucinatory, non-rational spheres of
madness."[72] Even more than her predecessors, Terry's sleepwalking scene was
the defining moment of the performance. Not only did Irving resist cutting
lines within the scene, giving it particular prominence in a heavily edited rendition of the play, but the Lyceum's well-read audiences likely would have been
familiar with Charcot's work on neuropathologies and hypnosis.[73] In her article
"Lady Macbeth and the Daemonologie of Hysteria," Joanna Levin pronounces:
"The play never mentions *hysterica passio*, but somnambulism was in fact one
of the symptoms of the 'Suffocation of the Mother.'"[74] And so it was into this
anachronistic historical moment that Terry's Lady Macbeth glided, wearing
a dressing gown and clutching a lamp. Critics praised the poeticized beauty
of Terry's distressed somnambulist, and it was not by mistake that her Lady
Macbeth was visually arresting. In rehearsal Irving urged that the image of Terry
convey Lady Macbeth's fractured mental state: "Lady M should certainly have
the appearance of having got out of bed," Irving wrote, "to which she is returning when she goes off. The hair to my mind should be wild and disturbed, and
the whole appearance as distraught as possible and disordered."[75]

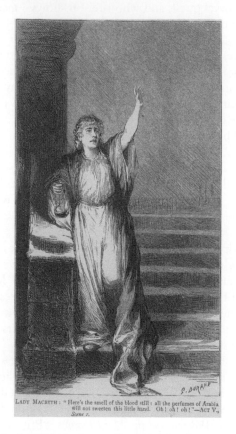

LADY MACBETH : " Here's the smell of the blood still : all the perfumes of Arabia will not sweeten this little hand. Oh ! oh ! oh ! "—ACT V., *Scene 1.*

Figure 5.4 Lady Macbeth, "Here's the smell of blood still." *Graphic*, January 2, 1889. Courtesy of Folger Shakespeare Library.

In an illustration printed in January 12's *Graphic*, it would seem that—at least from the artist's perspective—Terry satisfied Irving's vision of the "disordered" queen (Figure 5.4). In dressing gowns that vaguely traced the actress's shape like a Grecian statue, curled hair disheveled, Terry is pictured descending a staircase from her bedchamber holding her left hand aloft, an iconographic gesture of madness. The actress's furrowed brow, unfocused eyes, and downturned, open mouth mark the queen's psychological distress. According to the *Globe*: "Not more easily will pass from the memory the vision of the pallid figure … with the worn, spiritualised features, the abiding ache, and the senses locked, which glides like a vision, and wrings the long, pale hands in a vain attempt to wash out the imaginary stain." Once Terry reached the stage floor her walk continued in a "quiet, unconscious" fashion; even when her feet stopped moving, Lady Macbeth's body swayed incessantly, her eyes "vacant yet sorrowful." The embodied composition, *London Figaro* asserted, was that of a "broken" woman.[76]

Opinions were mixed on Terry's intonations of Lady Macbeth's nocturnal mutterings. The *Daily News* was impressed by the control Terry possessed over her speeches, observing that "a pretty trait was the delivery of the words 'One, two,' with a pause between, in a bell-like tone; again, the occasional lapses into a more dreamy vein as if sleep were hovering near, ready to reassert its power over her weary brain."[77] According to *The Graphic*, "In the sleep-walking scene she looked charming – some may say too charming for a woman on the brink of death – but she also, with her broken, impassioned utterances, conveyed a vivid sense of the mental terrors (and possibly remorse also) by which she was tortured."[78] Others judged Terry's voice as too monotone, weak, or cooing to express the character's spectrum of emotions, though the *London Figaro* characterized the "moaning cadence of her voice" as appropriate for Lady Macbeth's disordered ramblings.[79] Transfigured by Terry into a caressing and cajoling wife of limitless fidelity, the Lady Macbeth of the Lyceum was revolutionary but not revelatory. She was, however, a madwoman fit for Victorian sensibilities; Lady Macbeth trespassed into the masculine realm and suffered dearly for it.

Lucy Ashton, 1890

Of course, Terry's performances of mental illness were not restricted to Shakespeare's canon. One of her lesser-known roles, Lucy Ashton in *Ravenswood* (1890) was, in the eyes of critics as well as the actress herself, a character of limited dramatic potential. However, Lucy serves as important example of how female madness could be reduced, both onstage and within the Victorian zeitgeist, to a single source: an essential, inexorable weakness of the sex. In *Ravenswood*, a retelling of Sir Walter Scott's *The Bride of Lammermoor* (1819), Lucy's fidelity to the play's hero, the Master of Ravenswood (Edgar), is no match for her domineering mother, a grasping schemer bent on uniting her daughter with the rich Laird of Bucklaw. Believing her mother's lie that Edgar abandoned her and renounced their love, a heartbroken Lucy agrees to marry Bucklaw, but when Edgar returns to confront his onetime paramour on her wedding day, Lucy's fragile mind snaps from the sudden revelation of her betrayal. With a blast of hysterical laughter (of which critics made much ado) and a cry for Edgar, Lucy dies.[80] *Ravenwood*'s adaptor, Herman Merivale, removed the demented Lucy's stabbing of Bucklaw in their bridal chamber, a brutal assault that in Scott's novel signals her full break with sanity and immediately precedes her death. One critic lamented this reworking, stating: "Hysterical frenzy of this sort is exactly what Miss Ellen Terry most excels in, and she might have made a great and tragic effect with the words, 'Take up your bonny bridegroom,' uttered with a maniac laugh, over the body of Bucklaw."[81] The character of Lucy Ashton demanded that Terry be beautiful, virtuous, gullible, and most fundamentally to her performance of illness, physically and mentally inferior to every other character within the play. In a theatre review in *Murray's Magazine* (1890), J. Murray dismissed Lucy as colorless and submissive heroine who "can hardly be described as an interesting character." Even the story's most unquestioning readers, Murray claimed (emphasis added):

> [would] find it difficult to understand how so pliable a nature could, even when distraught with terror and madness, have tried to murder Hayston of

Bucklaw her 'bonny bridegroom.' It is true that it is pathologically the case that when a person loses his senses, he or *oftener she*, becomes the direct antithesis of the former self; and thus a pure-minded Ophelia is made in her madness to use language of astonishing coarseness. Yet from the point of view of art and not from medical science, it is not unnatural to wish that Lucy Ashton had been made of sterner stuff.[82]

Of the abrupt onset of Lucy's insanity in the fourth act, several reviewers remarked that, while not objectionably unrealistic (for women's minds were more liable to snap without warning), it prohibited Terry from doing—for any length of time, anyway—what she did very well: embodying a madwoman.[83] "Whether it would have been judicious to introduce a scene illustrative of Lucy's madness is a point upon which opinions may differ," wrote one critic. "Remembering Miss Terry's Ophelia, many will be inclined to regret the omission."[84] The single signifier of Lucy's precipitous derangement, her maniacal laugh, was reported by the newspapers as being compelling and frighteningly naturalistic, though none detailed its aural and visual effects. "Ah! That awful laugh –" proclaimed *Punch*, "far more tragic than the one secured by *Bucklaw!* It is *Lucy* going mad!"[85] The maiden's collapse followed, with a "flickering return to reason" preceding her sudden death.[86] "[I]f we were not permitted to see Lucy's mad scene," noted one newspaper, "we saw her touching and poetic death."[87] Though Terry was charged with playing a "lifeless heroine," something she often bemoaned about in her memoirs, Michael Holroyd claims that as Lucy Ashton, Terry "found some relief [from more taxing roles] in going insane like Ophelia and dying before a Turneresque landscape."[88] That a young woman of robust physical health could be felled by a sudden shock (or perhaps a resulting cardiac arrest) drew no commentary from critics.

In her Lyceum years, Ellen Terry composed a set of mental illness roles that affirmed symbolic and clinical figurations of female hysteria and insanity, calibrating them and their aesthetic leverage for the Victorian popular stage. A comparative analysis of these performances yields several crucial findings. First, the actress's fetchingly feminine embodiments of hysteria and madness reinforced the nineteenth-century notion that mental illness was a commonly occurring and not entirely dreadful condition in women: a normal abnormal state-of-being. Unlike Ibsen's new stage hysterics who struggled within and through their psychoses, Terry's characters grew increasingly beautiful, natural, and pathetic after madness commandeered their corporealities: minds, nerves, and/or reproductive organs. Each embodiment also corroborated medicocultural assumptions about the causes of female madness. Lady Macbeth's fatal choice to breach the masculine sphere's barriers—a move fully at odds with her maternalistic, nervous depiction—was rendered exceedingly topical by Terry's portrayal. Her ceremonious (but half-hearted) unsexing was abortive; she remained resolutely feminine throughout her participation in Duncan's murder and the ensuing public duplicity, as well as her private, sensual coddling of Irving's milksop Macbeth. Because these deeds were not executed from a position of appropriated masculinity, the gentlewoman's mental and reproductive health were immutably ruined, echoing the threats of Darwinian psychiatrists lobbed at the ambitious New Woman. That Terry's Lady Macbeth may have also experienced the anguish of losing an infant child only strengthens her likeness to the Victorian hysteric. Unanticipated emotional traumas (Charcot's *le grand ébranlement psychique*) also intensified the already fragile states (*tare nerveuse*) of both Ophelia and Lucy. As performed by Terry, Ophelia's vulnerability to hysterical attacks and insanity was linked to male subjugation and the repression of sexual desires, while Lucy's appears to be embedded in her genetic makeup, thanks to her unbalanced mother. All three characters exhibited classic indicators of hysteria and madness and all were presented as wretchedly weak in mind and body. Finally, Terry's performances of illness confirmed the morbid Victorian illation, no doubt influenced by pervasive cultural representations of incurable madwomen, that female insanity was far more intractable than that of men. Ophelia, Lady Macbeth, and Lucy Ashton pay the ultimate price for their slip off the precipice of mental health: death.

Notes

1 "The Rose Norreys Fund," *The Era*, Sept 14, 1895.
2 "Miss Rose Norreys," *The Era*, Sept 14, 1895.
3 The Lunacy Act of 1845, which together with the Country Asylums Act classified the mentally ill as patients requiring institutionalizing or professional monitoring, distinguished between idiots (those born with severe and permanent mental deficiencies), lunatics (those who suffered bouts of madness interposed between times of lucidity), and people of unsound minds (those who because of a "morbid condition of intellect" were incapable of self-management and sensible judgments). Quoted in David Wright, *Mental Disability in Victorian England: The Earlswood Asylum, 1847–1901* (Oxford: Oxford University Press, 2001), 16.
4 Andrew Scull, *The Most Solitary of Afflictions: Madness and Society in Britain, 1700–1900* (New Haven: Yale University Press, 1993), 2–3. There are a wealth of cultural histories of mental illness, institutionalization, and psychiatry in the Victorian period, including Lisa Appignanesi, *Mad, Bad and Sad: Women and the Mind Doctors* (New York: W.W. Norton, 2008), 53–180; Marlene A. Arieno, *Victorian Lunatics: A Social Epidemiology of Mental Illness in Mid-Nineteenth-Century England* (Selinsgrove: Susquehanna University Press, 1989); Joseph Melling and Bill Forsythe, eds., *Insanity, Institutions and Society, 1800–1914: A Social History of Madness in Comparative Perspective* (London: Routledge, 1999); Roy Porter, *A Social History of Madness: Stories of the Insane* (London: Weidenfeld and Nicolson, 1987); Andrew Scull, ed., *Madness in Civilization: A Cultural History of Insanity, from the Bible to Freud, From the Madhouse to Modern Medicine* (Princeton: Princeton University Press, 2015); Anna Shepherd, *Institutionalizing the Insane in Nineteenth-Century England* (London: Pickering & Chatto Ltd, 2014); and Jennifer Wallis, *Investigating the Body in the Victorian Asylum: Doctors, Patients, and Practices* (London: Palgrave Macmillan, 2017).
5 Scull, *Most Solitary of Afflictions*, 8. See also Janet Oppenheim, *"Shattered Nerves": Doctors, Patients, and Depression in Victorian England* (New York: Oxford University Press, 1991) Foucault's arguments are found in his *Madness and Civilization: A History of Insanity in the Age of Reason* (New York: Vintage, 1988), while Szasz's are in *The Myth of Mental Illness: Foundations of a Theory of Personal Conduct* (New York: Harper, 1984) and *The Manufacture of Madness: A Comparative Study of the Inquisition and the Mental Health Movement* (Syracuse, NY: Syracuse University Press, 1997).

6 Because of the Lyceum's location, I have chosen largely to focus on British and continental European understandings and treatments of "mental disease," though I periodically draw on pertinent American sources, such as George Miller Beard's pioneering concept of neurasthenia. The United States developed its mental health care systems primarily in the nineteenth and early twentieth centuries, including a vast network of public hospitals designed to cure the curable and care for patients unresponsive to therapies, as well as the robust discipline of psychiatry. Influenced by European science (particularly German) and the Enlightenment and rooted in the moral tenets of Christian Protestantism and American exceptionalism, the country's mental health care system was both an outgrowth of European models and a distinctive, culturally bound approach. The push for a nonrestraint system in English mental institutions in the 1830s, for example, did not take hold in the United States for a number of reasons, leading to a fierce debate between American and British asylum doctors over medical ethics, patient safety, and race slavery. Lynn Gamwell and Nancy Tomes, *Madness in America: Cultural and Medical Perceptions of Mental Illness Before 1914* (New York: Cornell University Press, 1995), 46.

7 See Shepherd's *Institutionalizing the Insane* and Melling and Forsythe, eds., *Insanity, Institutions and Society*.

8 Jane E. Kromm, "The Feminization of Madness in Visual Representation," *Feminist Studies* 20, no. 3 (Autumn 1994): 507–535.

9 Michael Holroyd, *A Strange Eventful History: The Dramatic Lives of Ellen Terry, Henry Irving, and Their Remarkable Families* (New York: Farrar, Straus and Giroux, 2009), 115. This biographical sketch of Terry was composed from Holroyd's history as well as the following sources: Nina Auerbach, *Ellen Terry: Player in Her Time* (New York: W.W. Norton, 1987); Michael R. Booth, "Ellen Terry," in *Bernhardt, Terry, Duse: The Actress in Her Time* (Cambridge: Cambridge University Press, 1988); Roger Manvell, *Ellen Terry* (New York: G.P. Putnam, 1968); Russ McDonald, *Look to the Lady: Sarah Siddons, Ellen Terry, and Judi Dench on the Shakespearean Stage* (Athens: University of Georgia Press, 2005); and Joy Melville, *Ellen Terry* (London: Haus Books, 2006).

10 Terry's other two marriages were to actors Charles Kelly (real name Wardell) and James Carew.

11 The Lyceum Theatre toured the United States and Canada eight times during Irving's management, with openings in 1883, 1884, 1887, 1893, 1895, 1899, 1901, and 1903. Terry was no longer with the company for the final tour, as she had begun her own management of the Imperial Theatre alongside her son in 1903.

12 Charles Hiatt, *Ellen Terry and Her Impersonations* (London: George Bell, 1898), 266.

13 "Landing and Reception at New York," *New York Herald*, reprinted in *Mr. Henry Irving and Miss Ellen Terry in America: Opinions of the Press* (Chicago: John Morris, 1884), V&A.

14 Anorexia nervosa and nymphomania, both believed to predominantly strike women, were either conflated with or acknowledged to be components of hysteria, and physicians often considered a patient's hysterical condition a chilling harbinger of full-blown insanity.

15 Mark S. Micale, *Hysterical Men: The Hidden History of Male Nervous Illness* (Cambridge: Harvard University Press, 2008), 159 and 160.

16 Micale, *Hysterical Men*, 129.

17 Robert Brudenell Carter, *On the Pathology and Treatment of Hysteria* (London: John Churchill, 1853), 33.

18 Mark S. Micale's *Approaching Hysteria: Disease and Its Interpretations* (Princeton: Princeton University Press, 1995) covers this ongoing debate.

19 Hysteria's list of possible causes included the following: a wandering womb or uterine suffocation; erotic urges, masturbation or an excessively passionate soul; sexual abstinence; a humoral imbalance; illnesses such as scarlet fever, the flu, and rheumatism; witchcraft; demonic or animal spirit possessions; any and all aspects of a woman's lifecycle; sundry venereal diseases; reproductive barrenness, miscarriages, or stillbirths; a cerebral affliction; melancholy; exorbitant bodily processes (including fasting, bleeding, purging, and evacuations); overindulgence of foods rich in animal fat; a nervous disorder; extreme

sensibility; the repression of emotional or sexual desires; and sudden shocks. Though nearly all scholarly treatments of hysteria provide an account of the various etiological theories, Ilza Veith's coverage in *Hysteria: The History of a Disease* (Chicago: University of Chicago Press, 1965) is the most comprehensive.

20 Elisabeth Bronfen, *The Knotted Subject: Hysteria and Its Discontents* (Princeton: Princeton University Press, 1998), xi. For other (often contradictory) inquiries into the historical subject of hysteria and its elusive but crucial role in nineteenth-century culture, see Laura Briggs, "The Race of Hysteria: 'Overcivilization' and the 'Savage' Woman in Late Nineteenth-Century Obstetrics and Gynecology," *American Quarterly* 52, no. 2 (2000): 246–273; Elin Diamond, *Unmaking Mimesis: Essays on Feminism and Theater* (London: Routledge, 1997); Elizabeth J. Donaldson, "The Corpus of the Madwoman: Toward a Feminist Disability Studies Theory of Embodiment and Mental Illness," *Feminist Formations* 14, no. 3 (Fall 2002): 99–119; Sander Gilman et al., *Hysteria Beyond Freud* (Berkeley: University of California Press, 1993); Diane Price Herndl, *Invalid Women: Figuring Feminine Illness in American Fiction and Culture, 1840–1940* (Chapel Hill: University of North Carolina Press, 1993); R. A. Houston, "Madness and Gender in the Long Eighteenth Century," *Social History*, 23, no. 3 (2002): 309–326; Micale, *Approaching Hysteria* and *Hysterical Men*; Andrew Scull, *Hysteria: The Biography* (Oxford: Oxford University Press, 2009); Elaine Showalter, *The Female Malady: Women, Madness, and English Culture, 1830–1980* (New York: Pantheon, 1985); Showalter, *Hystories: Hysterical Epidemics and Modern Media* (New York: Columbia University Press), 1997); and Joanna Townsend, "Elizabeth Robins: Hysteria, Politics and Performance," in *Women, Theatre, and Performance: New Histories, New Historiographies*, eds. Maggie B. Gale and Viv Gardner (Manchester: Manchester University Press, 2000).
21 Roy Porter, "The Body and the Mind, the Doctor and the Patient: Negotiating Hysteria," *Hysteria Beyond Freud*, 225–285, 251, and 253.
22 Porter, "Body and the Mind," 254.
23 Elaine Showalter, "Victorian Women and Insanity," in *Madhouses, Mad-Doctors, and Madmen: The Social History of Psychiatry in the Victorian Era*, ed. Andrew Scull (Philadelphia: University of Pennsylvania Press, 1981), 313–338, 332.
24 Porter, "Body and the Mind," 243.
25 Oppenheim, "*Shattered Nerves*," 152.
26 Showalter, *Female Malady*, 123.
27 Ibid., 184.
28 Herndl, *Invalid Women*, 21.
29 Porter, *Social History of Madness*, 113.
30 Diamond, *Unmaking Mimesis*, 10. For Diamond, hysteria has the potential to disrupt "traditional epistemological methods of seeing/knowing," whether it is situated empirically as a historical medical disorder, or discursively as a part of a feminist reclamation of the condition's symbolic force. While I agree with Diamond's assertion, it is also crucial to recognize hysteria's significance to the process of feminizing mental illness in the nineteenth century. The condition's deployment in feminist and anti-feminist discourses is one of its most intriguing, vexing qualities.
31 Micale, *Hysterical Men*, 141.
32 Appignanesi, *Mad, Bad and Sad*, 136.
33 Ibid., 137–138.
34 For American physician A.F.A. King, women only felt one thing following exhibitions of hysterical phenomena: shame. King, *Hysteria* (New York: William Wood & Co., 1891), 7.
35 Kromm, "Feminization of Madness," 515.
36 Phyllis Chesler, *Women and Madness* (Garden City: Doubleday, 1972), 37; and Porter, "Body and the Mind," 229.
37 Jane Wood, *Passion and Pathology in Victorian Fiction* (Oxford: Oxford University Press, 2001), 6–7.
38 Ellen Terry, *Story of My Life* (London: Hutchinson, 1908), 153.

39 Quoted in Showalter, *Female Malady*, 92.
40 Terry, *Story of My Life*, 154–155.
41 Ibid., 157.
42 Ibid., 155–157.
43 Holroyd, *Strange and Eventful History*, 117.
44 Kimberly Rhodes, *Ophelia and Victorian Visual Culture: Representing Body Politics in the Nineteenth Century* (Aldershot: Ashgate, 2008), 51. Both images are available in Rhodes's book.
45 Ellen Terry, *Four Lectures on Shakespeare*, ed. Christopher St. John (New York: Benjamin Blom: 1969), 165.
46 Auerbach, *Ellen Terry*, 237.
47 Terry, *Story of My Life*, 279.
48 This debate on agency, feminism, and nineteenth-century invalidism is recorded in the following: Chesler, *Women and Madness*; Rachel Fensham, "On Not Performing Madness," *Theatre Topics* 8, no. 2 (1998): 149–171; Showalter, "Hysteria, Feminism, and Gender," in *Hysteria Beyond Freud*, 286–344; Sandra M. Gilbert and Susan Gubar, *The Madwoman in the Attic: The Woman Writer and the Nineteenth-Century Literary Imagination* (New Haven: Yale University Press, 1979); Donaldson, "The Corpus of the Madwoman"; Marta Caminero-Santangelo, *The Madwoman Can't Speak: Or, Why Insanity is Not Subversive* (Ithaca: Cornell University Press, 1998); and Shoshana Felman, "Women and Madness: The Critical Phallacy," in *Feminisms: An Anthology of Literary Theory and Criticism*, eds. Robyn R. Warhol and Diane Price Herndl (New Brunswick, NJ: Rutgers University Press, 1997), 7–20.
49 *Baltimore Day*, reprinted in "Mr Irving and Miss Terry in America," unidentified newspaper clipping, Henry Irving Scrapbook – Freeman, Henry Irving Biographical File, personal box 51, V&A.
50 "Hamlet at the Lyceum," *Punch*, Jan 11, 1879, Henry Irving Scrapbook – Peters, V&A.
51 *Boston Traveller*, reprinted in unidentified newspaper, Oct 21, 1884, V&A. See also *Chicago Times*, reprinted in "Mr Irving and Miss Terry in America," unidentified newspaper clipping, Henry Irving Scrapbook – Freeman, Henry Irving Biographical File, personal box 51, V&A.
52 Alan Hughes, *Henry Irving, Shakespearean* (Cambridge: Cambridge University Press, 1981).
53 "Lyceum Theatre," *Dramatic Notes* (Dec 1879): 13–18; Henry Irving Scrapbook – Peters, V&A, 14.
54 Booth, "Ellen Terry," in *Bernhardt, Terry, Duse*, 100.
55 Rhodes, *Ophelia and Victorian Visual Culture*, 146.
56 Ibid., 146.
57 *Boston Globe*, reprinted in unidentified newspaper, Oct 21, 1884, V&A.
58 "*Macbeth*:—Shakespearian Criticism and Acting," *Westminster Review* 41, no. 1 (Aug 12, 1843): 1–72, 65.
59 Letter from Ellen Terry to William Winter, reprinted in Auerbach, *Ellen Terry*, 259. I have retained Terry's punctuation but have removed her copious underlines.
60 Terry, *Four Lectures on Shakespeare*, 125; and Melville, *Ellen Terry*, 144.
61 Booth, "Ellen Terry," in *Bernhardt, Terry, Duse*, 107.
62 Quoted in Auerbach, *Ellen Terry*, 256.
63 McDonald, *Look to the Lady*, 97.
64 *Pall Mall Gazette*, Dec 31, 1888, reprinted in *The Era*, Jan 26, 1889, V&A.
65 *The People*, Dec 30, 1888, reprinted in *The Era*, Jan 26, 1889, V&A.
66 *The World*, Jan 2, 1889, reprinted in *The Era*, Jan 26, 1889, V&A.
67 Terry, *Story of My Life*, 306.
68 *The Graphic*, January 5, 1889, Lyceum 1888, box 1436, V&A.
69 *Sporting and Dramatic News*, Jan 5, 1889, Lyceum 1888, box 1436, V&A. Emphases added.
70 *The Star*, Dec 31, 1888, reprinted in *The Era*, Jan 26, 1889, V&A.
71 *The Times*, Dec 31, 1888, reprinted in *The Era*, Jan 26, 1889, 16, V&A.

72 Appignanesi, *Mad, Bad and Sad*, 148. Charcot published a case history of "hysterical sleepwalking" in January 1893.

73 Charcot's research was often published in English in the *Lancet* and *BMJ*, and he periodically traveled to Britain for medical congresses and to deliver keynote addresses in English. Charcot's fame in England, at least within the scientific communities, was on full display at 1881's International Medical Congress in London, where Charcot presented on neuropathic joint disease. The congress's main hall featured his bust alongside the busts of Pasteur and Virchow, and his face was blasted into the sky over the Crystal Palace with fireworks on the congress's final night. Raymond Hierons, "Charcot and His Visits to London," *BMJ* (December 13, 1993): 1589–1591, 1590.

74 Joanna Levin, "Lady Macbeth and the Daemonologie of Hysteria," *ELH* 69, no. 1 (Spring 2002): 21–55, 43.

75 Quoted in Melville, *Ellen Terry*, 144.

76 *The Globe*, Dec 31, 1888, reprinted in *The Era*, Jan 26, 1889, V&A; and "Before and Behind the Curtain," *London Figaro*, Jan 5, 1889, Lyceum 1888, box 1436, V&A.

77 *Daily News*, Dec 31, 1888, reprinted in *The Era*, Jan 26, 1889, V&A.

78 "'Macbeth' at the Lyceum Theatre," *The Graphic*, undated, personal box 54, Henry Irving and Ellen Terry, Theatre Museum Biographical File, V&A.

79 "Before and Behind the Curtain," *London Figaro*, Jan 5, 1889, Lyceum 1888, box 1436, V&A.

80 Elaine Showalter relates the physical manifestations of Lucy's violent madness in Scott's *The Bride of Lammermoor*: "But on her wedding night, the guests hear shrieks coming from the bridal chamber. Rushing to the room, they discover the bridegroom stabbed on the threshold and Lucy huddled in a corner, 'her head-gear disheveled; her night-clothes torn and dabbled with blood, – her eyes glazed, and her features convulsed into a wild paroxysm of insanity. When she saw herself discovered, she gibbered, made mouths, and pointed at them with her bloody fingers, with the frantic gestures of an exulting demoniac.'" Showalter, *Female Malady*, 14.

81 "The Theatre," unidentified newspaper clipping, box 54, Henry Irving and Ellen Terry, Theatre Museum Biographical File, V&A.

82 W. L. C., "The Lyceum 'Ravenswood,'" *Murray's Magazine* 8 (1890): 696–703, 701.

83 Of the reviews I consulted, the critic at *Punch* was the only reviewer that thought Terry's Lucy "already show[ed] signs of incipient insanity" before the telltale snap of raving laughter. ("Scott-Free, or Ravenswood-Notes Wild," *Punch*, Oct 4, 1890, 160, *Ravenswood* production file, V&A).

84 Unidentified newspaper clipping, box 54, Henry Irving and Ellen Terry, Theatre Museum Biographical File, V&A.

85 "Scott-Free, or Ravenswood-Notes Wild," *Punch*, Oct 4, 1890, *Ravenswood* production file, V&A. Terry later revealed just how predictable her seemingly impulsive laugh was, according to biographer Joy Melville. "Ellen [came] off stage one night, after a scene with Irving in which she had to burst into hysterical laughter, to find Irving waiting for her, much put out, to ask why she had finished laughing early. She said she had laughed as usual. 'No you didn't,' said Irving. 'You always say Ha-ha 17 times. You only said it 14 times tonight.'" Melville, *Ellen Terry*, 147–148.

86 W. L. C., "The Lyceum 'Ravenswood,'" 702.

87 Unidentified newspaper clipping, box 54, Henry Irving and Ellen Terry, Theatre Museum Biographical File, V&A.

88 Holroyd, *Strange and Eventful History*, 223.

Bibliography

Appignanesi, Lisa. *Mad, Bad and Sad: Women and the Mind Doctors*. New York: W.W. Norton, 2008.

Arieno, Marlene A. *Victorian Lunatics: A Social Epidemiology of Mental Illness in Mid-Nineteenth-Century England*. Selinsgrove: Susquehanna University Press, 1989.

Auerbach, Nina. *Ellen Terry: Player in Her Time*. New York: W.W. Norton, 1987.

Booth, Michael R. "Ellen Terry." In *Bernhardt, Terry, Duse: The Actress in Her Time*, edited by John Stokes, Michael R. Booth, and Susan Bassnett, 65–118. Cambridge: Cambridge University Press, 1988.

Briggs, Laura. "The Race of Hysteria: 'Overcivilization' and the 'Savage' Woman in Late Nineteenth-Century Obstetrics and Gynecology." *American Quarterly* 52, no. 2 (2000): 246–273.

Bronfen, Elisabeth. *The Knotted Subject: Hysteria and Its Discontents*. Princeton: Princeton University Press, 1998.

C., W. L. "The Lyceum 'Ravenswood.'" *Murray's Magazine* 8 (1890): 696–703.

Caminero-Santangelo, Marta. *The Madwoman Can't Speak: Or, Why Insanity is Not Subversive*. Ithaca: Cornell University Press, 1998.

Carter, Robert Brudenell. *On the Pathology and Treatment of Hysteria*. London: John Churchill, 1853.

Chesler, Phyllis. *Women and Madness*. Garden City: Doubleday, 1972.

Diamond, Elin. *Unmaking Mimesis: Essays on Feminism and Theater*. London: Routledge, 1997.

Donaldson, Elizabeth J. "The Corpus of the Madwoman: Toward a Feminist Disability Studies Theory of Embodiment and Mental Illness." *Feminist Formations* 14, no. 3 (Fall 2002): 99–119.

Felman, Shoshana. "Women and Madness: The Critical Phallacy." In *Feminisms: An Anthology of Literary Theory and Criticism*, edited by Robyn R. Warhol and Diane Price Herndl, 7–20. New Brunswick, NJ: Rutgers University Press, 1997.

Fensham, Rachel. "On Not Performing Madness." *Theatre Topics* 8, no. 2 (1998): 149–171.

Foucault, Michel. *Madness and Civilization: A History of Insanity in the Age of Reason*. New York: Vintage, 1988.

Gamwell, Lynn and Nancy Tomes. *Madness in America: Cultural and Medical Perceptions of Mental Illness Before 1914*. New York: Cornell University Press, 1995.

Gilbert, Sandra M. and Susan Gubar. *The Madwoman in the Attic: The Woman Writer and the Nineteenth-Century Literary Imagination*. New Haven: Yale University Press, 1979.

Gilman, Sander, L., Helen King, Roy Porter, G. S. Rousseau, and Elaine Showalter. *Hysteria Beyond Freud*. Berkeley: University of California Press, 1993.

Herndl, Diane Price. *Invalid Women: Figuring Feminine Illness in American Fiction and Culture, 1840–1940*. Chapel Hill: University of North Carolina Press, 1993.

Hiatt, Charles. *Ellen Terry and Her Impersonations*. London: George Bell, 1898.

Hierons, Raymond. "Charcot and His Visits to London." *BMJ* (Dec 13, 1993): 1589–1591.

Holroyd, Michael. *A Strange Eventful History: The Dramatic Lives of Ellen Terry, Henry Irving, and Their Remarkable Families*. New York: Farrar, Straus and Giroux, 2009.

Houston, R. A. "Madness and Gender in the Long Eighteenth Century." *Social History* 23, no. 3 (2002): 309–326.

Hughes, Alan. *Henry Irving, Shakespearean*. Cambridge: Cambridge University Press, 1981.

King, A.F.A. *Hysteria*. New York: William Wood & Co., 1891.

Kromm, Jane E. "The Feminization of Madness in Visual Representation." *Feminist Studies* 20, no. 3 (Autumn 1994): 507–535.

Levin, Joanna. "Lady Macbeth and the Daemonologie of Hysteria." *ELH* 69, no. 1 (Spring 2002): 21–55.

"*Macbeth*:—Shakespearian Criticism and Acting," *Westminster Review* 41, no. 1 (Aug 12, 1843): 1–72.

Manvell, Roger. *Ellen Terry*. New York: G.P. Putnam, 1968.

McDonald, Russ. *Look to the Lady: Sarah Siddons, Ellen Terry, and Judi Dench on the Shake-spearean Stage*. Athens: University of Georgia Press, 2005.

Melling Joseph and Bill Forsythe, eds. *Insanity, Institutions and Society, 1800–1914: A Social History of Madness in Comparative Perspective*. London: Routledge, 1999.

Melville, Joy. *Ellen Terry*. London: Haus Books, 2006.

Micale, Mark S. *Approaching Hysteria: Disease and Its Interpretations*. Princeton: Princeton University Press, 1995.

Micale, Mark S. *Hysterical Men: The Hidden History of Male Nervous Illness*. Cambridge: Harvard University Press, 2008.

Oppenheim, Janet. *"Shattered Nerves": Doctors, Patients, and Depression in Victorian England*. Oxford: Oxford University Press, 1991.

Porter, Roy. *Bodies Politic: Disease, Death, and Doctors in Britain, 1650–1900*. Ithaca: Cornell University Press, 2001.

Porter, Roy. "The Body and the Mind, the Doctor and the Patient: Negotiating Hysteria." In *Hysteria Beyond Freud*, edited by Sander L. Gilman, Helen King, Roy Porter, G. S. Rousseau, and Elaine Showalter, 225–285. Berkeley: University of California Press, 1993.

Porter, Roy. *A Social History of Madness: Stories of the Insane*. London: Weidenfeld and Nicolson, 1987.

Rhodes, Kimberly. *Ophelia and Victorian Visual Culture: Representing Body Politics in the Nineteenth Century*. Aldershot: Ashgate, 2008.

Scull, Andrew. *Hysteria: The Biography*. Oxford: Oxford University Press, 2009.

Scull, Andrew. *Madness in Civilization: A Cultural History of Insanity, from the Bible to Freud, From the Madhouse to Modern Medicine*. Princeton: Princeton University Press, 2015.

Scull, Andrew. *The Most Solitary of Afflictions: Madness and Society in Britain, 1700–1900*. New Haven: Yale University Press, 1993.

Scull, Andrew, ed. *Madhouses, Mad-Doctors, and Madmen: The Social History of Psychiatry in the Victorian Era*. Philadelphia: University of Pennsylvania Press, 1981.

Shepherd, Anna. *Institutionalizing the Insane in Nineteenth-Century England*. London: Pickering & Chatto Ltd, 2014.

Showalter, Elaine. "Hysteria, Feminism, and Gender." In *Hysteria Beyond Freud*, edited by Sander L. Gilman, Helen King, Roy Porter, G. S. Rousseau, and Elaine Showalter, 286–344. Berkeley: University of California Press, 1993.

Showalter, Elaine. *Hystories: Hysterical Epidemics and Modern Media*. New York: Columbia University Press, 1997

Showalter, Elaine. *The Female Malady: Women, Madness, and English Culture, 1830–1980*. New York: Pantheon, 1985.

Showalter, Elaine. "Victorian Women and Insanity." In *Madhouses, Mad-Doctors, and Madmen: The Social History of Psychiatry in the Victorian Era*, edited by Andrew Scull, 313–338. Philadelphia: University of Pennsylvania Press, 1981.

Szasz, Thomas. *The Manufacture of Madness: A Comparative Study of the Inquisition and the Mental Health Movement*. Syracuse: Syracuse University Press, 1997.

Szasz, Thomas. *The Myth of Mental Illness: Foundations of a Theory of Personal Conduct*. New York: Harper, 1984.

Terry, Ellen. *Four Lectures on Shakespeare*. Edited by Christopher St. John. New York: Benjamin Blom: 1969.

Terry, Ellen. *Story of My Life*. London: Hutchinson, 1908.

Townsend, Joanna. "Elizabeth Robins: Hysteria, Politics and Performance." In *Women, Theatre, and Performance: New Histories, New Historiographies*, edited by Maggie B. Gale and Viv Gardner, 102–120. Manchester: Manchester University Press, 2000.

Veith, Ilza. *Hysteria: The History of a Disease*. Chicago: University of Chicago Press, 1965.

Wallis, Jennifer. *Investigating the Body in the Victorian Asylum: Doctors, Patients, and Practices.* London: Palgrave Macmillan, 2017.

Wood, Jane. *Passion and Pathology in Victorian Fiction.* Oxford: Oxford University Press, 2001.

Wright, David. *Mental Disability in Victorian England: The Earlswood Asylum, 1847–1901.* Oxford: Oxford University Press, 2001.

6 Neurotic princes and enfeebled kings

Stigmatizing male mental illness in Henry Irving's mad roles

If Victorians conceived of madwomen as organic creatures that had surrendered to their gender's foundational instability, they deemed madmen true perversions of nature. As the divinely and evolutionarily chosen vessels of reason, moderation, resourcefulness, and enterprise as well as physical muscularity (or so nineteenth-century ideologies maintained), men lacked the intrinsic emotionalism and intellectual fragility that tethered women to so-called "mind disorders." Their native potential squandered and thwarted by mental illness, madmen were among Victorian society's most tragic figures, both pitied and abhorred. Centuries past represented the male lunatic as a raging, aggressive, hyper-masculine beast; the modern emasculated madman, in contrast, was doubly enfeebled by the gradual feminization of mental illness in the nineteenth century and burgeoning *fin-de-siècle* theories of social and biological degeneration. Though the mentally ill male, so unnaturally trapped in his psychogenic cage, required intense medical treatment in order to be restored to sanity and balance, his biological sex assured physicians that rehabilitation was possible. Perhaps because of this gendered paradox, Victorian medicine was less inclined to lump all masculine mental ailments into one general diagnosis, as was sometimes the function of female hysteria. Attempts to clarify the origins and symptomatic borders of masculine mental illnesses, or to divide them into "partial" and "general" insanities or functional disorders, largely failed to advance medical knowledge or improve treatment. Still, cultural expressions of mental illness, including those generated in Victorian theatres, contributed to the deliberate gendering of mind disorders in incongruous ways; male mental patients were often stigmatized as burdensome or impotent anomalies of their sex, and yet they were also depicted as more capable of recovering their health and reason than women. During his tenure at the Lyceum Theatre, actor-manager Henry Irving constructed a repertoire of psychological illness roles that drew upon the expanding catalogue of masculine neuroses and psychoses forwarded by Victorian psychiatrists, while deepening the affiliations of mentally ill men (however sympathetically drawn) with aberrance, degeneration, and emasculation.

Born in 1838 in Somerset, England, John Henry Brodribb's early years were spent in Cornwall being looked after by his aunt Sarah and her violent-tempered husband and, in his happiest times, playing pretend with his Cornish chums. Financial hardships befell the Brodribbs soon after John's birth, necessitating his relocation, but by age eleven John was back with his parents, this time in London. Upon seeing his first play, *Hamlet*, at Samuel Phelps' Sadler's Wells, he resolved to become an actor. The adolescent John worked clerical jobs in order to fund his entrance into the craft of acting: fencing lessons, elocution classes, a fitness regimen that included daily swims in the Thames, and eventually private tutorials in comedy and pantomime. His hard work paid off when he secured a position in a provincial theatre under his new stage name, Henry Irving. Critics and audiences were quick to point out Irving's shortcomings: his broken speech patterns with strangely accented vowels, idiosyncratic gestures and facial expressions, and, writes Michael Holroyd, "the dragging gait on bent knees with which he unevenly perambulated the stage."[1] Despite Irving's best efforts, a severe childhood stutter returned in times of nervousness. And yet, even in his early years, there was something captivating about Irving onstage: intense, controlled, and both cerebrally and kinesthetically aware, he was dynamic without resorting to the artificial theatrics of the classical school of acting and uncommonly adept at manifesting his characters' psychological turmoil. Irving earned increasingly positive reviews while on tour, particularly as a character actor of ingenuity and wit. He married Florence O'Callaghan in 1869 and was shortly after hired by Hezekiah Bateman to be the leading actor opposite his daughter Isabel at London's Lyceum Theatre. The Irvings had two sons but lived apart completely from 1871 on when, after his thunderously applauded premiere in *The Bells*, a pregnant Florence asked him "Are you going on making a fool of yourself like this all your life?" Irving immediately exited the brougham carrying them home from the theatre and never spoke to his wife again, save the occasional letter.[2] Over the next seven years Irving became the preeminent London actor, and in 1878 he took over the Lyceum from the Bateman family, where his prodigious self-discipline expanded outward to encompass all of his duties as theatre manager and visionary.

Despite his probable belief to the contrary, Irving was not an immersive actor. Though he seemed to feel the emotions of his characters keenly, Irving nevertheless remained Irvingesque in all roles he embodied. As *Times* critic A. B. Walkley noted in 1892's *Playhouse Impressions*: "It was evident from the first that he had not the fluid or ductile temperament which makes your all-round actor, your Betterton, your Garrick … Mr. Irving's individuality is too strongly marked."[3] The actor's "profound intellectuality" was part of this individuality, Eden Phillpotts wrote when recalling Irving's Hamlet: "Irving was an embodied brain of the most subtle and radical clarity."[4] For some critics, Irving appeared too animated and affected, urging the actor to curb his mannerisms or risk jeopardizing his career. Even more censorious was 1877's *The Fashionable Tragedian*, an "anonymous" pamphlet penned by William Archer and Robert William Lowe, which chastised audiences for applauding "every jerk, every spasm, every hysteric scream – we had almost said every convulsion – in which [Irving] chose to indulge."[5] It was not uncommon for the press to label Irving "realistic," though the word remained ambiguously applied even in theatrical realism's peak decades.

The Brits behind *The Fashionable Tragedian* bemoaned "his tendency to carry realism to a ludicrous extent," and American dramatist and theatre manager Augustin Daly wrote of Irving's "frenzy – for it appears to be a frenzy with him, – to be realistic or NATURAL."[6] Besides his crowd-pleasing comedic turns that dwindled in number as he aged, Irving was best known for portraying men suffering from a guilty conscience, an overwhelming emotional trauma, or some other sorrow that—to the detriment of the characters' health—must be kept secret.

Irving's features were not classically handsome, but they matured together into a distinguished countenance that bore a considerable resemblance to period descriptions of neurasthenics and melancholics: thin figure, pale complexion (Irving portraitist Mortimer Menpes called it "iron-grey"), jet-black hair, piercing eyes, a forehead that sloped into a considerable brow bone and heavy eyebrows, and high cheekbones, narrow nose, and delicate mouth, which together made the lower half of his face a touch feminine.[7] His hands were long and thin-fingered, his shoulders were tapered and could be curled forward into a slouch or pressed back into a sharply erect posture depending on the role, and his softened knees made the actor appear to be in a sustained plié onstage. While his style was powerful and vigorous, it was not hypermasculine like the Forrests or Keans in decades prior. Irving approached character-building with an analytical mind, aiming to plumb the depths of his characters' psychologies, but he also relied upon gestural codes to communicate those psychologies to audiences. Commentators described Irving's cerebral and meticulous mode of acting as 'psychological,' 'hypnotic,' or 'nervous,' pronouncements befitting the modern age of psychiatry. Irving's art, the skillful conversion of mental states into perceptible actions, reveals as much about how Victorians conceived of and dealt with masculine mental illnesses as it does about nineteenth-century pictorial acting. While Ellen Terry's performances glided imprecisely along a feminized spectrum of hysteria and insanity, Irving's illness roles bore more definitive characteristics of discrete disorders, corroborating the perception that masculine mental illnesses—despite their nosological and theoretical slipperiness—were more deliberately delineated and rigorously combated than women's conditions. Like Terry's repertoire of madwomen and hysterics, Irving's madmen together advanced a bleak thesis: untreated mental illnesses marked men as inadequate or malignant leaders, providers, and partners, leading to tragic repercussions. Here I would like to reconstruct three of Irving's most scrutinized illness roles, examining the actor's script preparations and embodied practices in order to diagnose *The Bells*' Mathias, Hamlet, and King Lear, however tentatively, with Victorian mind disorders of medicocultural import.

Mathias, 1871

While still a hired player at the Lyceum, Irving lobbied Hezekiah Bateman to produce Leopold Lewis's translation of the French play *Le Juif Polonais*, or *The Polish Jew*, which had premiered in 1869 at the Théâtre Cluny.[8] The play tells the story of Mathias, who, as an impecunious young husband and father of an infant daughter, murdered a stranger for money. The crime was one of desperation and opportunity, the victim a Polish Jew who sought shelter in Mathias's hut from a Christmas Eve snowstorm. Mathias incinerated the body in a nearby limekiln and grew prosperous from the gold in the Jew's money belt, eventually becoming the town's burgomaster. During the course of the play's action, which begins on the fifteenth anniversary of the murder, Mathias's anxiety overtakes his reason: the bells of the victim's sleigh ring unabatedly in his ears and visions of the murder flash before his eyes. In the play's final act, Mathias dreams that he is being tried for murder and under the powers of a hypnotist is forced to act out his crime, after which the imagined court sentences Mathias to death by hanging. He awakens as full-blown mania overwhelms him and dies in anguish, imagining the hangman's noose tightening around his neck. Though Bateman was not entirely convinced of the play's virtues, he agreed to Irving's request. From his first performance as Mathias on November 25, 1871, to his last on the day before his death in October 1905, Irving played the role over 800 times, 151 of those in its opening season alone.[9]

The Lyceum's version of *The Bells* departed from *Le Juif Polonais* in ways that deepened Mathias's psychological trauma. With its emphasis on the mesmeric arts and the inclusion of a spectacular vision scene in which Mathias witnesses his younger self stalking the traveler's horse-drawn sleigh with a hatchet, *The Bells* blurred the distinctions between psychosomatic and supernatural phenomena far more than *Le Juif Polonais*. More importantly, however, the Lyceum's adaptation established Mathias's psychological deterioration as the dramatic action's catalyst, climax, and denouement. Whereas Mathias's criminality is only implied in *Le Juif Polonais* prior to his third act confession, *The Bells* reveals all by the end of act one, inviting theatregoers to witness Mathias's mental decline with the full knowledge of his guilt. *The Bells* is therefore less suspenseful but more moralistic than its source material. Furthermore, French and English performers conceived of the burgomaster's remorsefulness disparately. French actor Talien's Mathias appeared in *Le Juif Polonais* "a stout, coarse, prosperous, somewhat easy-going Alsatian innkeeper whose only fear was lest his crime should be discovered," according to Eric Jones-Evans; *The Daily Telegraph* similarly characterized M. Coquelin's Mathias as a "cheery little old gentleman [who] chuckles to himself that he has hoodwinked his neighbours and cheated the law," but Irving's was "a man whose nerves were unhinged by the action of awakened conscience."[10] The play's title change from *Le Juif Polonais* to *The Bells* concretized the centrality of Mathias's mental state for English audiences, as did Irving's addition of dying words for Mathias and his cutting from Lewis's script the play's final line (Father Walter's "Be comforted. He was a noble fellow, while he lived – and he has died without pain") so that the production ended with Mathias's death.[11]

Mathias's condition materializes in the play's first act and worsens alongside the developing plot to locate Koveski's murderer (the victim is only named in the third act's courtroom scene). In act one, a cheerful and snow-covered Mathias returns home to the village inn to find his wife Catherine in conversation with some of the inn's regular visitors. At mentions of the "Polish

Jew's winter" Mathias grows withdrawn and visibly agitated. Soon the jangles of sleigh bells ring out, detectable only to Mathias and the audience. Edward Gordon Craig wrote of Irving's reaction to the first sound of bells:

> He moves his head slowly from us – the eyes still somehow with us – and moves it to the right – taking as long as a long journey to discover a truth takes. He looks to the faces on the right – nothing. Slowly the head revolves back again, down, and along the tunnels of thought and sorrow, and at the end the face and eyes are bent upon those to the left of him ... A long pause, endless, breaking our hearts, comes down over everything, and on and on go these bells. Puzzled, motionless ... he glides up to a standing position ... With one arm slightly raised, with sensitive hand speaking of far-off apprehended sounds, he asks, in the voice of some woman who is frightened yet does not with to frighten those with her: "Don't you ... don't you hear the sound of sledge-bells on the road?"

After his companions answer in the negative, "suddenly he staggers, and shivers from his toes to his neck; his jaws begin to chatter; the hair on his forehead, falling over a little, writhes as though it were a nest of little snakes."[12] Thinking Mathias unwell, his companions bid him adieu and his wife and daughter exit into the kitchen to fetch warm wine. Bells continue to ring as he staggers once again and collapses into a chair. "I feel a darkness coming over me. A sensation of giddiness seizes me. Shall I call for help?" he asks. "No, no, courage, Mathias, courage. The Jew is dead – dead – ha ha ha – dead!" Mathias then hallucinates a vision of the murder, which is slowly revealed upstage; he turns and spies the appalling scene, cries out, and falls to the floor as the curtain is lowered.[13]

The methods by which Irving manifested Mathias's mental torment in the first act—glances, pauses in speech, moments of heavy stillness juxtaposed with nervous tremblings, and his physical collapse into the chair—received considerable attention in contemporary reviews. The *Chicago Inter-ocean* pronounced Irving successful in enacting Mathias's "mental action toward the collapse of reason and the destruction of vitality" through delicate shifts in facial expressions, while the *Brooklyn Union* marveled at the minute twitches of the actor's hands as part of his somatic portrait of paranoia.[14] "He looks into distance," reported another review, "and the story of his mental agitation is conveyed in his eyes, that seem to grow bloodshot as the face becomes haggard."[15] The second act begins with a doctor evaluating Mathias for his auditory hallucinations, head pains, and history of bad dreams, and ends with Mathias waltzing frenetically with a startled Catherine, bellowing at the bells only he can hear to "ring on! Ring on!" as partygoers stare.[16] What was once a manageable, largely private affliction is now a barely suppressed mania that pollutes even the joyous occasion of his daughter's marriage contract signing. Because of Irving's act two work, asserted amateur critic Winifred Callwall, "the fact that the man was a brutal murderer faded from the mind, [and] it was pity that was felt for his haunted condition of mind."[17] Bookended by acts that spectacularly stage Mathias's hallucinations, the second act builds tension more subtly by contrasting the furtherance of his domestic agenda (to marry his daughter—and fortune—off to a respected young Quartermaster) with the dissolution of his mental health. William Winter wrote of the actor's representation of Mathias's complex delusional state:

> The feverish alertness engendered by the strife of a strong will against a sickening apprehension, the desperate sense, now defiant and now abject, of impending doom, the slow paralysis of the feelings, under the action of remorse – these, indeed, were given with appalling truth.[18]

Mathias's periodic, at times extensive asides to the audience gave voice to this internalized strife; no other character used the audience as confidante.

"Appalling," declared Irving's reviewers of the third act's dream sequence and the burgomaster's subsequent death throes, as well as "spell-binding," "magnetic," "thrilling," "horrifying," and other hyperbolic descriptors typical of the period's dramatic critics. Under the spell of a mesmerist in the presence of an imagined jury, the somnambulistic Mathias confesses his crime by reenacting the murder and his disposal of the body, narrating his movements in a monologue inflected with rapid shifts in pacing, pitch, and emotional color. For the *New York Tribune*, the courtroom of Mathias's psyche resembled a laboratory of cruelty, with Irving as the living specimen: "No display of morbid spiritual vivisection has been seen upon the stage that approaches, or even resembles, the dream of Mathias as acted by Henry Irving."[19] Mathias's death at the play's conclusion was, according the critics, a piece of graphic realism signaling the "end of a man whose physical frame had broken under the strain of a tormented mind."[20] Irving's personal script chronicles the character's final moments:

> (MATHIAS *rushes on dressed as he was at the time he retired behind the curtains. His eyes are fixed, and his appearance deathly and haggard. He clutches the drapery convulsively, and staggers with a yell to* CATHERINE, *is caught in the arms of* CHRISTIAN, *who places him in chair brought forward to* CATHERINE *hastily by* HANS. MATHIAS *sinks in chair, holds one hand to* ANNETTE L. *then to* CHRISTIAN R.)
> MATH. Take the rope from my neck – take – the –rope – neck –
> (*Struggles and dies.*)[21] (See Figure 6.1.)

For famed *Times* critic John Oxenford, Irving excelled at physicalizing the battle being waged within Mathias's mind: "[His] own conscience torments him in form so palpable that it almost becomes a bodily persecution, and he finally dies under its pressure."[22] Though Irving executed Mathias's death scene with customary physical control, Ellen Terry voiced concerns that the part was too emotionally and physiologically taxing for the aging actor to undertake frequently. Convulsing, gasping, and growing pale, Irving engaged his entire corporeality (and at least part of his gray matter) to enact Mathias's

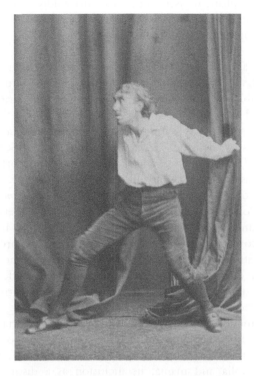

Figure 6.1 Photograph of Henry Irving as Mathias in *The Bells*, Lyceum Theatre, 1871, Guy
  Little Collection. Courtesy of Victoria and Albert Museum, London.

hallucinated asphyxiation. When Irving's personal physician advised him to
remove Mathias from his repertoire or face the medical consequences, the
actress admitted being relieved:

> It was clever of the doctor to see what a terrible emotional strain "The
> Bells" put upon Henry – how he never could play the part of Mathias
> with ease … Every time he heard the sound of the bells, the throbbing of
> his heart must have nearly killed him. He used always to turn quite white
> – there was no trick about it. It was imagination acting physically on the
> body. His death as Mathias – the death of a strong, robust man – was dif-
> ferent from all his other stage deaths. He did really almost die – he imag-
> ined death with such horrible intensity. His eyes would disappear upward,
> his face grow gray, his limbs cold.[23]

The *New York Times'* critic, who judged the first two acts of *The Bells* to be
"intolerably tedious," nevertheless marveled at Irving's *tour de force* in the final act:

> No violence of realism was wanting to the scene. There is no measure,
> no restraint. All is rant and paroxysm. He shouts, screams, hisses, moans;

he staggers, contorts himself, flings his arms wildly, grovels on his face in a manner the description of which would be most absurd, although in action nothing could be more keenly thrilling.[24]

If a Victorian alienist abreast of the latest mental disorders and their symptoms evaluated Irving's tormented burgomaster, what would be his diagnosis? Personal and public accounts of the performance from largely non-medical writers presented a wealth of contradictory hypotheses: the burgomaster's laughter was "hysterical" (Eric Jones-Evans, *Chicago Tribune*, and Callwall); he exhibited signs of "delirium" in the first act (Clement Scott) and "mania" in the second (*The Times*'s Oxenford); an excessively tortured conscience unhinged Mathias's highly strung "nerves" (*Boston Daily Advertiser* and *The Daily Telegraph*) or agitated his "nervous system" (*The Times*'s Walkley and Walter Herries Pollock); and his behavior during his daughter's nuptials as well as his overall countenance were "melancholic" (Callwall).[25] In addition to this imprecise inventory of diagnoses (which, at the very least, proves that reviewers perceived Mathias as mentally ill rather than simply remorseful), the character's visual and aural hallucinations would suggest he suffered from a form of guilt-induced dementia. But the script and Irving's performance controvert many of these speculations.

Though melancholia and dementia are plausible, Victorian medical literature suggests an altogether different diagnosis, that of monomania. In French alienist Jean-Etienne Dominque Esquirol's nosology, monomania resided between melancholia and mania, its inclusion as a disorder prompted by Esquirol's disapproval of the common conflation of all "manialike" illnesses. English physician J.C. Pritchard listed monomania as a subset of "intellectual insanity," meaning that the monomaniac, while partially or fully insane, still experienced feelings of guilt and paranoia following violent, criminal, or perverse acts.[26] Like the melancholic, the monomaniac was singularly obsessed by an *idée fixe*, an unhealthy preoccupation that was the source of their delusional state. However, the often prideful monomaniac expressed their partial madness through hyperactive, excessive, and at times cheerful fervency, not to mention exaggerated "moral and physical agitation." Though monomaniacs could experience spells of melancholia, their perceived physiognomy differed from those of the more muted or introspective disorders: they were "animated, expansive, hypermobile; the eyes are lively, sometimes shining and look 'injected', their walk has an energetic gait. They're noisy, garrulous, petulant, brave, [and] overcome all obstacles."[27] Restless, short-tempered, distrustful of others, and subject to hallucinations and delirium, monomaniacs were reputedly driven by greed or delusions of grandeur, the latter being the distinguishing characteristic of Esquirol's "ambitious monomaniac." The ambitious monomaniac, he claimed, was most likely a man who, because of the post-Revolutionary destabilizing of conventional hierarchies and chains of command, fancied himself more socially and politically mobile than he was in reality. According to Lisa Appignanesi, it was often difficult to differentiate the delusional monomaniac from the tenacious-but-sane overachiever. Indeed, "only when the subject of the monomaniac's delirium comes into focus does the mania grip him and become visible," thereby exposing the person's illness.[28] Similarly, monomania (potentially) receded if the sufferer could acknowledge his *idée fixe* with reason, introspection, and an awareness of actual magnitude, thereby breaking the obsession's hold. "Monomania" entered nineteenth-century colloquial speech as a term to describe extreme states of obsession or behaviors, whether asocial, subversive, or bizarre, that polite society found objectionable.[29]

Mathias's *idée fixe*, that of Koveski's fatal visit on Christmas Eve, induces his feverish fits, mood shifts, and nightmares. Furthermore, Lewis and Irving amplified the character's monomania in his backstory, in which ambition, desire for money, delusions of grandeur, and a false sense of invincibility both motivated Mathias's crime and preserved his sense of righteousness, even as guilt interfered with his sleep. If, as Esquirol theorized, monomania was a hybrid disorder uniting the pathologies of mania and melancholia, its sufferers could experience depression and euphoria, an apt description of Mathias's vacillating emotions. Note the character's antithetical statements in act one: "I feel a darkness coming over me. A sensation of giddiness seizes me." The progressive pathology of monomania also explains the rapid collapse of Mathias's mental faculties. As Appignanesi reminds us, the "partiality of the monomania—when the sufferer is able to reason well across a range of thought unrelated to the driving *idée fixe*—disappears" as his mania becomes unmanageable.[30] The moral and physical agitation afflicting the monomaniac was certainly apparent in Irving's performance, as was the irreparable nature of his madness once mania took hold. Oxenford arrived at the same diagnosis after witnessing Irving's premiere performance in 1871:

> Mr H. Irving has thrown the whole force of his mind into the character, and works out bit by bit, the concluding hours of a life passed in a constant effort to preserve a cheerful exterior, with a conscience tortured 'til it has become a monomania.[31]

Hamlet, 1878

While Mathias's psychopathology remains somewhat ambiguous, diagnosing Hamlet with melancholia seems a simple task. The Danish prince was, in the words of English psychiatrist and asylum superintendent John Charles Bucknill "morbidly melancholic," and visual and textual coverage of the Lyceum's *Hamlet* indicates that Irving was of a similar mind.[32] Moreover, the tenor of Irving's acting style—nervous, intellectual, temporally syncopated, and somatically expressive—administered to the Elizabethan-era Hamlet a decidedly Victorian-era nerve disorder: neurasthenia. To declare the madness of Irving's Hamlet feigned or genuine is the trickier diagnosis. Though Irving believed Hamlet to be a sane man who periodically succumbed to stress-induced fits, theatregoers seemed divided: some reported witnessing a high-strung royal in full possession of his mental faculties, others an ill man wrestling to keep his grip on reality.

Melancholia's history dates back to the time of Hippocrates, when the term typically described a state of protracted depression or worry.[33] Through the course of its 2,000-year existence, melancholia and its many cognates not only indicated a diagnosable illness but a spectrum of emotional states from sadness to acute despair. The most familiar etiological explanation for the disorder was biliousness. In Galenic terms, melancholics possessed an overabundance of black bile that overwhelmed their humoral systems, leading to a temperament of habitual low spirits and crippling anxiety. Eighteenth-century physicians categorized melancholia as yet another disorder of the nervous system, purportedly a product of depleted nerve forces or compressed nerves and blood vessels. Victorians often used the terms "depression" and "melancholia" interchangeably to describe the same general pathology, though the latter still predominated in medical discourse. During that same century, the presumed causes of melancholia gradually shifted away from the concretely anatomo-clinical and toward mental and affective explanations, a transition shared by nearly all types of what we now call mental illnesses; by 1917, Freud claimed melancholia developed as a pathological response to real or imagined loss (as opposed to the non-pathological state of mourning). Because melancholia was associated with brooding intellectuals and roguish romantics, it was also considered by many to be a masculine illness.

Prominent theories of melancholia converged on some points and diverged on others. On the whole, physicians and alienists were in agreement that, along with melacholia's affective symptoms (sadness, irritability, anxiety) and physical effects (constipation, appetite loss, sleeplessness, etc.), each sufferer was driven by an *idée fixe* similar to that of the monomaniac. Most also believed that the illness had some sort of pathological cause, from nutrient-deficient blood or poor cerebral blood flow to brain injury or overactive nerve functioning. Esquirol, Wilhelm Griesinger, and Henry Maudsley contended that the melancholic, though delusional, retained an awareness of his changed condition. Chief among the theorists' concerns was whether or not the melancholic was, by definition, insane. Esquirol defined melancholia as a "cerebral malady" with "partial, chronic delirium" but without a comprehensive and permanent separation from sanity. Melancholics, he argued, "are never unreasonable, not even in that sphere of thought which characterizes their delirium. They proceed upon a false idea, as well as wrong principles, but all their reasonings and deductions are conformable to the severest logic."[34] Maudsley also viewed clinical melancholia as a type of partial insanity along with monomania, while Richard von Krafft-Ebing—now notorious for his *Psychopathia Sexualis: eine Klinisch-Forensische Studie* (1886) that condemned sexual "deviances" like homosexuality, sadism, and masturbation—conceived of a spectrum of melancholic conditions ranging from mild to extreme. Krafft-Ebing also warned of conflating true melancholia(s) with the temporary melancholic state that manifested at the beginning of other neurological diseases. The men also differed on the melancholic's behavioral response to his condition. Esquirol's melancholic "dread[ed] obscurity, solitude, insomnia, the terrors of sleep, etc." and was therefore compelled to be more social, while Johann Christian Heinroth's "gradually [became] quiet, withdrawn, secretive … shy and fearful or suspicious, [and] withdr[awn] from the company of his friends and acquaintances."[35] Irving's appearance bore remarkable similarities to the melancholic's reputed look: black hair, slender build, pallid skin, contracted facial muscles, and a transfixed yet apprehensive gaze. Melancholic complaints often ran in multigenerational families, and while medical experts viewed melancholia as a temporary affliction, they also acknowledged the regularity with which relapses occurred. Early nineteenth-century treatments for depressive conditions included water immersion, diet and exercise, enemas, and vomiting; the late 1800s introduced talk therapy and (in the severest cases) lobotomies.

For Irving, Hamlet's baseline despondency (a product of aristocratic breeding as well as the family tragedies immediately preceding the play's action) mutated and sharpened with the introduction of the prince's ambition: revenge.[36] Before the ghost's visitation, Irving's Hamlet showed signs of a "profound melancholy" that, for the *Temple Bar*'s critic, demonstrated that "Hamlet's will [was] already puzzled"; the *Baltimore Day* pronounced it "an almost Rembrandt-like gloom with which he surrounds his shadowed heart."[37] Both Shakespeare and Irving differentiated Hamlet's general malaise (what Krafft-Ebing would categorize as the pre-illness "melancholic state" and Maudsley's non-pathological "simple melancholia") from the full-blown melancholia that assumed control after he received his spectral father's directive, a progression that echoed the Victorian melancholic's presumed pattern of illness: predisposition to disorder. Alan Hughes' 1981 study of Irving as Hamlet confirms the character's two-tiered melancholia, for he attests that the earliest court scene "was the only glimpse the audience would get of the Prince in something like his natural state; melancholy and suspicion had obliterated his former happiness, of course, but he had not yet seen the Ghost."[38] Irving augmented his already striking physical resemblance to the stock melancholic with stage makeup. "How pale his make-up made him look against the blue-black tone of his hair and how beautiful his haggard face appeared," Terry noted admiringly.[39] The actor's distinctive physicality (hunched shoulders, shuffling gait, bent knees), used in *The Bells* to communicate Mathias's fitful state, now signaled Hamlet's depressive state.

For the period's literary scholars and dramatic critics, gauging the severity of Hamlet's mental condition—and particularly whether his madness was feigned, partly feigned, or genuine—was of paramount concern.[40] In his *The Psychology of Shakespeare* (1859), Bucknill pathologized Hamlet's mad acts, arguing "the feint is so close to nature" that "in spite of ourselves" we must acknowledge we are witnessing "a mind fallen," because even in his sanest moments the suicidal Hamlet is "far from being in a healthy state of mind." He is not yet a lunatic but a "reasoning melancholiac," Bucknill theorized, free from true delusional thoughts and behaviors but tormented nonetheless, vulnerable to developing insanity.[41] The literary discourse of the 1870s on *Hamlet* generally advocated for a mad prince, and yet Irving (like Goethe) concluded that Hamlet never touches true insanity, his "sensitive imagination" prompts hysterical outbursts when he experiences stress.[42] In his analysis of Irving's Hamlet, Hughes identifies the character's first hysterical state in act one's ghost scene in which he "worked himself up for the first time" and "exhibited the psychological mechanism by which, in his view, Hamlet became distracted."[43] Irving intensified Hamlet's fits in the mousetrap scene, in which he famously crawled along the floor, the ghost's second visitation, and act three's Hamlet-Gertrude scene, but his crowning achievement was in the nunnery scene with Terry's Ophelia. In it, Irving feigned madness until Hamlet's discovery of Polonius and Claudius's machinations induced real psychological distress. In subsequent years, Irving embellished Hamlet's "frantic ebullition" in this scene by chasing Ophelia around the room while spouting insults. Then, "'with wild gestures and a burst of hysterical laughter' he rushed out of the room" only to return hurling fresh invectives.[44] Replicating the often cyclical patterns of anxiety and mood disorders, each time a fit of Hamlet's subsided the character returned to his fundamental state of mind: downcast, apprehensive, and romantic, yet logical.

Though reviews measured the depth of Hamlet's mental illness in different ways, on one point there was near consensus among Irving's critics: his Hamlet was most certainly not just a *compos mentis* simulator of madness. Nearly all reviewers acknowledged that Irving's Hamlet possessed an inordinately delicate nervous system that, like his depressive state, was rooted in a natural propensity and aggravated by loss and his current familial strife. Indeed, Irving's Danish prince appeared to be, by most accounts, a Victorian neurasthenic. The term "neurasthenia" is largely credited to American neurologist George Miller Beard, who first published an article on the subject in 1869, though "[a] language of 'nerves,' a popular bodily economy of nervous energy, an expanding medical culture of nerve management, and a belief that civilisation produced nervousness were all in place in Britain long before Beard coined [the term]."[45] Beard introduced neurasthenia as the medical appellation for "American nervousness," a functional disorder with purported somatic origins but no detectible pathology that affected the most harried, energy-depleted citizens of modern societies in general, and the United States in particular.[46] Modernity, Beard hypothesized, wreaked havoc on the populace's nerve forces, giving rise to widespread cases of neurasthenia.[47] A true spirit-of-the-age diagnosis, neurasthenia's list of symptoms appears both random and limitless: prolonged exhaustion, insomnia, headaches, dyspepsia, tooth decay, and blushing, among many others. Its intangible side-effects, including languor, irritability, and anxiousness, were shared with an older functional nervous disorder thought to disproportionately affect men, hypochondriasis.[48]

The diagnosis of neurasthenia was appealing to physicians and their patients on several levels. First, it originated the neurasthenic's atypical feelings and behaviors in the nerves, somatically legitimating the patients' complaints, no matter how vague, diverse, or peculiar.[49] Furthermore, as the diagnosis grew in popularity, it subsumed a host of affiliated conditions under its generalized umbrella.[50] Doctors often diagnosed patients with neurasthenia to avoid handing down far more defamatory medical verdicts. In particular, neurasthenia permitted men to suffer from a nervous disorder without being branded a degenerate weakling, and it allowed both women *and* men to evade the dreaded moniker of "hysteric." Charcot and others employed neurasthenia as a synonym for male hysteria, and for famed nerve-doctor Sir George Henry Savage, the man who diagnosed Virginia Woolf as a neurasthenic, "neurasthenia was no more than a convenient euphemism [for insanity,] to soothe – and retain – the patients in his lucrative private practice."[51] Not all physicians were accepting of neurasthenia as a new category of nerve disorder. British specialist Sir Andrew Clarke, for example, discredited the condition as "unscientific, inaccurate, and misleading."[52] Nervous conditions were generally thought to produce gaunt and angular bodies, sallow complexions, and a vocabulary of movements that spanned from unnerving jitteriness to weary listlessness. Irving's Hamlet—with his fitful pacing, constant level changes from sitting to standing, and "fidget[ing]" hands regularly touching his forehead—appeared to critics a modern neurasthenic. "He shows us a Hamlet of a highly nervous and sensitive disposition," wrote Clement Scott:

> The terrible events which occur have the effect of unhinging the man's mind, but have no power to alter his nature. He is overwhelmed, he is distressed, he is irritable, he is hysterical, he is reflective, he talks to himself; the strain on the nervous system is almost too great for nature to bear.[53]

Similarly, the *World*'s critic noted:

> The restlessness of expression and gesture which seems natural to [Irving], or not perfectly controllable, is of real service in representing Hamlet's exacerbated nervous condition … in Mr. Irving's Hamlet it is to be noted that a simulated insanity keeps pace with, and yet is distinct from, a mental excitement near akin to absolute disease of brain.[54]

The *World*'s hint that Irving's own nervous disposition was "not perfectly controllable" is intriguing, as it subtly medicalizes Irving as well as condenses the actor and character into a single illness role.

Whether or not the actor intended to only perform "a *kind* of hysteria" (in Hughes's words) during moments of intense stress, the majority of critics perceived Irving's Hamlet as drawing close to fully-fledged madness. "[A]t times, his madness is clearly feigned," J. Ranken Towse reported; "at others … it is, to all appearance, real."[55] Embracing the metaphorical mapping of madness into a divided landscape of sane and insane, a rhetorical premise already used in medical discourses, reviewers placed Irving's Hamlet on a perilous threshold. For *Punch*, "He shows us a mind ticklishly poised on the line between great wit and madness … Any great shock can send this unstably-poised mind over the boundary between sanity and insanity."[56] Another London critic claimed that Irving took Hamlet "to the very verge of the irrational, and all but carries him over the border-line. But when the business is done for which the madness was assumed, his mind recovers its supremacy, and shows again the meditative scholar."[57] The cumulative effects of the Dane's neurotic and raving behaviors were such that his mental state seemed the crux of Irving's entire composition. Lady Hardy, who viewed Irving's Hamlet "as neither wholly mad nor wholly sane," consolidated the character's sharp intelligence and his compromised mental state into a portrait of masculine neuroticism of which Hamlet was both architect and victim:

> [W]e feel that over-study, aided by an over-sensitive organization, has given his brain a slight twist, and sent it a pin's point awry … the thread of insanity which is running through his whole nature makes it so hard for him to unravel the tangled skein of his own life, and, with a cunning perfectly intelligible to those who have studied the working of a diseased brain, he professes that he only seems to be what he really is; the actual disturbance of his mind will show itself in spite of his efforts to hide it.[58]

Lacking the anger, resoluteness, and cunning that typified earlier portrayals, Irving's Hamlet retained the character's contemplative insight, but the actor's application of a nervous disorder in the vein of neurasthenia was something new: a modernized justification for the character's famed paranoia, depression, evasiveness, and fits of spontaneous action. Irving's Hamlet was equal parts Shakespearean and Charcotian, an avatar for the educated, privileged, nervous men of the nineteenth century.

King Lear, 1892

Victorian medicine considered neurasthenia, melancholia, and monomania both functional, meaning they did not alter the anatomical structures of the brain or body, and potentially curable. The majority of dementias, however, were thought to be neither physiologically benign nor reversible.[59] Though the word "dementia" could connote any mental and physical incompetencies identified with imbecility or "chronic brain disease," alienists and clinicians in France, Germany, and Britain endeavored to determine more precisely the illness's various compositions.[60] Set apart from the acute and chronic dementias was a long-suspected but never formally pathologized dementia with one single cause: aging. The concept that human bodies experienced wear and tear due to aging was ubiquitous in centuries past, but of whether the mind decayed within the deteriorating body people were less certain.[61] By the nineteenth century, the cognitive deficits that aging often induced in persons with no history of impairments were beyond question, and alienists joined physicians in the quest for a more concrete understanding of senility. Terminal dementias, including senile dementia, were thought at first to be caused by what French physician Bénédict Morel labeled "the law of decline of faculties," prompted by a decrease in the brain's competence and energy over time.[62] In short, when the human brain lost vitality, it subsequently forfeited its ability to maintain the body's advanced functionings. Soon neuropathological studies and increased observations with light microscopy introduced tissue decay, cerebral arteriosclerosis, and other structural abnormalities of the brain as root causes of senile dementia. In 1896, Ralph Lyman Parsons argued that along with the physical impairments brought on by advanced age (loss of muscle tone, hearing, manual dexterity, eyesight, and vascular functioning), there were significant mental changes with the potential to erase a person's temperament and behavioral patterns, including "irritability, imperiousness, excitability or diminution of normal emotional responses, loss of memory, diminished attention-span, diminished power of abstract thought, and fickleness or perversity of disposition."[63] For British neurologist John Hughlings Jackson, who claimed of the forms of insanity only dementia was entirely without positive symptoms, a "healthy senescence" was the closest nature came to reversing evolution.[64]

Memory loss, an inability to experience intense emotions, compromised judgment, a lack of extemporaneous actions and decision making, and a debilitating impassiveness (collectively referred to by neurologists as "brain softening") were considered hallmarks of senile dementia. Most physicians agreed that the weakening of mental faculties accompanying aging could range from the most mild of inconveniences to what amounted to late-onset insanity. In 1876, Krafft-Ebing called for a differentiation to be made between senile dementia, a cumulative illness which attacked the elderly *because* of their advanced age, and other forms of insanity acquirable by all segments of the population that *could* affect the elderly. Despite their certainty that demented conditions escalated in severity, scientists were unsure of the permanence of any of the dementias until the 1840s, when experts declared "vesanic dementia," or the cognitive impairments lingering after a bout with insanity, to be rarely reversible.[65] While the diagnosis of vesanic dementia eventually lost support in the medical community, its irremediable nature was observed in several other forms of insanity or pre-insanity, including senile dementia.

Late nineteenth-century men were purportedly diagnosed with senile dementia only slightly more than women; however, the condition proved more stigmatizing in men than in women, a conceptual asymmetry founded not on statistics, but on stereotypes. The purported naturalness of female insanity furnished the quaint image of what Jesse F. Ballenger calls the "Picturesque Grandma," whose simple-mindedness enhanced her domesticity and her role as nurturer. Warm and snug by the hearth with her knitting needles, the Picturesque Grandma was a welcomed and respected Victorian figure whose dotage harmed neither kingdom nor family. By contrast, the senile old man was—particularly when contextualized by degeneration theory—an undesirable drain on community resources and a menace to social Darwinism and patriarchal society-at-large. For George Miller Beard, the neurologist who equated American nerve disorders with modern productivity,

> senile mental deterioration could hold no consolation − it signified only the start of the gradual, vegetative process of death ... failing to fulfill the

complex intellectual and moral tasks required of the individual in modern society, such people were ultimately an obstruction of progress.[66]

Reports that reckless hard living could act as a catalyst for senile dementia solidified the disease's connection to masculinity. Though most physicians claimed that the natural aging process was enough to bring about senile dementia, others believed the condition was not inevitable for all elderly individuals, only for those who "squandered the fund of vitality" through "the habits of dissipation – excessive drink and sexual activity, an immoderate diet, [and] chronic over- or underwork."[67] This moralistic perspective, coupled with a growing hostility toward the elderly, together forged the stereotyped *non compos mentis* geriatric who is perhaps now reaping what he imprudently sowed in his youth. Even Ignatz Leo Nascher, the founder of geriatrics, often portrayed the senile elderly man as self-absorbed and nagging:

> When the mind becomes impaired he neglects his person in every direction until he becomes obnoxious to those around him … He demands constant attention and complains of the slightest neglect. The firm insistence upon hygienic measures for his benefit and welfare, which necessarily impose some exertion on this part, is resented as a hardship and creates a dislike of those who are most interested in his welfare.[68]

More unpleasant than the old man's clinginess and contrariness, Nascher insinuated, was his sexual perversion, a product of "weakened mentality, diminished control over the emotions and some circumstances producing intense emotional excitement."[69] This objectionable patient with senile dementia joined the male neurasthenic, monomaniac, and melancholic as medicocultural symbols of failed masculinity.

Historians often cite the Lyceum's ambitious mounting of *King Lear* as one of the theatre's failures, but the three-month run of a play Victorians generally regarded as "too uncompromisingly tragic, unrelievedly bleak and overfull of horrors" suggests it was not a true catastrophe.[70] Still, Irving's premiere in the titular role disappointed audiences. He was "slow, laboured, mannered, uninspired, screechy, forcibly feeble, failing chiefly where all representations of Lear fail," wrote playwright Henry Arthur Jones.[71] Despite reports that by his fifth night Irving had corrected many of his missteps (particularly in making his Lear audible), he was unable to fully reverse the portrayal's initially poor reception. Irving's conception of Lear—visually, aurally, textually—revolved around the monarch's deepening senility, one that seems to confirm the correlational ties of aging, dementia, and insanity. Unlike Hamlet, there was never any question of Lear's insanity (apart from *when* it arose), and Irving's performance of madness followed the same basic trajectory as other actors' Lears: his epic rage was triggered by the desertions of his daughters and climaxed in the eye of the storm; the fury then ebbed, leaving a less savage insanity in its wake; he recovered his senses with the recognition of Cordelia; and the heartbreaking trauma of Cordelia's death spelled the king's demise.

In 1892, literary criticism of *King Lear* focused particularly upon why an experienced and heretofore effective royal would so obtusely divide his kingdom and give away the pieces. One school of thought argued that Lear acted on impulse without weighing the consequences; the other alleged that Lear was already slipping into madness long before the storm on the heath. For advocates of the latter theory, Lear's forgetfulness, impaired judgments, rash decisions, and his egotism and irritability were acknowledged behavioral symptoms of senile dementia. Physician Bucknill claimed that those who regarded Lear as sane at the play's opening based their judgments on flawed medical theories of insanity as manifesting in the intellect, not in the emotions. In the 1991 article "Dementia in Shakespeare's *King Lear*," J. G. Howells asserts that Lear "displays the composite of two clinical conditions—firstly, dementia resulting from old age, and secondly, emotional illness resulting from the anguish of filial ingratitude—each impinging on the other. His condition is worsened by exposure during his wanderings."[72] Howells's conviction, then, acknowledges in Lear a preexisting condition of senile dementia while allowing for the character's excessive psychological strain after being abandoned by his progeny. Responses indicate Irving was of the same mind. Reckoning that Lear was already "half insane" when he split his kingdom, the *Illustrated London News* argued that Irving's Lear was a man "whose half-unseated reason is gradually toppled over under the shocks of incredible treacheries, who presents the frightful spectacle of madness" that progresses from unbridled fury to "peaceful incoherence [and] chattering imbecility, into which the shattered man subsides."[73]

As part of his pictorial art, fifty-four-year-old Irving carefully curated his appearance as the grizzled sovereign. The Lyceum's Lear was, according to the *Daily Telegraph*:

> A tall, gaunt, supple, and kingly figure, the thin and attenuated frame weighed down with a swathing load of regal garments. A splendid head, indeed, with the finely-cut features, the restless eyes, and the yellow parchment skin set in a frame of snowy white hair and silvered straggling beard; and, of course, those eloquent hands which have been so often discussed and so frequently described … Henry Irving – not to speak it profanely, but in all reverence – in his character of Lear, might have stood for Moses on Mount Sinai or Noah at the hour of the flood. His appearance is patriarchal, not theatrical. The stage vanishes, and we seem to be in the presence of the sublimest instances of hoary senility.[74]

"He looked the character to perfection," remarked Henry Norman of *Illustrated London News*, "and behind the grey, lined face and tangled, grizzly locks of the King the familiar features of the great actor could not be discerned."[75] Irving's wig (which *The Times* described as "tawny gray" and not the typical pristine white) was employed as an important part of his performance of senile dementia; the actor tousled his hair with his hand as Lear grappled with confusion or forgetfulness.[76] As was often the case, some reviewers found Irving's voice too erratic in volume and peculiar in pronunciation and cadence to be truly effective. In an otherwise commendatory review, *Pick-Me-Up* ridiculed Irving's elocution:

> *King Lear*, who wanted his hair cut rather, sat back in his chair of state and snapped and growled and spoke in a series of short barks, as if his growing madness was about to take the form of hydrophobia. Once I caught the words, "Hear me!" and I heard as far as my ears would go, but I hadn't the faintest idea of what he was saying.[77]

Ironically, despite *Pick-Me-Up's* irritation at Irving's vocal weaknesses, the actor's propensity for odd articulations and brief moments of unintelligibility potentially served to reinforce the advanced stage of Lear's illness.

Irving's established Lear's dementia with his first entrance. Following the pageantry of the royal procession and the king's welcome from his warriors, Irving's Lear sat upon his throne to address his subjects. At that moment "one saw that the old man was wandering," offers Hughes, "not stark gibbering mad, but decidedly senescent and queer. He used his sword as a walking-stick, plucked at his beard and toyed with his hair."[78] Exhibiting in the early acts what A. Acton-Bond labeled "a distinct suggestion of incipient madness," Lear was shown to be in his dotage, ineffectual as a sovereign but not completely dysfunctional. For Augustin Filon, Irving displayed Lear's "predisposition of madness" in his first scene by juxtaposing the "infantine [with the] senile" in the king's hasty actions: he is an "impetuous and spoiled old child."[79] In a juxtaposition furnished by Shakespeare's text, Edgar's pledge to evade capture by playing "Poor crazy Tom," a dirty, raving, and self-harming lunatic who escaped the asylum (2.3.1-21), directly precedes Lear's refusal to acquiesce to Regan and Goneril's orders (which they claim are necessary safeguards against the king's failing mind), and the subsequent banishment of Lear and his entourage from Regan's house. As the dramaturgical tipping point for Lear's mental deterioration, the second act featured prominently in Irving's performative rendering of senile dementia. Irving's personal acting edition, which can be studied at the British Library, demonstrates both in textual edits and handwritten performance notations how Irving centralized the king's dementia in the Lyceum production. In it, Irving underlined several key phrases that conveyed Lear's confusion and emotional agony in his act two, scene four discussion with Regan, including "Fool me not so much" (2.4.316) and "I have full cause of weeping" (2.4.325). He also deliberately struck from the script the final conversation of the conspiring daughters, Cornwall, and Gloucester so that act two closed with a distracted and sobbing Lear confessing to his fool: "O Fool, I shall go mad" (2.4.327).[80] In employing Lear's pronouncement as the act's curtain line, Irving encouraged audiences to linger upon the character's mental decline as the scene shifted to the blustery heath.

In Lear's mad scenes, Irving avoided simplified and exaggerated spectacles of staged insanity, preferring instead to moderate the violence of Lear's outbursts through a devitalized body and voice. Hughes notes that Irving rejected the metaphorical linking of the tempest raging in the king's mind with the environmental tempest whipping through the heath; for him, Lear was not a universal Man who crises radiated outward into the cosmos, but an individual man suffering from a debilitating illness caught in a powerful storm. Several Hawes Craven illustrations in the souvenir program for *King Lear* confirm this claim. In one, Irving's Lear is centrally positioned but dwarfed by the immensity of the storm surrounding him. His arms are held aloft (again, a nineteenth-century iconographic gesture of insanity), but his glazed stare is cast outward, not up to the skies, as if regretting his own absurd challenge to the storm's power.[81] In another illustration of the storm scene, an enfeebled Lear leans on his Fool for support (Figure 6.2). Clad in billowing robes, Lear clutches the Fool's arm with spindly fingers while holding the back of his other hand to his brow in a decidedly effeminate display of mental confusion. Irving's muted performance of distraction while "battling" the elements prompted the *National Observer* to state that he was "hopelessly outplayed by the storm." This tottering and "unintelligible" old man, the critic continued, walked with "ancient difficulty"

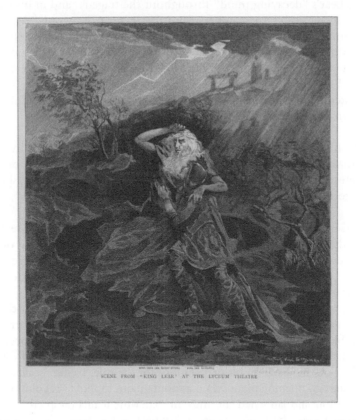

SCENE FROM "KING LEAR" AT THE LYCEUM THEATRE

Figure 6.2 Scene from "King Lear" at the Lyceum Theatre. Courtesy of Folger Shakespeare Library.

and constantly clutched at his beard or clothes, seeming more the "village idiot" than the reigning monarch.[82]

Even as Lear succumbed to senile dementia, Irving desired for the old man to retain a portion of his faded regality. "Lear is quite mad," the *Standard* observed of Irving's character following the act three, scene four entrance of Edgar's Poor Tom o' Bedlam, "and yet there is much of dignity as well as of pathos in the face and figure of the old King, as he sinks on the floor by the rude couch, playing with the straws or rushes that litter it."[83] Lear's simpleminded diversion not only mimicked an inmate tearing at his bedding (Irving claimed in a letter to Terry that he too had visited an insane asylum for research), but it also unveiled the juvenile living within the elderly man. This understated bit of stage business reflected Hughlings Jackson's assertion that senile dementia was the only disease capable of reversing human evolution. According to *The Times*, Irving performed unmitigated madness in the central acts of *King Lear*: "He croons like a Bedlamite, his eye is bright but unsteady, and his crown of poppies and cornflowers stuck on awry completes a remarkable exhibition of witlessness."[84] As described by E. R. Russell at the *Nineteenth Century*, Irving signaled Lear's "decaying mind" throughout the tragedy, and in his exit from act four, scene six "'Lear scampers from the stage at the words 'you shall get it by running', as only a lunatic could run – with utter indifference to appearances, to grace, to everything', fleeing imaginary dangers 'with wild, suffering, pathetic eyes.'"[85] Once reunited with his beloved Cordelia, Irving's Lear recovered much of his reason but surrendered to emotionalism. For *The Times*, Lear's interactions with his daughter together composed a "splendid example of overwrought senility," while the *Standard* reported:

> Mr. Irving is here, as already said, at his very best; he, too, lives in the part, and the episode ends most fittingly with Cordelia supporting and protecting the feeble old man, who clings so lovingly to her as she guides his tottering footsteps.[86]

Of course, Lear's restoration to sanity was fleeting; Cordelia's death dealt his already damaged mind its final blow. Like the medical theory of pathological permanence in cases of dementia, Lear's illness was progressive and indefinite, lending even more pathos to the tragedy's final scene and the king's death.

Irving once pronounced Lear "the most difficult undertaking in the whole range of the drama" because the lead actor "has to represent the struggles of an enfeebled mind with violent self-will, a mind eventually reduced to the pathetic helplessness of a ruin in which some of the original grandeur can still be traced."[87] Looking back on his preparations for the role, Irving recalled standing in the wings on opening night when a spontaneous thought "revolutionized the impersonation and launched me into an experiment unattempted at rehearsal. I tried to combine the weakness of senility with the tempest of passion." By the performance's end, Irving had concluded that this was "a perfectly impossible task … Lear cannot be played except with the plentitude of the actor's physical powers, and the idea of representing extreme old age is futile."[88] Despite Irving's proclamation that merging senile weakness with the violence of passion was unworkable, reviews suggest Irving did just that:

> [T]hrough all the paroxysms of rage, the almost inarticulate curses, the rare moments of unnatural self-control, to the gentle, cynical imbecile who jokes Gloster [sic] on his sightlessness, and the last dying touches of the hand upon Cordelia's hair … Mr. Irving's Lear [epitomizes the phrase] 'violent and weak.'[89]

Given Irving's reputation as an actor with a penchant for flamboyant physicalities, it is significant that he received repeated commendation for his measured performance of senile dementia. Wrote the *Illustrated London News*:

> His Lear will be wondered at as a very remarkably subtle and detailed analysis and minute portrayal of a character of colossal intellectual interest, and that interest, too, consisting chiefly of intellectual aberration … [T]he thousand transitions of mind which pull the outraged man backwards and forwards till his recurring passion and relapse finally tear his body to pieces had evidently been studied by Mr. Irving with the most scrupulous delicacy, and were portrayed with a ceaseless faithfulness so great as almost to become a fault.[90]

The *Daily Telegraph* concurred, remarking: "There have been wild Lears, Bedlamite Lears, Lears frenzied from the outset; here was a Lear who from first to last emphasized the chord of human affection."[91]

Irving's emasculated madmen

Unlike Terry's naturalized madwomen, the psychological disorders plaguing Irving's madmen designated them as aberrant, impotent, or dangerous.[92] Variously regarded as self-indulgent egotists, high-strung neurotics, physical or intellectual weaklings, hedonists, and, particularly those with senile dementia, unproductive parasites, mentally ill men posed a threat to Western colonialist patriarchies even as their presence indexed the triumph of British and American modernity. The most common stigmatizing tactic, and one that is pervasive in the performance of and responses to Irving's madmen, was the feminization of the male mental patient. Irving's Hamlet endured the most thorough emasculation, both at the hands of the actor and his critics. *Temple Bar* disparaged the actor's hypersensitive prince for his "limpness" and categorized his condition as a sort of effeminate impotence: "Where one expects wild mirth one finds hysterical depression."[93] The *Baltimore Day*'s notice, which judged Irving's construction of Hamlet as "marvelous in texture, delicate in treatment, and almost pre-Raphaelite in its attention to even the smallest detail," strikes the ear as a review equally suited to his costar's turn as Ophelia. "He has brought out far more clear than before his view of the intensely affectionate nature of Hamlet," observed another critic, "and shows how this exquisite sensitiveness is a main factor in the wreck of his life."[94] Identifying Hamlet's finely tuned nerves as his hamartia both feminized the character and trivialized his psychological suffering. Even modern criticism adopts a similar vocabulary when describing Hamlet's real or feigned madness, such as Hughes's use of the term "hysteria" for the character's fits of frenzy.

The senility that crippled Irving's Lear also emasculated the king. Kaara L. Peterson argues that the feminine label of "hysteric" has been misapplied (particularly by psychoanalytic theorists) to the masculine Lear because of his exclamation "hysterica passio" (2.4.55).[95] And yet, misapplication or not, audiences likely linked Lear's self-diagnosis with the oft-feminized pathology of hysteria; at the very least, Irving referenced props, gestures, and movement associated with the institutionalized madwoman, including scampering youthfully across stage and donning a wildflower crown. Printed alongside a *Punch* review titled "His Mad-jesty at the Lyceum," one cartoon captioned "Rather mixed. Irving as 'Ophe-Lear'" satirized Lear's emasculating illness

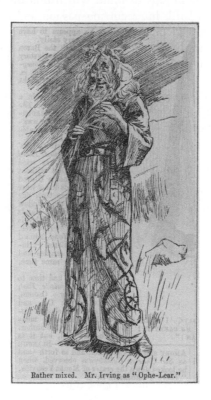

Rather mixed.   Mr. Irving as " Ophe-Lear."

Figure 6.3 "Rather Mixed. Mr. Irving as Ophe-Lear." *Punch*, November 19, 1892. Courtesy of Folger Shakespeare Library.

(Figure 6.3). In it, Lear's signature robes are cut similar to a lady's kimono, accentuating Irving's thin frame; the actor's angled left foot peaks out coyly from beneath the hem. On his nest of tangled hair sits the wildflower and straw crown. Straw also makes up a spiky bouquet held in his right hand, an obvious allusion to Ophelia's remembrances and perhaps even to Terry's well-circulated Window & Grove photograph (see Figure 5.2). Irving's eyes are absurdly crossed, and his left-hand fingers absentmindedly worry the tips of his straw bouquet.[96] In suggesting that Irving's lighter touch in portraying Lear's senility aligned it more with Terry's delicate madwomen than with the seething Lears of decades past, "Ophe-Lear" lampoons the actor's approach and bolsters the Victorian association of madness with the female sex. Finally, Mathias's feminization resulted not from any one pronounced source but from a composite of characteristics taken both from Lewis's script and Irving's performance: his inconstancy in behavior and moods, neglect of his patriarchal duties, hysterical outbursts and extreme emotionality, susceptibility to hypnotic suggestion, and acute sensitivity to stimuli. It is notable that Mathias's somnambulistic reenactment of his crime and its cover-up, complete with the character gazing at his bloodied hands, is itself haunted by Lady Macbeth's famous sleepwalking scene. A period caricature of Irving's Mathias by Frederick Waddy forges a link between the actor's psychological roles while further emasculating the character. Evoking Ophelia's description of Hamlet's discordant mind, which by the nunnery scene rings "Like sweet bells jangled, out of tune and harsh," Mathias swats at a clanging chorus of bells encircling him.[97]

The doctor is out: The closing of the Lyceum laboratory

> If, then, you wish an emotion, go to the *Medicine Man*.
> He hypnotises all the audience, except the critics.
>
> *Judy*, May 18, 1898[98]

Acting opposite one another for twenty-four years (and on several continents), Henry Irving and Ellen Terry devised some of the late Victorian period's most widely publicized and celebrated illness roles. Photographers, portraitists, cartoonists, dramatic critics, journalists, trained physicians, and recreational theatregoers together formed a multimedial record of the portrayals so vast and diverse that it impacted the age's collective imaginary. The press, who medicalized Irving and Terry as sensitive aesthetes prone to exhaustion and breakdowns, represented the actors as singularly equipped, physically and temperamentally, to embody mentally ill characters. Both performers actualized and elaborated upon gendered notions of psychological disorders already present in medical science and in extant theatrical scripts. In general, such theories limited the effects of female mental illness to the domestic sphere, which contained the sufferings of Ophelia and Lady Macbeth and concealed their offstage deaths; even Lucy Ashton's public demise proved a matter of lasting consequence only for her loved ones. Critics applauded Terry for performing her characters' symptomatologies with grace and restraint (save an alarming laugh or fainting spell), techniques likely informed both by social protocols and by the actress's awareness of her own proficiencies. Lacking appreciable autonomy or sociopolitical authority, Terry's hysterical and mad characters grew more pure, beautiful, and feminine even as their behavior transgressed the boundaries regulating white bourgeois womanhood.

The illnesses and deaths of Irving's madmen (all of which occurred center stage), toppled kingdoms, enfeebled patriarchies, and challenged the foundational stability of the male sex. Despite suffering from masculine varieties of mind disorders, Irving's embodied performances of Hamlet, Mathias, and King Lear hystericized the characters' emotionalism, introspectiveness, and paranoia, an approach reflective of configurations of male mental illness as degenerative and potentially injurious to society-at-large. His characters remained sympathetic, however, due to Irving's tortured depictions, the men's potential to recover from ill health, and their privileged whiteness and sociopolitical prestige. Unlike Ophelia, Lady Macbeth, and Lucy Ashton, who experienced immediate, permanent breaks with sanity, Irving's neurotic and senile men were both aware of their deepening conditions and actively struggled to manage or alleviate their symptoms. However, as they sank into their illnesses his madmen fell from advantaged heights of wealth and esteem, binding each character's mental health crisis to his inadequacies as a civic, familial, or moral leader. Installed within and reified by Irving's performative body, mental illness and its accompanying symptoms signaled the displacing of his characters from the epicenters of their own environments into weakened social positions (akin to those normally held by women). If Terry's roles harnessed the power of pathos, Irving's harnessed the tragic.

In May 1898, the Lyceum premiered *The Medicine Man*, a new play by H. D. Traill and Robert Hichens that was performed only twenty-two times before it was consigned to the back-alley dustbin.[99] A blatant attempt to capitalize on the success of Herbert Beerbohm Tree's 1895 production of *Trilby* at the Haymarket, *Medicine Man* featured Irving (in his only Lyceum role in modern dress) as Dr. Tregenna, a brain doctor, hypnotist, and private asylum proprietor with more than a passing resemblance to one Dr. Charcot. The plot revolves around Dr. Tregenna exacting revenge on Lord Belhurst, the widower of the doctor's old flame, using as his weapon the couple's beautiful daughter Sylvia. In the men's first encounter at a ball in Mayfair, we learn that Belhurst's beloved wife had gone mad before her death and, on the eve of Sylvia's marriage to a handsome officer, Belhurst is bent on learning if his daughter inherited her mother's proclivity for lunacy. Tregenna promises to assess Sylvia's mental health by taking her to his asylum in Hampstead for sessions of hypnosis. Though Tregenna finds Sylvia to be entirely sane, he forces her through hypnotic suggestion to perform the symptomatic behaviors of insanity. Remarked S. R. Littlewood of the *Morning Leader*: "[L]earning everything that the mother did in her madness – her little Ophelia-like ways of pulling roses petal by petal and such trifles – Tregenna watches with fiendish delight while Sylvia, under the domination of his will, does the same things."[100] When the doctor learns that Lord Belhurst knew nothing of him when he married Sylvia's mother, Tregenna sends the young woman back to her father (relatively) unharmed. In the play's strangest twist, Tregenna is murdered by one of his own mental patients, a burly Eastender who disapproved of the doctor's manipulation of Sylvia.

While *Medicine Man's* plot alone offers countless reasons why it failed to attract an audience, it was only one of several factors responsible. First, early modernism's invasion of British theatre in the 1890s gradually rendered the Lyceum and its standard repertoire antiquated. More closely resembling the mid-century melodramas of Boucicault than the dramas of Ibsen or even Pinero, the *Medicine Man* script served only to accentuate the Lyceum's increasingly old-fashioned aesthetic. The pictorial acting of Irving and Terry, hailed in recent decades by London's critics as "naturalistic," now appeared to border on the histrionic when compared with the styles of Elizabeth Robins and Mrs. Patrick Campbell. Second, though Irving was enthusiastic about *Medicine Man*, a play he himself commissioned from Hichens and Traill, Terry regarded Sylvia as a frivolous character with little to offer an actress of her experience and intelligence. "Poor [Robert] Taber has such an awful part in the play, and mine is even worse," wrote Terry in her diary. "It is short enough, yet I feel I can't cut too much of it."[101] To her frequent penpal, George Bernard Shaw, Terry wittily confessed: "It 'lunatics' me to watch Henry at these rehearsals. Hours and hours of loving care on this twaddle!"[102] Sylvia, who Terry's niece Kate Terry Gielgud rightly labeled "invertebrate" in her handwritten review of the piece, seemed to the actress just one more vapid heroine on whom her talents were squandered.[103] It is also conceivable that Sylvia's ersatz performance of female madness while under hypnosis felt to the actress like a thin metatheatrical parody of her own Ophelia. Whatever the reason for her displeasure, the actress's transferring of matinee performances to Miss Dorothea Baird (the lead actress in Beerbohm Tree's *Trilby*, no less), defended publicly as a tactic for warding off exhaustion, telegraphed the actress's spurning of the role to Victorians adept at reading between the lines. Third and most importantly, the play premiered during a paradigmatic shift in modern psychological and psychiatric practice. The gestation and birth of psychoanalysis in the 1890s upended earlier theories of psychopathological illnesses and their treatment, and the publication of Freud and Breuer's *Studien über Hysterie* in 1895 reshaped medicocultural representations of female madness. The visually arresting hysterical attacks of Charcot's clinic/theatre, triggered by hypnotic suggestion and enacted by a bevy of sexualized and seemingly self-aware patients, were eventually displaced by Freud and Anna O's collaborative explorations of the subconscious through therapeutic dialogues. Ultimately, theatricality—once an integral element on the stage *and* in the clinic—was denounced in both domains as prohibitive to innovation, truthfulness, and progress. In such a climate, perhaps, *The Medicine Man* could not have hoped to succeed. No other new performances of illness premiered at the Lyceum for the remainder of Irving and Terry's partnership, and three years later, Irving sold the theatre. Though the Lyceum's doors are still open at 21 Wellington Street, those on Irving's laboratory closed long ago.

Notes

1   Michael Holroyd, *A Strange Eventful History: The Dramatic Lives of Ellen Terry, Henry Irving, and Their Remarkable Families* (New York: Picador, 2009), 98.

2   Jeffrey Richards, *Sir Henry Irving: A Victorian Actor and His World* (London: Hambledon and London, 2005), 152.

3   A.B. Walkley, *Playhouse Impressions* (London: T. Fisher Unwin, 1892), 259.

4   Eden Phillpotts, "Irving as Hamlet," in *We Saw Him Act: A Symposium on the Art of Sir Henry Irving*, eds. H.A. Saintsbury and Cecil Palmer (New York: Benjamin Blom, 1969), 84.

5   William Archer and Robert William Lowe, *The Fashionable Tragedian: A Criticism* (Edinburgh and Glasgow: Thomas Gray & Co., 1877), 3 and 4–5. Archer's critique of Irving continued in his *Henry Irving, Actor and Manager, A Critical Study*, published in 1883.

6   Archer and Lowe, *Fashionable Tragedian*, 21 and quoted in Laurence Irving, *Henry Irving, the Actor in His World, by His Grandson* (London: Faber and Faber, 1951), 309–310.

7   Mortimer Menpes, *Henry Irving* (London: Adam and Charles Black, 1906), 10.

8   The French original was penned by Emile Erckmann and Pierre Alexandre Chatrian; the score was composed by Etienne Singla. The Erckmann-Chatrian play was itself an adaptation of an opera by Camille Erlanger.

9   Richards, *Sir Henry Irving*, 402.

10 Eric Jones-Evans, "The Centenary of 'The Bells,'" printed in "'The Bells' Centenary Exhibition," Bournemouth Museums Bulletin, Russell-Cotes Art Gallery and Museum and the Rothesay Museum, Bournemouth 36, no. 3 (Nov 1971), 36, *The Bells* production file, V&A; and *The Daily Telegraph*, Nov 8, 1887, reprinted in *Henry Irving and The Bells*, ed. David Mayer (Manchester: Manchester University Press, 1980), 106. Amusingly, in a letter to the editor of *The Times*, Margot Oxford described taking her friend Coquelin to see Irving's interpretation of the role. When she asked him what he saw as the difference between their two performances, "He replied that there was all the difference in the world as the stupidest detective would have arrested Irving at once, whereas he (Coquelin) would never have been caught." *The Bells* production file, V&A.

11 David Mayer, "Notes," ed. Mayer, *Henry Irving and* The Bells, 95n23.

12 Edward Gordon Craig, *Henry Irving* (New York: Benjamin Blom, 1969), 60–61. Clara Morris describes Mathias's "wild bound" upon clearly hearing the phantom bells, as if his nerves had been electrocuted by a sudden shock. Her account of Irving's characterization, while somewhat contradictory in details to Craig's description, nevertheless confirms that the most enthralling action of the scene was the character's listening for the bells. James L. Ford, "'Listening' on the Stage," *Scribner's Magazine* 42 (July–Dec 1907): 500–505.

13 In another departure from *Le Juif Polonais*, Mathias's mental unrest manifests in *The Bells* by way of his companions' conversations and the jangling sleigh bells, rather than being visual triggered by a similarly featured Polish Jew entering the inn in the first scene.

14 *Chicago Inter-ocean* and *Brooklyn Union*, reprinted in *Mr. Henry Irving and Miss Ellen Terry in America: Opinions of the Press* (Chicago: John Morris, 1884), V&A.

15 Unidentified newspaper clipping, July 4, 1881, in Henry Irving Scrapbook – Freeman, Henry Irving Biographical File, personal box 51, V&A.

16 Lewis, *The Bells*, in Mayer, *Henry Irving and* The Bells, 61.

17 Winifred Callwall, "Descriptions of Performances by Henry Irving," Scrapbook 1904–1905, V&A.

18 William Winter, *New York Tribune*, Oct 31, 1883.

19 *New York Tribune*, reprinted in *Mr. Henry Irving and Miss Ellen Terry in America: Opinions of the Press* (Chicago: John Morris, 1884), V&A.

20 Callwall, "Descriptions of Performances by Henry Irving," V&A.

21 Lewis, *The Bells*, in Mayer, *Henry Irving and* The Bells, 76.

22 Oxenford, *The Times*, Nov 28, 1871, in Walter Calvert, "Souvenir of Sir Henry Irving" (London: Henry J. Drane, Chant & Co., n.d.), 6, V&A.

23 Ellen Terry, *Story of My Life* (London: Hutchinson, 1908), 338.

24 "Mr. Irving's Debut in New York," *The Standard*, Oct 30, 1883, Henry Irving Scrapbook – Freeman, Henry Irving Biographical File, personal box 51, V&A.

25 Eric Jones-Evans, "Notes," ed. Mayer, *Henry Irving and The Bells*, 88n14; *Chicago Tribune* reprinted in *Mr. Henry Irving and Miss Ellen Terry in America*, V&A; Callwall, "Descriptions of Performances by Henry Irving," V&A; Scott, *The Observer*, Nov 26, 1871, in Scott and Irving, *From 'The Bells' to 'King Arthur,'* 5; Oxenford, *The Times*, Nov 28, 1871; *Boston Daily Advertiser* reprinted in *Mr. Henry Irving and Miss Ellen Terry in America*, V&A; *The Daily Telegraph*, Nov 8, 1887; Walkley, *Playhouse Impressions*, 258; and Walter Herries Pollock, *Impressions of Henry Irving: Gathered in Public and Private During a Friendship of Many Years* (London: Longmans, Green and Co., 1908).

26 The nineteenth-century designation "moral insanity," forwarded by both Pritchard and Thomas Mayo, described a condition of "morbid perversion" and moral degeneracy that may or may not include intellectual impairments. John Macpherson, *Mental Illness: An introduction to the Study of Insanity* (London: Macmillan and Co., 1899), 300–301.

27 Lisa Appignanesi, *Mad, Bad and Sad: Women and the Mind Doctors* (New York: W.W. Norton, 2008), 66.

28 Ibid.

29 Valerie Pedlar, *"The Most Dreadful Visitation": Male Madness in Victorian Fiction* (Liverpool: Liverpool University Press, 2006), 121.

30 Appignanesi, *Mad, Bad and Sad*, 66.

31 John Oxenford, *The Times*, Nov 28, 1871 in Walter Calvert, "Souvenir of Sir Henry Irving" (London: Henry J. Drane, Chant & Co., n.d.), 6, V&A.

32 John Charles Bucknill, *The Psychology of Shakespeare* (London: Longman, Brown, Green, Longmans, and Roberts, 1859), 58.

33 Stanley W. Jackson, *Melancholia and Depression: From Hippocratic Times to Modern Times* (New Haven: Yale University Press, 1986), 4. My summary of melancholia in the nineteenth century is drawn primarily from Jackson's work.

34 Etienne Esquirol, *Mental Maladies; a Treatise on Insanity*, trans. E. K. Hunt (Philadelphia: Lea and Blanchard, 1845), 203 and 209.

35 Jackson 178, 152, and 156.

36 For lengthy contemporary analyses of Irving's Hamlet see Baron Edward Richard Russell, *Irving as Hamlet* (London: King, 1875); Austin Brereton, *The Life of Henry Irving*, v 1 (London: Longmans, Green, 1908), BL; Austin Brereton, *Henry Irving: A Biographical Sketch* (London: David Bogue, 1883), BL; J. Ranken Towse, "Henry Irving," in *The Century* 27 (London: Century Co, 1884): 660–688, 666; Lady Hardy, [description of Irving's Hamlet], 1879, Henry Irving Scrapbook – Peters, V&A; and "Mr. Irving's Hamlet," *Temple Bar* (March 1879): 398–403, 398, Henry Irving Scrapbook – Peters, V&A.

37 "Mr. Irving's Hamlet," *Temple Bar* (March 1879): 398–403, Henry Irving Scrapbook – Peters, V&A and *Baltimore Day*, reprinted in "Mr. Henry Irving and Miss Ellen Terry in America: Opinions of the Press," V&A.

38 Alan Hughes, *Henry Irving, Shakespearean* (Cambridge: Cambridge University Press, 1981), 43.

39 Terry, *Story of My Life*, 126.

40 As Alan Hughes tells it, the question of Hamlet's insanity "was the burning question in Irving's time. It is the only interpretive issue given a section entirely to itself in the Variorum edition of 1877, where the debate covers forty-one closely printed pages." Hughes, *Henry Irving, Shakespearean*, 36.

41 Bucknill, *Psychology of Shakespeare*, 58 and 101.

42 Ibid., 36.

43 Hughes, *Henry Irving, Shakespearean*, 51.

44 Ibid., 56.

45 Mathew Thomson, "Neurasthenia in Britain: An Overview," in *Cultures of Neurasthenia From Beard to the First World War*, eds. Marijke Gijswijt-Hofstra and Roy Porter (New York: Rodopi, 2001), 77–96. Oppenheim notes that Beard's introductory article was published the same year that E. H. Van Deusen applied the term "neurasthenia" on "diverse manifestations of nervous collapse." Oppenheim, *"Shattered Nerves": Doctors, Patients, and Depression in Victorian England*. Oxford: Oxford University Press, 1991, 92. For other histories of neurasthenia in nineteenth-century Britain see Oppenheim's *Shattered Nerves* and Chandak Sengoopta, "'A Mob of Incoherent Symptoms'? Neurasthenia in British Medical Discourse, 1860–1920," in Gijswijt-Hofstra and Porter, *Cultures of Neurasthenia*, 97–116.

46 Sengoopta, "Incoherent Symptoms," 97.

47 Oppenheim, *Shattered Nerves*, 93. While Beard's version of the disorder targeted mostly middle-class male professionals, other nerve specialists expanded neurasthenia's reach to include women and members of the working class.

48 Sengoopta, "Incoherent Symptoms," 97; and Oppenheim, *Shattered Nerves*, 142.

49 Thomson, "Neurasthenia in Britain," 79.

50 Sengoopta, "Incoherent Symptoms," 98.

51 Mark S. Micale, *Hysterical Men: The Hidden History of Male Nervous Illness* (Cambridge: Harvard University Press, 2008), 129; and Sengoopta, "Incoherent Symptoms," 108.

52 Sengoopta, "Incoherent Symptoms," 103.

53 "Lyceum Theatre," *The Times*, Nov 2, 1874; and Clement Scott, unidentified review of *Hamlet*, reprinted in "Souvenir of Sir Henry Irving" by Walter Calvert (London: Henry J. Drane, Chant & Co., n.d.), 14.

54 "'Hamlet' at the Lyceum," *The World*, Jan 18, 1879, Henry Irving Scrapbook – Peters, V&A.

55 Hughes, *Henry Irving, Shakespearean*, 36 and Towse, "Henry Irving," 666.

56 "Hamlet at the Lyceum," *Punch*, Jan 11, 1879, Henry Irving Scrapbook – Peters, V&A.

57 "Mr. Irving at the Lyceum," unidentified newspaper clipping, Jan 4, 1879, *Hamlet* (1878) production file, V&A.

58 Lady Hardy, [description of Irving's Hamlet], 1879, Henry Irving Scrapbook – Peters, V&A.

59 A number of early nineteenth-century alienists, including Esquirol, Philippe Pinel, and Johann Christoph Hoffbauer, distinguished between acute (reversible) and chronic (often irreversible) dementias.

60 G. E. Berrios and H. L. Hoffman, "Introduction" in *Alzheimer and the Dementias*, eds. G. E. Berrios and H. L. Hoffman (London: Royal Society of Medicine Services Ltd., 1991), 2 and 12.

61 G. E. Berrios, *The History of Mental Symptoms: Descriptive Psychopathology Since the Nineteenth Century* (Cambridge: Cambridge University Press, 1996), 191.

62 Berrios and Hoffman, "Dementia Before the Twentieth Century," in *Alzheimer and the Dementias*, 16.

63 Ralph Lyman Parsons, "Practical Points Regarding the Senile Insanities, with Special Reference to Prophylaxis and Management," 1896, quoted in Jesse F. Ballenger, *Self, Senility, and Alzheimer's Disease in Modern America* (Baltimore: Johns Hopkins University Press, 2006), 17.

64 J. Hughlings Jackson, "Croonian Lectures on Evolution and Dissolution of the Nervous System," *Lancet* 1 (1884): 555–558, 649–652, and 739–744.

65 G.E. Berrios provides a summary of the different theoretical viewpoints on the vesanic dementias: "According to the unitary insanity view, vesanic dementia was a terminal stage (the end point in the sequence mania– melancholia–); according to degeneration theory, it was the final expression of a corrupted pedigree; and according to post-1880s nosology, it was a final common pathway to all the insanities" (Berrios, *The History of Mental Symptoms*, 190).

66 Ballenger, *Self, Senility, and Alzheimer's*, 21.

67 Ibid., 17.

68 I. L. Nascher, *Geriatrics; the Disease of Old Age and Their Treatment: Including Physio-logical Old Age, Home and Institutional Care, and Medico-legal Relations* (Philadelphia: P. Blankinson, 1916), 489.

69 Nascher, *Geriatrics*, 514–515.

70 Richards, *Sir Henry Irving*, 136.

71 Laurence Irving, *Henry Irving*, 551.

72 Bucknill, *Psychology of Shakespeare*, 133; and J. G. Howells, "Dementia in Shakespeare's King Lear," in *Alzheimer and the Dementias*, eds. G. E. Berrios and H. L. Freeman (London: Royal Society of Medicine Services Ltd., 1991), 101–109.

73 Henry Norman, "Shakspere's 'King Lear' at the Lyceum Theatre, *Illustrated London News*, Nov 19, 1892, *King Lear* 1892 production file, V&A.

74 "'King Lear' at the Lyceum," *Daily Telegraph*, undated newspaper clipping, Henry Irving Scrapbook – Peters, V&A.

75 Norman, "Shakepere's 'King Lear' at the Lyceum Theatre," *Illustrated London News*, Nov 19, 1892.

76 "'King Lear' at the Lyceum," *The Times* (London), undated newspaper clipping, Henry Irving Scrapbook – Peters, V&A.

77 "Through the Opera Glass: From Drop-Scene to Curtain," *Pick-Me-Up*, Dec 17, 1892, *King Lear* 1892 production file, V&A.

78 Hughes, *Henry Irving, Shakespearean*, 122.

79 A. Acton-Bond, "Irving as *King Lear*," in *We Saw Him Act*, 296; and Augustin Filon, review from "Le Journal des Débates," *King Lear at the Lyceum, Produced November 10, 1892, Some Extracts from the Press on the Performances of Mr. Henry Irving and Miss Ellen Terry* (London: Chiswick Press, 1893), 106–118, 113.

80 William Shakespeare, *King Lear*, Irving acting edition, BL. In Irving's script, the lines were not numbered. I have included line numbers from the Folger digital edition of *The Tragedy of King Lear*, eds. Barbara A. Mowat and Paul Werstine (Washington: Folger Shakespeare Library, nd).

81 Souvenir of Shakespeare's Tragedy *King Lear*, presented at the Lyceum Theatre, 10th November, 1892, by Henry Irving. Illustrated by J. Bernard Partridge and Hawes Craven. (London: The "Black and White" Publishing Company, Ltd, 1892).

82 "Two Views of Irving's Lear," *Current Opinion* 12 (Jan 1893): 182–183.

83 "'King Lear' at the Lyceum," *The Standard*, Nov 11, 1892, Henry Irving Scrapbook – Peters, V&A.

84 "'King Lear' at the Lyceum," *The Times*, undated newspaper clipping, Henry Irving Scrapbook – Peters, V&A.

85 E. R. Russell, "King Lear," in *King Lear at the Lyceum*, 5–14, 10 and 12.

86 "'King Lear' at the Lyceum," *The Times* (London) undated newspaper clipping, Henry Irving Scrapbook – Peters, V&A; and "'King Lear' at the Lyceum," *The Standard*, Nov 11, 1892, Henry Irving Scrapbook – Peters, V&A.

87 Henry Irving, "My Four Favorite Parts," *The Forum* 16 (Sept 1893): 33–37, 36–37.

88 Ibid.

89 Henry Norman, "Shakepere's 'King Lear' at the Lyceum Theatre, *Illustrated London News*, Nov 19, 1892, *King Lear* 1892 production file, V&A.

90 Ibid.

91 "'King Lear' at the Lyceum," *Daily Telegraph*, undated newspaper clipping, Henry Irving Scrapbook – Peters, V&A.

92 The illness roles analyzed above are representative of three character types often played by Irving: the guilt-stricken pseudo-villain (Mathias, Eugene Aram, Edward Mortimer in the *Iron Chest*), the neurotic romantic (Hamlet, Cardinal Richelieu), and the senile old man (King Lear, Louis XI).

93   "Mr. Irving's Hamlet," *Temple Bar*, March 1879, 398–403, 400, Henry Irving Scrapbook – Peters, V&A.

94   *Baltimore Day*, reprinted in "Mr. Henry Irving and Miss Ellen Terry in America: Opinions of the Press," 8, V&A; and "Lyceum Theatre," unidentified newspaper clipping, May 2, 1885[?], Henry Irving Scrapbook – Freeman, Henry Irving Biographical File, personal box 51, V&A.

95   Kaara L. Peterson, "Historica Passio: Early Modern Medicine, *King Lear*, and Editorial Practice," *Shakespeare Quarterly* 57, no. 1 (spring 2006): 1–22. Peterson argues instead that Lear's exclamation should be perceived as the king's misprision, not the playwright's blunder.

96   "His Mad-Jesty at the Lyceum," *Punch*, Nov 19, 1892, *King Lear* 1892 production file, V&A.

97   Frederick Waddy, *Cartoon Portraits and Biographical Sketches of Men of the Day* (London: Tinsley Brothers, 1873), 52–53.

98   "At Play," *Judy*, May 18, 1898, 236, BL.

99   For reviews of *The Medicine Man*, see "'The Medicine Man' at the Lyceum," *Sketch*, May 11, 1898, *Medicine Man* production file, V&A; *Standard*, May 5, 1898, *Medicine Man* production file, V&A; "The Medicine Man," *The Era*, May 7, 1898; "The Medicine Man," W. Moy Thomas, *The Graphic*, May 14, 1898; "'Medicine Man' at the Lyceum," *Pall Mall*, May 5, 1898; and S. R. Littlewood, *Morning Leader*, May 5, 1898, reprinted in *We Saw Him Act: A Symposium on the Art of Sir Henry Irving*, 1939, eds. H. A. Saintsbury and Cecil Palmer (New York: Benjamin Blom, 1969), 367.

100 Littlewood, *Morning Leader*, May 5, 1898.

101 Terry, *Story of My Life*, 324.

102 Letter from Ellen Terry to George Bernard Shaw, quoted in Bingham, *Henry Irving*, 287.

103 Kate Terry Gielgud, handwritten description of *The Medicine Man*, in *Plays I Have Seen*, BL.

Bibliography

Acton-Bond, A. "Irving as *King Lear*." In *We Saw Him Act: A Symposium on the Art of Sir Henry Irving*, edited by H. A. Saintsbury and Cecil Palmer, 296. New York: Benjamin Blom, 1969.

Appignanesi, Lisa. *Mad, Bad and Sad: Women and the Mind Doctors*. New York: W.W. Norton, 2008.

Archer, William and Robert William Lowe. *The Fashionable Tragedian: A Criticism*. Edinburgh and Glasgow: Thomas Gray & Co., 1877.

Ballenger, Jesse F. *Self, Senility, and Alzheimer's Disease in Modern America*. Baltimore: Johns Hopkins University Press, 2006.

Berrios, G.E. *The History of Mental Symptoms: Descriptive Psychopathology Since the Nineteenth Century*. Cambridge: Cambridge University Press, 1996.

Berrios, G. E. and H. L. Freeman. "Dementia Before the Twentieth Century." In *Alzheimer and the Dementias*, edited by G. E. Berrios and H. L. Freeman, 9–27. London: Royal Society of Medicine Services Ltd., 1991.

Bingham, Madeleine. *Henry Irving: The Greatest Victorian Actor*. New York: Stein and Day, 1978.

Brereton, Austin. *Henry Irving: A Biographical Sketch*. London: David Bogue, 1883.

Brereton, Austin. *The Life of Henry Irving*, v 1. London: Longmans, Green, 1908.

Bucknill, John Charles. *The Psychology of Shakespeare*. London: Longman, Brown, Green, Longmans, and Roberts, 1859.

Craig, Edward Gordon. *Henry Irving*. New York: Benjamin Blom, 1969.

Esquirol, Etienne. *Mental Maladies; a Treatise on Insanity*. Trans. E. K. Hunt. Philadelphia: Lea and Blanchard, 1845.

Filon, Augustin. Review from "Le Journal des Débate." In *King Lear at the Lyceum, Produced November 10, 1892, Some Extracts from the Press on the Performances of Mr. Henry Irving and Miss Ellen Terry*, 106–118. London: Chiswick Press, 1893.

Ford, James L. "'Listening' on the Stage," *Scribner's Magazine* 42 (July–Dec 1907): 500–505.

Gijswijt-Hofstra, Marijke and Roy Porter, eds. *Cultures of Neurasthenia from Beard to the First World War*. New York: Rodopi, 2001.

Holroyd, Michael. *A Strange Eventful History: The Dramatic Lives of Ellen Terry, Henry Irving, and Their Remarkable Families*. New York: Farrar, Straus and Giroux, 2009.

Howells, J. G. "Dementia in Shakespeare's *King Lear*." In *Alzheimer and the Dementias*, edited by G. E. Berrios and H. L. Freeman, 101–109. London: Royal Society of Medicine Services Ltd., 1991.

Hughes, Alan. *Henry Irving, Shakespearean*. Cambridge: Cambridge University Press, 1981.

Irving, Henry. "My Four Favorite Parts," *The Forum* 16 (Sept 1893): 33–37.

Irving, Laurence. *Henry Irving, the Actor in His World, by His Grandson*. London: Faber and Faber, 1951.

Jackson, J. Hughlings. "Croonian Lectures on Evolution and Dissolution of the Nervous System," *Lancet* 1 (1884): 555–558, 649–652, and 739–744.

Jackson, Stanley W. *Melancholia and Depression: From Hippocratic Times to Modern Times*. New Haven: Yale University Press, 1986.

King Lear at the Lyceum, Produced November 10, 1892, Some Extracts from the Press on the Performances of Mr. Henry Irving and Miss Ellen Terry. London: Chiswick Press, 1893.

Macpherson, John. *Mental Illness: An Introduction to the Study of Insanity*. London: Macmillan and Co., 1899.

Mayer, David, ed. *Henry Irving and* The Bells. Manchester: Manchester University Press, 1980.

Menpes, Mortimer. *Henry Irving*. London: Adam and Charles Black, 1906.

Nascher, I. L. *Geriatrics; the Disease of Old Age and Their Treatment: Including Physiological Old Age, Home and Institutional Care, and Medico-legal Relations*. Philadelphia: P. Blankinson, 1916.

Oppenheim, Janet. *"Shattered Nerves": Doctors, Patients, and Depression in Victorian England*. Oxford: Oxford University Press, 1991.

Pedlar, Valerie. *"The Most Dreadful Visitation": Male Madness in Victorian Fiction*. Liverpool: Liverpool University Press, 2006.

Peterson, Kaara L. "Historica Passio: Early Modern Medicine, King Lear, and Editorial Practice." *Shakespeare Quarterly* 57, no. 1 (spring 2006): 1–22.

Phillpotts, Eden. "Irving as Hamlet." In *We Saw Him Act: A Symposium on the Art of Sir Henry Irving*, edited by H. A. Saintsbury and Cecil Palmer, 83–88. New York: Benjamin Blom, 1969.

Pollock, Walter Herries. *Impressions of Henry Irving: Gathered in Public and Private During a Friendship of Many Years*. London: Longmans, Green and Co., 1908.

Richards, Jeffrey. *Sir Henry Irving: A Victorian Actor and His World*. London: Hambledon and London, 2005.

Russell, Baron Edward Richard. *Irving as Hamlet*. London: King, 1875.

Russell, E. R. "King Lear." In *King Lear at the Lyceum, Produced November 10, 1892, Some Extracts from the Press on the Performances of Mr. Henry Irving and Miss Ellen Terry*, 5–14. London: Chiswick Press, 1893.

Sengoopta, Chandak. "'A Mob of Incoherent Symptoms'? Neurasthenia in British Medical Discourse, 1860–1920." In *Cultures of Neurasthenia From Beard to the First World War*, edited by Marijke Gijswijt-Hofstra and Roy Porter, 97–116. New York: Rodopi, 2001.

Shakespeare, William. *The Tragedy of King Lear*. Edited by Barbara A. Mowat and Paul Werstine. Washington: Folger Shakespeare Library, n.d.

Terry, Ellen. *The Story of My Life*. London: Hutchinson, 1908.

Thomson, Mathew. "Neurasthenia in Britain: An Overview." In *Cultures of Neurasthenia From Beard to the First World War*, edited by Marijke Gijswijt-Hofstra and Roy Porter, 77–96. New York: Rodopi, 2001.

Towse, J. Ranken. "Henry Irving." *The Century*. Vol. 27. London: Century Co., 1884: 660–688.

"Two Views of Irving's Lear," *Current Opinion* 12 (Jan 1893): 182–183.

Waddy, Frederick. *Cartoon Portraits and Biographical Sketches of Men of the Day*. London: Tinsley Brothers, 1873.

Walkley, A.B. *Playhouse Impressions*. London: T. Fisher Unwin, 1892.

Conclusion

Armed with acerbic wits and exacting tastes, the best of the Victorian dramatic critics were not known for pulling punches when reviewing plays. Still, the gloves officially came off and battle lines were drawn when on March 13, 1891, Henrik Ibsen's *Ghosts* premiered in England at London's Royalty Theatre.[1] A dramatic meditation on the maxim "the sins of the father will be visited upon the son," *Ghosts* follows Oswald Alving's descent into debilitating insanity from syphilis, a disease that unbeknownst to the young man was inherited from his depraved father, now deceased. Oswald believes his only hope for happiness and recovery can be found in marrying Regina, the family's attractive house-servant. However, the ghosts of the late Captain Alving's past haunt his son's every step, as Regina is actually Oswald's illegitimate half-sister, born of the Captain's lecherous pursuit of his wife's former maid. Oswald's romantic designs on Regina force his mother to reveal the Captain's misdeeds, toppling the pedestal upon which Oswald had placed his father. In the play's final scene, Oswald entreats his mother, now his only source of tenderness and succor, to give him a fatal dose of morphine pills should his disease overtake his mind. Mrs. Alving's reluctant promise to do so is tested at the curtain's close, when Oswald's nonsensical mutterings and vacant eyes signal to audiences his permanent mental degeneration. Providing the counterpoint to Captain Alving's deliberate indiscretions are the sins of Mrs. Alving, whose attempts to conceal her husband's dissolute behavior from the public and Oswald lead her son indirectly to his ruin.

The Norwegian play ignited a firestorm of controversy in England, and debates between rapturous Ibsenites and their outraged adversaries dominated newspaper and magazine pages for many months following. Over 500 reviews and editorials were published in response to the production, an astronomical number that is all the more astounding considering the unlicensed play was only performed twice for a private subscription audience by J. T. Grein's newly formed Independent Theatre. At the height of the dispute, *Ghosts* commentators discarded the rules governing civilized Victorian debate, developing a confrontational style even more unprincipled than the play's reputedly objectionable themes. Appropriating what they deemed to be the contaminated language of Ibsen's drama, many of the production's harshest detractors attacked the play and playwright as diseased, infectious, fetid, and hazardous to the English people and their theatre. Anti-Ibsenites engaged in this graphic epidemiological discourse in the hopes of repulsing polite society, sullying "Dr. Ibsen's" reputation, and dissuading even the vaguely curious from patronizing his plays. Though the majority of reviewers adopted this critical tactic, Clement Scott, the incontestable leader of the anti-Ibsenite movement, incorporated the diseased rhetoric of pathology with unmatched authority and gusto. In his "anonymous" editorial in the *Daily Telegraph* the morning after *Ghosts* premiered, Scott called the play,

> simple only in the sense of an open drain; of a loathsome sore unbandaged; of a dirty act done publicly; or of a lazar-house with all its doors and windows open … Even the *Lady of the Camelias* – that hectic harlot – coughed her frail soul away with some external propriety; but Ibsen's patients expectorate, if we may venture to say so, in public, and air on the stage matters that a blind beggar would hide under his patches.[2]

Profanity, pollution, and pathology seemed to breed in the same metaphorical cesspool for *Ghosts'* harshest critics, who coupled their pathological language with heavy doses of moralizing.

I turn to Ibsen's modernist drama now not just because its plot unites contagious disease, insanity, and a physician-endorsed drug overdose in a dark convergence of heredity and environment, or because it sparked a contentious debate using the rhetoric of pathology. *Ghosts* indicates the path theatrical representations of illness will take in the twentieth century. Nineteenth-century popular dramas were seldom explicit or comprehensive in their written descriptions of illness roles, whether in dialogue or stage directions, nor did they provide instructions to actors on how to embody these characters. Even *Sherlock Holmes's* relatively long stage direction describing the detective's cocaine injection was penned by Gillette, the role's originator. Building upon the scripts' minimal treatments of medical conditions, actors were the true architects of their illness roles, selecting the physiological symptoms and emotional tones that in their estimation best expressed "an illness lived." However, at century's close there rose a breed of playwrights acutely fascinated with the natural sciences, modern psychology, and human experiences of illness. In their works, the illness-processes of the *dramatis personae* were given prominence not just in plots and exchanges of dialogue, but in stage directions and character descriptions. Ibsen was one such playwright. Though ill characters appear throughout his oeuvre—the tubercular Lynstrand in *Lady From the Sea*, the syphilitic Dr. Rank in *A Doll's House* (though the doctor claims he's suffering from spinal tuberculosis), and the neurotic-hysteric Hedda in *Hedda Gabler*, to name three—*Ghosts* offers one of the playwright's most detailed representation of illness. The final moments of Oswald's syphilitic insanity, for example, are carefully drawn:

> (*With his back toward the distant view,* OSVALD *sits motionless in the armchair.*)

OSVALD *(abruptly):* Mother, give me the sun.

MRS. ALVING *(by the table, looks at him, startled):* What did you say?

OSVALD *(repeats in a dull monotone):* The sun. The sun.

MRS. ALVING *(moves over to him):* Osvald, what's the matter?

(OSVALD appears to crumple inwardly in the chair; all his muscles loosen; the expression leaves his face; and his eyes stare blankly.)

MRS. ALVING *(shaking with fear):* What is it? *(In a shriek.)* Osvald! What's wrong! *(Drops to her knees beside him and shakes him.)* Osvald! Osvald! Look at me! Don't you know me?

OSVALD *(in the same monotone):* The sun – the sun.[3]

Unlike the Camilles, Lears, and Lucy Ashtons of the period, those who took the role of Oswald Alving received explicit instructions from the playwright on how to embody his illness: an expressionless face, nonsensical mutterings in monotone, and an unnatural stillness that gives way to muscular slackening. Such specifications, which expanding copyright protections in the late nineteenth century safeguarded from removal or revision, had the potential to lessen the actor's creative autonomy in embodying ill characters.

My detection of a shift from performer-devised to playwright-defined illness roles finds authentication in the broader assertions of Gay Gibson Cima, who argues that acting styles, once named for the actors or acting families who popularized them (Garrick, Kemble, Macready), began to be associated with playwrights whose works demanded innovations in performance techniques: the Ibsenite actor, the Brechtian actor, the Pinteresque actor. The nineteenth-century dramatic script, Cima writes, "was customarily viewed as a detailed skeleton, easily understood and visualized, requiring only the flesh and emotion of the actor to be brought to life." Pre-Ibsen repertoires demanded little from actors in the way of penetrating textual analyses, and so the majority of working performers did not view such intellectual exercises as being "the crux of the art of acting." Rather, they fleshed out the dramaturgical skeletons provided by playwrights through the discerning and creative use of conventional performance codes. However, the plays of Ibsen, Zola, Shaw, and their contemporaries, boasting a complex network of secrets, hints, and revelations for the studious actor to discover and interpret, "engendered a new attitude toward the necessary collaboration between playwright and actor."[4] Critics increasingly credited playwrights as the authoritative crafters of characters, a shift perceptible in the grand pillorying of Ibsen for the character of Oswald after *Ghosts'* London premiere with only brief mentions of Frank Lindo, the actor who embodied him. Interestingly, the rhetorical transfer of acting styles from performer to playwright coincided with a time when female performers like Eleonora Duse and Elizabeth Robins were acknowledged as pioneers of new performance trends. It is not surprising, given that theatrical realism and naturalism were inspired in part by the natural and medical sciences, that the transition to playwright-centric performance practices mimicked the distinctive shift to physician-centric healthcare. In this way, those who observed and defined illnesses displaced those who subjectively experienced illness as the dominant makers of meaning at the century's end.

The actors contained within these case studies marked their characters' afflictions with an inventory of physical and vocal techniques. Trembling hands, vacant stares, sighs, coughs, furrowed brows, feverish complexions, fainting spells, convulsions, grasping at furniture for support, and agonized cries constitute a fraction of the methods used to perform pathologies. This lexicon of embodied illness, as I have proposed, was flexible in two ways. First, it successfully traversed generic divides and theatrical movements, from Shakespearean tragedy (*Hamlet*) to Romantic thesis play (*La dame aux camélias*), from Victorian melodrama (*Ravenswood*) to *fin-de-siècle* thriller (*Dr. Jekyll and Mr. Hyde*). Second, the performative lexicon's components could be adapted, reordered, or deconstructed to fit the symptoms of the entire catalogue of stage illnesses. Hysterical laughter, for example, could signify to audiences mental illnesses ranging from monomania (Mathias) to female insanity (Lucy Ashton, Ophelia), but it was also employed by Richard Mansfield to indicate Jekyll/Hyde's drug-fueled illusion of invincibility. Practically all of the performances of illness analyzed in *Playing Sick* featured manifestations of physical or mental agitation: the melancholic trudge of Hamlet, the worrying hands of Lady Macbeth, the restless eyes of Sherlock Holmes, and the quavering voice of Camille. Though these symptoms all operate under the same emotive umbrella of "nervousness," marking illness as a psychophysical state-of-being, they deviate from one another in bodily location as well as tone, severity, and duration. Similarly, according to nineteenth-century performance traditions, the epileptic seizure became erroneously symptomatic of disease, addiction, *and* madness. Unlike Dr. Cyrus Edson, who lamented in 1893 that actors used epileptic fits too habitually and imprecisely to signify a veritable spectrum of illnesses, performers recognized the undeniable value in the seizure's theatrical versatility. After all, convulsions—however inaccurately or insensitively performed—communicated more swiftly than any other performative strategy the sufferer's loss of physical control and intellectual self-mastery. A well-executed fit intensified the gravity of any expression of illness and could unite in one extraordinary moment several prized elements of late nineteenth-century theatre: suspense, pathos, and spectacle. The lexicon of embodied illness was also surprisingly durable, persisting through the latter half of the nineteenth century even as pictorial acting waned in influence. Indeed, it was forged through an effective blend of neo-romantic emotionalism and proto-realistic authenticity; this delicate balance of theoretical and technical approaches to acting mimicked a similar blending of subjective experience and objective science maintained within the period's guiding notions of illness.

At the *fin de siècle*, however, once theatrical realism's dominance was secured, the lexicon used by decades of actors grew noticeably antiquated. In yet another example of the interconnectedness of medicine and theatre, as theories of human psychology evolved so too did the theatre's mimetic conventions. While nineteenth-century alienists sought to identify somatic origins for mental disorders and treated patients' maladies from the outside in (a path echoed by the demonstrative physical renderings of illness by the period's actors), Freudian psychoanalysis fundamentally altered psychopathological definitions and treatment strategies. The subconscious suppression of traumatic memories became the focus for psychologists and their innovative talk therapies, reversing the flow of analysis to an inside-out approach. Not surprisingly, a parallel shift occurred within the realm of acting technique. The internality of the acting process and the subtle expressivity of onstage appearances, including reenactments of illnesses, epitomized the modern performer's craft. Conspicuous shows of suffering, from labored gasps to spasmodic fits, from the rapturous postures of the hysteric to the delirium tremens of the alcoholic, were rendered outdated and too elaborate in their externality. Moreover, they were deemed obstructive to the pursuit of artistic authenticity. The spectacular had no place within the realist's vision and, even if they were earnestly drawn from real-life observations, most pronounced embodiments of illness were thrown out with the proverbial bath water. Just as Freud's contained and couch-bound hysteric superseded the histrionic Charcotian hysteric, the nineteenth-century actor's explicit performances of illness were replaced by the modern actor's minutely drawn embodiments. While it is true that Gillette's Sherlock Holmes, Bernhardt's Camille, and other nineteenth-century performances of illness appeared onstage well into the twentieth century, contemporaneous reviews imply that such offerings were regarded as relics of the past, praiseworthy not in spite of but *because* of their charming obsolescence.

In 1928 Bertolt Brecht pronounced *Ghosts* an irrelevant museum piece. "While Ibsen was writing *Ghosts*, Ehrlich was working to find a cure for syphilis," he mused. "The devil that Ibsen painted on the wall for the hypocrites, was wiped out by Ehrlich."[5] Ehrlich was Dr. Paul Ehrlich who, assisted by Dr. Hata Sahachirō, developed the spirochete-destroying drug Salvarsan. For Brecht, medical science had obliterated *Ghosts*'s dramatic power and social purpose. At the risk of simplifying a man of noted profundity, Brecht's argument for retiring *Ghosts* relies upon the foregrounding of syphilis's materiality. If we conceive of illness primarily as a pathological condition, the discovery of the cure for syphilis would indeed render its continued cultural referencing worthless. But illness was not merely a bacterial strain breeding on a microscope slide; it was a complex construction of interfacing scientific, societal, and cultural meanings. Just as *Camille* is not the story of tuberculosis, *Ghosts* is not the story of syphilis. It is about the "devil on the wall" that Ibsen paints in clashing hues and diverse brushstrokes, an entity that draws sufferers and witnesses alike into its chaotic composition. It is the story of human relationships, societal divisions, and selfhoods rescripted through illness. As I have attempted to demonstrate in this book, the direct relevance of a pathological performance text to its audiences necessarily evolves along with advances in medical science, and yet its longevity ultimately depends upon how actors embody the experience of being ill, in all its dizzying complexities. Furthermore, despite its stylistic broadness, commercialism, and limiting depictions of women, people of color, the poor, and other disenfranchised and non-normative identities, the popular stage performed restorative work in the age of Victorian medicine. Because the period's medical establishment, both in the United States and Britain, defined itself largely through techno-centric research and healthcare practices, increasing institutionalization, and the enlarging of physician authority, the ill patient became a figure of diminished visibility. The microscopes that brought germs, cells, and the human biome into sharp focus also blurred the distinctive identities of the sufferers and trivialized their testimonies. Ill characters often lived (and died) onstage as individuals not defined by their diagnoses, but redefined by their experiences of physiological and psychological suffering. Playing sick, for some of the nineteenth century's most honored actors, required threading together multiple "truths"—those of objective medical science and those of subjective human experience—to create multidimensional beings of consequence whose stories endured, even if their imagined bodies could not.

Notes

1 For information on *Ghosts'* English premiere see Gretchen P. Ackerman, *Ibsen and the English Stage, 1889–1903* (New York: Garland, 1987); William Archer, *William Archer on Ibsen: The Major Essays, 1889–1919*, ed. Thomas Postlewait (Westport: Greenwood Press, 1984); Miriam Alice Franc, *Ibsen in England* (Boston: Four Seasons Co., 1919).
2 [Clement Scott], editorial in *Daily Telegraph*, March 14, 1891.
3 Henrik Ibsen, *Ghosts*, trans. Rolf Fjelde, in *Plays Onstage: An Anthology*, Ronald Wainscott and Kathy Fletcher, eds. (Boston: Pearson, 2006), 264–294.
4 Gay Gibson Cima, *Performing Women: Female Characters, Male Playwrights, and the Modern Stage* (Ithaca: Cornell University Press, 1996), 23, 24, and 26.
5 Bertolt Brecht, quoted in Toril Moi, *Henrik Ibsen and the Birth of Modernism: Art, Theater, Philosophy* (Oxford: Oxford University Press, 2006), 348, n79.

Bibliography

Ackerman, Gretchen P. *Ibsen and the English Stage, 1889–1903*. New York: Garland Publishing, 1987.
Archer, William. *William Archer on Ibsen: The Major Essays, 1889–1919*. Edited by Thomas Postlewait. Westport: Greenwood Press, 1984.
Cima, Gay Gibson. *Performing Women: Female Characters, Male Playwrights, and the Modern Stage*. Ithaca: Cornell University Press, 1996.
Franc, Miriam Alice. *Ibsen in England*. Boston: Four Seasons Co., 1919.
Ibsen, Henrik. *Ghosts*. Trans. Rolf Fjelde. In *Plays Onstage: An Anthology*, edited by Ronald Wainscott and Kathy Fletcher, 264–291. Boston: Pearson, 2006.
Moi, Toril. *Henrik Ibsen and the Birth of Modernism: Art, Theater, Philosophy*. Oxford: Oxford University Press, 2006.

Index

Page numbers in *italic* denote figures

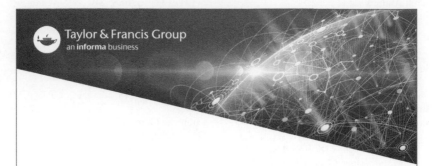